Mechanical Support for Cardiac and Respiratory Failure in Pediatric Patients

Mechanical Support for Cardiac and Respiratory Failure in Pediatric Patients

edited by

Brian W. Duncan

Children's Hospital and Regional Medical Center and
University of Washington School of Medicine
Seattle, Washington

CRC Press
Taylor & Francis Group
Boca Raton London New York

CRC Press is an imprint of the
Taylor & Francis Group, an **informa** business

CRC Press
Taylor & Francis Group
6000 Broken Sound Parkway NW, Suite 300
Boca Raton, FL 33487-2742

First issued in paperback 2019

ISBN-13: 978-0-8247-0275-5 (hbk)
ISBN-13: 978-0-367-39755-5 (pbk)

Visit the Taylor & Francis Web site at
http://www.taylorandfrancis.com

and the CRC Press Web site at
http://www.crcpress.com

Foreword

It has now been more than 60 years since Robert Gross pioneered surgery for congenital heart disease by ligation of the patent ductus arteriosus in 1938. Following the introduction of cardiopulmonary bypass by Gibbon in 1954, however, advances in the surgical care of children with heart disease made relatively slow progress in comparison with the spectacular advances for adults with coronary artery and valve disease. The principal reason for the lag of decades in providing equal care for children was that engineering efforts were focused on heart–lung machines for adults. The deleterious effects of early cardiopulmonary bypass circuits were intolerable to the infant and small child. Barratt-Boyes and Castaneda employed circulatory arrest to minimize exposure of the child to the damaging effects of bypass and demonstrated that primary repair of even complex congenital heart problems could be accomplished if one could avoid the damage inflicted on small bodies and immature organ systems by machines designed for adults. The discovery of prostaglandin E_1 in the mid-1970s opened the field of congenital heart surgery even further, since now even the neonates with ductal-dependent life-threatening heart disease could undergo careful diagnosis and a planned operation. But the medical device industry, which by now was reaping massive profits from coronary artery surgery, required considerable goading to become interested in development of bypass circuits specifically meant for infants and neonates. The first neonatal oxygenator was not released for sale until the 1990s, more than 35 years after heart–lung machines were first developed for adults. The small size of the pediatric ''market'' simply did not appeal to those in search of corporate profit.

And now the story is being repeated in the development of ventricular assist devices. Remarkable progress has been made over the last 10 years on ventricular devices for adults with failing ventricles. Several devices are currently available for adults as a bridge to transplantation and even for long-term implantation. But no U.S. company is presently interested in developing a specific pediatric ventricular assist device.

This remarkable book, which has been beautifully assembled and edited by Brian Duncan, pleads the case for the importance of cardiac assist devices for the neonate, infant, and child. No area could more aptly demonstrate that children are not simply small adults and that the challenges in developing pediatric cardiac assist devices are not simply engineering challenges to downsize chambers and inflow and outflow cannulae. The differences are in fact legion and are beautifully presented in this book. Dr. Duncan has brought together many of the leading figures in the field. The exciting progress with the two pediatric pulsatile assist devices presently being developed in Europe is of particular interest.

Although many of the challenges associated with the management of congenital heart disease have already been met, there are many that remain unsolved, and undoubtedly new challenges will emerge as our successes create new populations of patients, for example, long-term survivors of single ventricle surgery. This group in particular is very likely to benefit enormously from a concerted effort by industry in partnership with dedicated physician researchers to develop auxiliary implantable cardiac pump support designed for the long term. Hopefully this book will help to stimulate interest in making this possible.

Richard A. Jonas, M.D.
Cardiovascular Surgeon-in-Chief
Children's Hospital and
William E. Ladd Professor of Child Surgery
Harvard Medical School
Boston, Massachusetts

Preface

Pediatric patients with cardiorespiratory disease who require mechanical circulatory support after failing routine medical management represent the most critically ill subset of an already challenging patient population. As in adult patients, pediatric patients can now benefit from some of the exciting advances that are occurring in the field of mechanical support for cardiorespiratory failure. However, there remain substantial differences (size constraints and cardiac pathophysiology) that make many of the considerations regarding mechanical circulatory support unique in pediatric patients.

Mechanical circulatory support occupies an increasingly important role in the treatment of pediatric cardiac disease. In the acute care setting, advances in extracorporeal membrane oxygenation (ECMO), ventricular assist devices, and intra-aortic balloon counterpulsation have contributed to the continually improving outcomes of children who undergo surgery to correct congenital heart disease. In fact, postoperative mechanical circulatory support has become a necessary tool in the successful management of these patients. Similarly, the use of mechanical circulatory support for nonsurgical pediatric cardiac disease such as myocarditis has resulted in continued improvement in outcomes for these conditions as well. In addition to the use of mechanical circulatory support in the acute setting, an expanding patient population with congenital heart disease exists that may benefit from chronic mechanical circulatory support. As results of operative repair of congenital heart lesions have improved, there is an increasingly large population of patients with congenital heart disease who survive to adulthood. Many of these patients who possess palliated cardiovascular physiology may ultimately require implantable circulatory support devices as a bridge to transplantation or as definitive cardiac replacement.

This book attempts to fill a void in the current literature by concisely summarizing the state-of-the-art of mechanical circulatory support for pediatric cardiac patients in a single volume. All of the currently available modalities of mechanical support—ECMO, ventricular assist devices, and intra-aortic balloon pumps—are covered to demonstrate the specific clinical settings where each modality might be best utilized. Special topics in which these modes of support have been effective, for example, resuscitation after cardiac arrest, support of patients with myocarditis, and circulatory support of pediatric patients without cardiac disease, such as those with overwhelming sepsis, are also covered.

The care of this most critically ill subset of pediatric cardiac patients requires expertise from a wide range of medical specialties and medical professionals. This book aims to serve as a guide for management issues that arise in the pediatric intensive care setting when mechanical circulatory support is utilized. Sections covering management issues that pediatric intensivists, cardiologists, cardiac surgeons, nursing personnel, and perfusionists might face have been included to cover the unique clinical features that arise during the care of these children. The backgrounds of the authors of this text reflect the diverse nature of the skills that are necessary for creating a successful team to manage these patients. It is hoped that this book will satisfy the need for a concise reference for health professionals of all backgrounds who provide care for these patients.

The increasingly important field of long-term mechanical support in pediatric patients is also covered. This includes topics related to the existing experience with implantable ventricular assist devices and the long-term follow-up of pediatric cardiac patients supported with ECMO or ventricular assist devices. Because of their importance in preoperative and postoperative support of transplant patients, issues of mechanical circulatory support in the perioperative period of cardiac and pulmonary transplantation are also covered. Finally, a glimpse into the future of mechanical circulatory support for pediatric cardiorespiratory disease is provided by reviewing early clinical experience with a number of new devices that may lead to improved results and by examining some of the exciting new areas of research in the field.

Pediatric cardiac patients who require mechanical circulatory support deserve the attention and focus that this book provides. These patients represent an expanding patient population and require unique management techniques when compared to the management of adult patients in this setting. In addition, the outcome for these patients would be uniformly fatal without the availability of mechanical circulatory support options. Successfully supporting these patients through their critical illness is one of the most gratifying aspects of pediatric cardiac care. The authors hope this text enables more successful outcomes to be realized for affected children.

Brian W. Duncan

Contents

Contributors

Vladimir Alexi-Meskishvili, M.D., Ph.D. Department of Cardiovascular and Thoracic Surgery, German Heart Institute, Berlin, Germany

Melvin C. Almodovar, M.D. Cardiac Intensive Care Unit, Children's Hospital and Harvard Medical School, Boston, Massachusetts

Emile A. Bacha, M.D. Department of Cardiovascular Surgery, Children's Hospital and Harvard Medical School, Boston, Massachusetts

Dorothy M. Beke, R.N., B.S.N. Cardiac Intensive Care Unit, Children's Hospital, Boston, Massachusetts

Desmond Bohn, M.B., F.R.C.P.C. Department of Critical Care Medicine, The Hospital for Sick Children, Toronto, Ontario, Canada

Harvey S. Borovetz, Ph.D. Department of Bioengineering and Surgery, McGowan Center for Artificial Organ Development, University of Pittsburgh, Pittsburgh, Pennsylvania

Lynne K. Bower, C.C.P., R.R.T. Children's Hospital, Boston, Massachusetts

Kenneth C. Butler, M.S. Nimbus Inc., Rancho Cordova, California

Pedro J. del Nido, M.D. Department of Cardiovascular Surgery, Children's Hospital and Harvard Medical School, Boston, Massachusetts

Brian W. Duncan, M.D. Division of Cardiac Surgery, Children's Hospital and Regional Medical Center and University of Washington School of Medicine, Seattle, Washington

David M. Farrell, M.A., C.C.P. Department of Cardiovascular Surgery, Children's Hospital, Boston, Massachusetts

Mark E. Galantowicz, M.D. Columbia-Presbyterian Medical Center and College of Physicians and Surgeons of Columbia University, New York, New York

Allan Goldman, M.B.B.Ch.B., M.R.C.P. Great Ormond Street Hospital for Children, London, England

Bartley P. Griffith, M.D. Department of Surgery, McGowan Center for Artificial Organ Development, University of Pittsburgh, Pittsburgh, Pennsylvania

John A. Hawkins, M.D. Department of Cardiothoracic Surgery, Primary Children's Medical Center, and Department of Surgery, University of Utah, Salt Lake City, Utah

David N. Helman, M.D. Columbia-Presbyterian Medical Center and College of Physicians and Surgeons of Columbia University, New York, New York

Roland Hetzer, M.D., Ph.D. Department of Cardiovascular and Thoracic Surgery, German Heart Institute, Berlin, Germany

Patricia A. Hickey, M.S., R.N. Cardiovascular Program, Children's Hospital, Boston, Massachusetts

Stephen B. Horton, C.C.P. Department of Cardiac Surgery, Royal Children's Hospital, Melbourne, Australia

Robert J. Howe, C.C.P. Department of Cardiovascular Surgery, Children's Hospital, Boston, Massachusetts

Charles B. Huddleston, M.D. Division of Cardiothoracic Surgery, Department of Surgery, St. Louis Children's Hospital and Washington University School of Medicine, St. Louis, Missouri

Andra E. Ibrahim, M.D. Department of Anesthesiology, University of Washington School of Medicine, Seattle, Washington

Jill E. Ibrahim, M.D. Division of Pediatric Cardiology, St. Louis Children's Hospital and Washington University School of Medicine, St. Louis, Missouri

Marina V. Kameneva, Ph.D. Department of Surgery, McGowan Center for Artificial Organ Development, University of Pittsburgh, Pittsburgh, Pennsylvania

Tom R. Karl, M.D. Department of Cardiothoracic Surgery, Children's Hospital of Philadelphia, Philadelphia, Pennsylvania

Caroline Killick, M.B.B.Ch.B., M.R.C.P. Great Ormond Street Hospital for Children, London, England

Wolfgang F. Konertz, M.D., Ph.D. Department of Cardiovascular Surgery, Charité, Humboldt University, Berlin, Germany

Robert A. LaPierre, C.C.P. Department of Cardiovascular Surgery, Children's Hospital, Boston, Massachusetts

Peter C. Laussen, M.D. Cardiac Intensive Care Unit, Children's Hospital and Harvard Medical School, Boston, Massachusetts

Philip Litwak, D.V.M., Ph.D. Department of Surgery, McGowan Center for Artificial Organ Development, University of Pittsburgh, Pittsburgh, Pennsylvania

Matthias Loebe, M.D. Department of Cardiovascular and Thoracic Surgery, German Heart Institute, Berlin, Germany

Mahendar Macha, M.D. Department of Surgery, McGowan Center for Artificial Organ Development, University of Pittsburgh, Pittsburgh, Pennsylvania

Timothy R. Maher, M.S. Nimbus Inc., Rancho Cordova, California

Gregory S. Matte, C.C.P. Department of Cardiovascular Surgery, Children's Hospital, Boston, Massachusetts

Eric N. Mendeloff, M.D. Division of Cardiothoracic Surgery, Department of Surgery, St. Louis Children's Hospital and Washington University School of Medicine, St. Louis, Missouri

L. LuAnn Minich, M.D. Department of Pediatrics, Primary Children's Medical Center and University of Utah, Salt Lake City, Utah

Paula J. Moynihan, R.N., B.S.N., C.C.R.N. Cardiac Intensive Care Unit, Children's Hospital, Boston, Massachusetts

Patricia O'Brien, R.N., M.S.N., P.N.P. Department of Cardiology, Children's Hospital, Boston, Massachusetts

Mehmet C. Oz, M.D. Columbia-Presbyterian Medical Center and College of Physicians and Surgeons of Columbia University, New York, New York

Michael A. Portman, M.D. Division of Pediatric Cardiology, Children's Hospital and Regional Medical Center and University of Washington School of Medicine, Seattle, Washington

Evgenij Potapov, M.D. Department of Cardiovascular and Thoracic Surgery, German Heart Institute, Berlin, Germany

Kim Reiser, R.N., B.S.N., C.C.R.N. Cardiac Intensive Care Unit, Children's Hospital, Boston, Massachusetts

Dominique Shum-Tim, M.D., C.M., F.R.C.S.C. Department of Cardiothoracic Surgery, Montreal Children's Hospital and McGill University, Montreal, Quebec, Canada

Leslie Smoot, M.D. Department of Cardiology, Children's Hospital and Harvard Medical School, Boston, Massachusetts

Brigitte Stiller, M.D. Department of Congenital Heart Disease, German Heart Institute, Berlin, Germany

Lynn P. Taylor Department of Quality Assurance, Nimbus Inc., Rancho Cordova, California

Douglas C. Thomas, M.S. Department of Engineering, Nimbus Inc., Rancho Cordova, California

Yuguo Weng, M.D. Department of Cardiovascular and Thoracic Surgery, German Heart Institute, Berlin, Germany

David L. Wessel, M.D. Cardiac Intensive Care Unit, Children's Hospital and Harvard Medical School, Boston, Massachusetts

Mechanical Support for Cardiac and Respiratory Failure in Pediatric Patients

1

Extracorporeal Membrane Oxygenation for Children with Cardiac Disease

Brian W. Duncan
Children's Hospital and Regional Medical Center and University of Washington School of Medicine, Seattle, Washington

I. INTRODUCTION

The provision of mechanical circulatory support when other forms of treatment have failed is increasingly common in the therapeutic approach to patients with cardiac disease. For adults in the acute setting, left ventricular failure due to coronary artery disease has been managed with intraaortic balloon pumping (IABP) and left ventricular assist device (LVAD) insertion. For chronic circulatory support, the success of implantable LVAD systems has led to their increasing use in the management of patients with end-stage ventricular failure. In children, however, isolated left ventricular failure is relatively rare, while right ventricular failure, pulmonary hypertension, and hypoxemia often contribute significantly to circulatory failure in pediatric heart disease. Due to these physiological differences isolated support of the left ventricle by IABP or LVAD has more limited application in children. Extracorporeal membrane oxygenation (ECMO) provides biventricular cardiopulmonary support and has emerged as the dominant modality of mechanical circulatory assistance in children with heart disease who have failed conventional medical treatment. This chapter will address the current status of ECMO in these patients by examining historical aspects of its development, technical issues related to management of the circuit, and unique clinical features of pediatric cardiac ECMO such as indications and contraindications for support.

II. HISTORICAL ASPECTS

A. The Development of ECMO for Pediatric Cardiac Support

The use of ECMO as a means of providing support for cardiorespiratory failure in pediatric cardiac patients arose as a natural extension of work in the 1970s that established the efficacy of ECMO in treating respiratory failure in children. Baffes is credited with the first use of prolonged extracorporeal circulation in congenital heart disease, although the duration of support was relatively brief for each patient in this series (1). However, significant innovations were introduced by these investigators including the use of the circuit for resuscitation from cardiac arrest and provision of support for perioperative stabilization at the time of palliative cardiac procedures. The first reported use of ECMO for extended periods in a pediatric heart patient was supplied by Soeter, who described the successful use of ECMO to support a 4-year-old girl with severe hypoxemia after repair of tetralogy of Fallot (2). The system described employed a rotary pump with a membrane oxygenator and a heat exchanger. The patient was weaned from support within 48 hours, was extubated 2 days later, and was discharged on the 13th postoperative day.

Other landmark studies in the development of ECMO for pediatric cardiac support include those by Hill and Bartlett and colleagues (3–5). Although these reports focused on patients with respiratory failure, they also included descriptions of the successful use of ECMO for postoperative support in children undergoing repair of congenital heart defects. Important contributions provided by these early studies included the careful consideration of those aspects of management that make ECMO for cardiac support unique from those required for respiratory failure. Some of the issues that were addressed included how best to handle anticoagulation issues in fresh postoperative cardiac surgical patients, the development of guidelines for indications and contraindications for support, and identification of the importance of appropriate patient selection. It is a testimony to the remarkable foresight of these pioneers that the same issues still retain central importance to the success of ECMO used for pediatric cardiac support, as we shall discuss below.

B. Current Status of Pediatric Cardiac ECMO from the Extracorporeal Life Support Organization Registry

The Extracorporeal Life Support Organization (ELSO) was founded in 1989 as the organized body to facilitate the study of the clinical use of ECMO. One of the most important functions of the organization is the maintenance of the ELSO

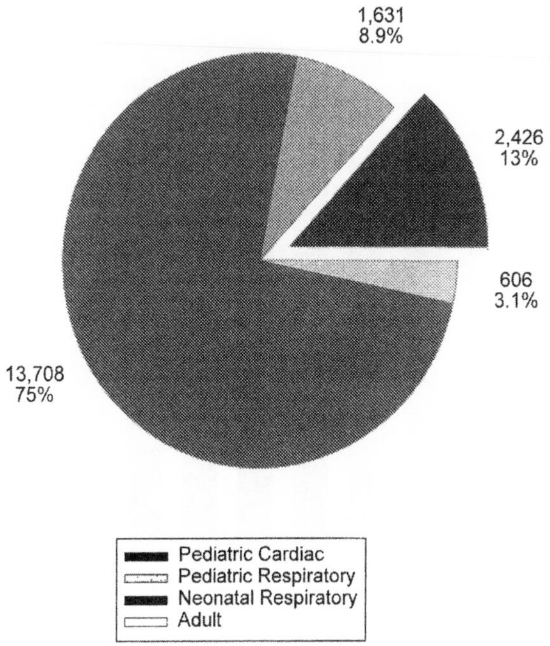

Fig. 1 ELSO data for total number of patients requiring support by diagnostic group.

Registry, which compiles data on the use of ECMO by participating institutions and currently contains records for over 12,000 cases worldwide dating back to 1986 (6). The ELSO Registry maintains cases recorded according to each of four diagnostic groups—neonatal respiratory, pediatric respiratory, neonatal/pediatric cardiac, and adult. Examination of the Registry demonstrates that pediatric cardiac support has comprised approximately 13% of total ECMO utilization overall (7) (Fig. 1). However, during the period covered by the Registry there has been a steady increase in the proportion of neonatal/pediatric cardiac cases in comparison to all other patient groups requiring ECMO (Fig. 2). This change reflects both the greater utilization of ECMO in the treatment of pediatric heart disease as well as decreased utilization of ECMO for respiratory failure owing to the success of other respiratory support measures such as nitric oxide administration and high-frequency jet ventilation. With these changes in utilization patterns in mind, a greater understanding of the issues that lead to successful support of pediatric cardiac patients becomes increasingly important for all ECMO services.

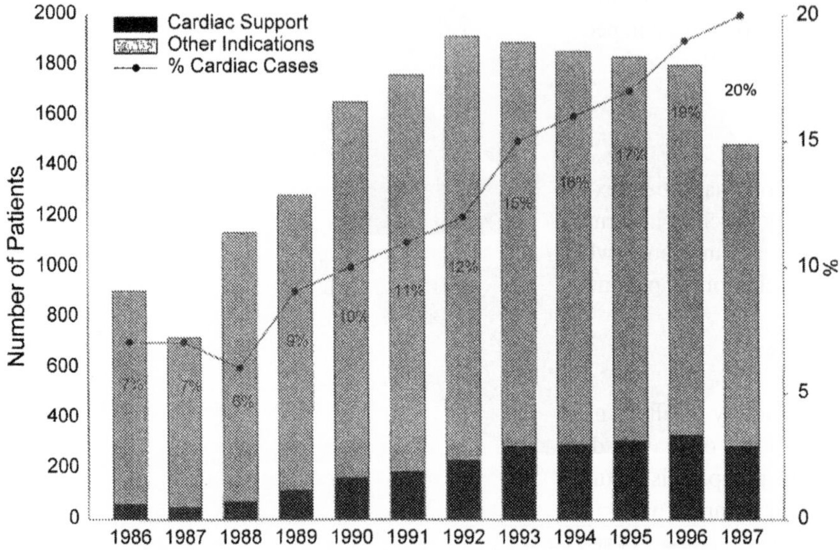

Fig. 2 Comparison of ELSO data for annual number and percentage of total for pediatric cardiac support patients versus all other diagnostic categories.

III. CIRCUIT-RELATED AND OTHER TECHNICAL ASPECTS

A. Components of the Circuit

Precise details regarding the components of the ECMO circuit will be covered in other chapters of this book, while the following summary will address theoretical aspects of circuit design for pediatric cardiac patients. For children with cardiac disease, technical considerations related to the circuit are similar to those utilized for the support of respiratory failure with some important modifications. Most patients with cardiac disease require a venoarterial mode for full cardiopulmonary support. However, several reports have described the successful use of venovenous ECMO for pediatric patients with heart disease (8,9). Since a substantial amount of morbidity in congenital heart disease is due to hypoxia, pulmonary hypertension, and right ventricular failure, venovenous ECMO may currently be an underutilized modality in pediatric cardiac patients. Although not providing cardiac pump support, the use of venovenous ECMO may lead to improved right ventricular function by eliminating hypoxia and decreasing pulmonary vascular resistance. A particularly ingenious approach to venovenous support is the AREC system (assistance respiratoire extra-corporelle) described by Chevalier, which utilizes a single venous cannula driven by a nonocclusive rotary pump with tidal flow in the circuit provided by alternating clamps (10). This system has been successfully used in pediatric cardiac patients with hypoxia and pulmonary hypertension as the primary indication for ECMO support (8).

Most centers utilize a standard ECMO circuit that employs a membrane oxygenator, roller pump, and heat exchanger. Membrane oxygenators are currently utilized by the majority of centers, however, the use of hollow fiber oxygenators has been explored recently (11–13). Hollow-fiber oxygenators are highly efficient in terms of gas exchange and are easy to prime, which is especially advantageous when rapid institution of support is critical such as for the resuscitation of patients from cardiac arrest (13). A major impediment to more widespread use of hollow-fiber oxygenators, however, arises from their limited longevity due to plasma leak requiring frequent replacement with prolonged use (14). Although most centers continue to use roller pumps, several groups report satisfactory results using a centrifugal pump, which maintains venous inflow independent of gravity drainage so that the patient may be at any height relative to the pump. This feature of the centrifugal pump has been found to be especially useful in larger patients to maintain adequate venous return at higher flow rates (15–18). An additional advantage of the centrifugal pump is that occlusion of arterial outflow from the pump does not generate excessive arterial line pressure, reducing the risk of ''blow-out'' of the arterial limb of the circuit if distal occlusion occurs. The chief disadvantage of the centrifugal pump is the high negative pressure that may be generated on the venous side of the circuit potentially leading to hemolysis and cavitation (19).

Circuit flow is controlled by a servoregulatory mechanism, comprised of an in-line distensable bladder that compresses a spring-loaded mechanical switching device that turns the pump off if venous inflow is inadvertently interrupted. Although employed in the majority of circuits utilized worldwide, this system is subject to a number of problems related to the sensitivity of the switching device, which may be difficult to adjust. In addition, the bladder is an area in the circuit with relative stasis of blood flow that may be the site of thrombus formation. New electronic systems may provide a more accurate approach to pump servoregulation and may be utilized more widely in the future (19).

B. Anticoagulation

The status of each patient's anticoagulation is monitored by the whole blood activated clotting time (ACT). Achieving an ACT of 180–200 seconds with a continuous heparin infusion maintains the circuit with a minimal risk of important thrombosis (9,12,16,17,20–22). Platelets are maintained above 100,000 per dL and in patients requiring postoperative support where bleeding is a critical problem, above 150,000 per dL. Clotting factors are supplied with infusions of fresh frozen plasma or cryoprecipitate to maintain fibrinogen levels above 100 mg/dL.

For patients who require intraoperative support after cardiopulmonary bypass, we have not reversed the heparin effect with protamine, but allow the ACT to drift to the 180–200 second range as factor levels and platelets are repleted (9). Instituting the heparin infusion may be safely deferred for several hours until the ACT drifts downward in the bleeding postoperative patient.

Recently, heparin-bonded hollow-fiber oxygenators and heparin-bonded tubing have been utilized in an attempt to decrease the amount of systemic heparin required (11). Since 1990 we have utilized epsilon amino caproic acid (AMIKAR; Lederle Parenterals, Carolina, Puerto Rico) to diminish the risk of important postoperative hemorrhage (9,23). AMIKAR is administered as an intravenous bolus of 100 mg/kg, maintained as a continuous intravenous infusion of 30 mg/kg/h for the initial 48 hours of support and then discontinued. Maintaining the infusion for longer periods is usually unnecessary due to abatement of postsurgical bleeding as well as increasing problems with circuit thrombosis resulting from prolonged administration. A recent multicenter trial failed to demonstrate an improvement in rate of significant intracranial hemorrhage or surgical site bleeding with AMIKAR infusion for neonates requiring ECMO for respiratory failure, however, the number of patients enrolled in the study was small (24).

C. Cannulation

The approach to cannulation should be flexible and based on the setting in which the need for ECMO arises. Transthoracic cannulation of the right atrial appendage and the ascending aorta is most appropriate for cases that require intraoperative support for failure to wean from cardiopulmonary bypass. In the immediate postoperative period chest cannulation provides the most expeditious route to institute support, especially in patients that suffer cardiac arrest. Adequate venous drainage and excellent arterial perfusion are assured by chest cannulation, however, significant hemorrhage remains the chief disadvantage making peripheral cannulation sites preferable in most other settings. In addition, the risk of mediastinitis is significantly increased with transthoracic cannulation, which is itself a potential source of morbidity and, should the need arise, may make cardiac transplantation impossible. Cannulation of the right internal jugular vein and the common carotid artery provides excellent venous drainage and perfusion and is the preferred cannulation site in neonates and children below approximately 15 kg in weight. Cannulation of the femoral vessels provides adequate venous drainage and perfusion for larger children. A second venous drainage cannula placed in the right internal jugular vein may be added if venous drainage through the femoral route alone is inadequate. The risk of lower extremity ischemia can be minimized by placing a perfusion cannula in the distal femoral artery from a side arm brought off of the arterial limb of the circuit (9,21). Venous congestion of the lower extremity may be prevented by placement of a "saphenous sump" catheter at the time of femoral venous cannulation (15). The axillary artery and iliac vessels may represent additional cannulation sites in difficult access cases, however, we have not had to utilize either of these sites. Based on these considerations we prefer transthoracic cannulation only for cases that require the institution of support in the operating room or in cases of cardiac arrest in the immediate postoperative period. We perform peripheral cannulation for virtually all other cases including severe cardiogenic shock in postcardiotomy patients to limit the amount of postoperative bleeding.

D. Left Ventricular Decompression

Left ventricular distension must be assiduously avoided during ECMO especially in cases of severe left ventricular dysfunction. We carefully monitor for the development of left-sided distension with echocardiography and direct measurement of left atrial pressure when available. If left-sided distension is discovered, we aggressively treat this with left atrial venting, which can be easily performed in patients who have undergone transthoracic cannulation by cannulating the right pulmonary veins at the atrioventricular groove or via the left atrial appendage. In patients cannulated by the peripheral route, left-sided decompression may be achieved by balloon atrial septostomy performed in the cardiac catheterization laboratory or preferably, at the patient's bedside under echocardiographic guidance (25,26). An innovative experimental approach utilizing a percutaneously placed spring that renders the pulmonary valve incompetent effectively provided left-sided decompression but has not been utilized clinically due to the success of direct venting or the creation of an atrial level communication (27). Some authors state that left-sided distension can be effectively dealt with by increasing ECMO flow, which maintains little blood flow through the lungs and minimizes pulmonary venous return (28). We agree with other reports that propose an aggressive stance toward left-sided decompression using direct venting or balloon atrial septostomy to diminish the risks of left ventricular distension injury and optimize the chances for return of ventricular function (16–18,21,22).

E. Other Management Points

We maintain ECMO flow rates generally in the range of 80–150 cc/kg/min until patients are considered ready for weaning. Regarding inotropic support during ECMO, we substantially decrease our dosages but routinely maintain these patients on low-dose dopamine and vasodilators. This combination hopefully improves peripheral and renal perfusion as well as encouraging some degree of ventricular emptying in a further attempt to limit left-sided distension. We have routinely utilized total parenteral nutrition for patients on ECMO due to concerns about splanchnic perfusion and ileus in these critically ill patients to avoid septic gastrointestinal complications such as necrotizing enterocolitis. Recent reports, however, indicate that enteral nutrition may be utilized safely in these patients (29,30). These reports will probably alter our current practice to include the use of enteral feeding in a larger percentage of ECMO-supported patients due to the well-recognized beneficial effects of enteral nutrition in patients in the critical care setting.

We feel that it is important to maintain moderate levels of ventilatory support for the cardiac patient that requires ECMO support. Several studies have shown that coronary perfusion is primarily derived from the left ventricle during ECMO if there is any appreciable cardiac function (31,32). Therefore, blood returning from the pulmonary veins should be fully saturated to maintain adequate myocardial oxygenation and optimize the chances for ventricular recovery. With the exception of patients who have severe pulmonary parenchymal disease, fully saturated pulmonary venous blood is easily provided by maintaining moderate levels of ventilatory support during ECMO. We maintain the majority of our ECMO-supported cardiac patients with a fractional inspired oxygen of 40%, a respiratory rate of 16 breaths per minute, positive end expiratory pressure of 5 cm of H_2O, and a tidal volume of 10 cc/kg.

F. Weaning from Support

Weaning is performed under echocardiographic guidance to assess ventricular filling and function. We do not routinely place pulmonary arterial catheters for cardiac output and pulmonary capillary wedge pressure determination but would do so in borderline cases. At the time of weaning, flows are gradually turned down over a several hour period until flows of 25–40 cc/kg/min are achieved. Concurrently ventilatory support and inotrope dosages are increased to appropriate levels. We then clamp the arterial and venous lines, maintaining full anticoagulation, and intermittently flush the cannulas (every 15–20 minutes) until the patient is clearly stable off ECMO. We routinely perform decannulation at the patient's bedside. We have maintained borderline patients off ECMO for 1–2 hours with intermittent flushing of the cannulas until it is clear that support is no longer needed, however, we have not capped the cannulas for periods of 24 hours or more as some groups have described for respiratory failure patients. A strategy that we have found useful in cases of profound ventricular dysfunction is to spread out the weaning period over 48–72 hours with gradual reduction in flows over that period. It is our observation that especially fragile patients who may have failed with more rapid weaning may benefit from this approach by gradually accommodating to lower flows.

IV. CLINICAL ASPECTS

A. Cardiac Diagnoses

We recently reviewed the experience at Children's Hospital, Boston, for pediatric cardiac patients that required mechanical circulatory support with either ECMO or ventricular assist devices (VAD) (9). There were 67 ECMO supported patients spanning a 10-year period, which represents a relatively large single institution experience. The diagnostic categories for the ECMO supported patients are presented in Table 1, demonstrating that more than one half of these cases were patients with complex cyanotic heart disease possessing either increased (33% of the total patients) or decreased (25% of the total patients) pulmonary blood flow. Reviewing reports from other centers reveals this to be a generally representative make-up of patient diagnoses. In Walters' report of a large series of patients requiring postoperative support after cardiac surgery, complete atrioventricular canal (20%), complex single ventricle anatomy (17%), and tetralogy of Fallot (14%) were the most common diagnoses (33). Meliones in his 1991 review of ELSO Registry data for pediatric cardiac patients found patients with left-to-right shunt (24%), cyanosis with decreased pulmonary blood flow (22%), and cyanosis with increased pulmonary blood flow (17%) to be the most commons diagnostic groups (34). Comparing the two modalities, we found ECMO to be superior to VAD for the support of most children with complex cyanotic heart disease where hypoxia, pulmonary hypertension, or biventricular failure contributes significantly to the pathophysiology necessitating mechanical circulatory support. Due to the presence of an oxygenator in the circuit, ECMO more directly addresses the underlying pathophysiology and provides greater flexibility than VAD in these instances (see chapter 4) (9).

Table 1 Diagnostic Groups and Survival for ECMO Support

Diagnosis	Survivors (% survival)	Nonsurvivors (% nonsurvival)	Total (% of all diagnostic groups)
Left-to-right shunt	1 (14%)	6 (86%)	7 (11%)
Left-sided obstruction	5 (42%)	7 (58%)	12 (18%)
Right-sided obstruction	1 (100%)	0 (64%)	1 (1.5%)
Cyanosis, ↑ pulmonary blood flow	8 (36%)	14 (64%)	22 (33%)
Cyanosis, ↓ pulmonary blood flow	7 (41%)	10 (59%)	17 (25%)
ALCAPA	1 (100%)	0	1 (1.5%)
Cardiomyopathy	3 (75%)	1 (25%)	4 (6%)
Other	1 (33%)	2 (67%)	3 (4%)
Total	27 (40%)	40 (60%)	67

ALCAPA = Anomalous left coronary artery from pulmonary artery.

B. Indications for Support

Reviewing several large clinical series confirms that indications for support differ according to whether ECMO is required in the preoperative or postoperative period of cardiac surgery. Studies that summarize the preoperative use of ECMO demonstrate that hypoxia and pulmonary hypertension are the most common indications leading to ECMO support (8,35). Postoperative support is most commonly initiated for failure to wean from cardiopulmonary bypass, cardiogenic shock, or cardiac arrest occurring in the intensive care unit after cardiac surgery (15–18,20–22,28,33,36,37).

Our experience, which combined preoperative, postoperative, and cardiac medical patients, demonstrated that hypoxia (36%), cardiac arrest (24%), and failure to wean from cardiopulmonary bypass (14%) were the most common indications for ECMO support (9) (Table 2). Although hypoxia was the single largest indication in our experience, innovative therapies such as nitric oxide administration and high-frequency jet ventilation may decrease the need for ECMO support in the treatment of pediatric patients with cardiac disease and

Table 2 Indications for ECMO Support and Survival

Indication	Survivors (% survival)	Nonsurvivors (% nonsurvival)	Total (% of all indications)
Hypoxia	11 (44%)	14 (56%)	25 (36%)
Preop cardiac failure	1 (100%)	0	1 (1.4%)
Postop cardiac failure	2 (29%)	5 (71%)	7 (10%)
Cardiac arrest	7 (41%)	10 (59%)	17 (24%)
Bridge to transplant	2 (67%)	1 (33%)	3 (4.4%)
Failure to wean from CPB	1 (10%)	9 (90%)	10 (14%)
Pulmonary hypertension	1 (25%)	3 (75%)	4 (5.8%)
Cardiac failure no operation	2 (67%)	1 (33%)	3 (4.4%)
Total	27 (39%)	43 (61%)	70

CPB = Cardiopulmonary bypass.

Note: The total number of indications (70) in this table exceeds the total number of diagnoses (67) in Table 1 due to two ECMO runs that were performed in three patients. Each run is considered to have its own indication, while there is a single diagnosis per patient.

refractory respiratory failure (38–40). Kocis reported the use of high-frequency jet ventilation in patients that would have otherwise required ECMO for refractory respiratory failure. Seven of eight patients treated with high-frequency jet ventilation had their respiratory failure reversed, with only a single patient subsequently requiring ECMO (40). Goldman used nitric oxide to treat 10 patients with severe pulmonary hypertension after surgery for congenital heart disease, including 5 patients who could not be weaned from cardiopulmonary bypass. They were able to avoid ECMO in 8 of these 10 patients, with 80% of the total patients surviving to hospital discharge (38).

In our experience, the need for ECMO for failure to wean from cardiopulmonary bypass had a significant negative impact on survival with only 1 of 10 (10%) patients surviving to hospital discharge (9). Several other studies also report failure to wean from cardiopulmonary bypass as a negative prognostic indicator in these patients (12,18,33). However, a number of studies have not found inability to wean from bypass to be a risk factor (21,28). In fact, these latter studies stress the importance of early institution of ECMO before prolonged periods of low cardiac output in the postoperative patient result in end organ damage. The importance of early institution of ECMO support cannot be over emphasized, however, we have observed that patients who are unable to wean from cardiopulmonary bypass without ECMO fare poorly due to excessive mediastinal hemorrhage and often possess greater degrees of ventricular dysfunction.

C. Contraindications

As the use of ECMO for cardiac patients has increased, those clinical features defined as contraindications for the institution of support have evolved. There is universal agreement that certain conditions constitute absolute contraindications including incurable malignancy, advanced multisystem organ failure, extreme prematurity, and severe central nervous system damage (9,16,33,37). Various reports have stressed that residual cardiac lesions after cardiac surgery should be viewed as a contraindication to support due to the poor outcome of patients with residual defects in these studies (12,15). Any patient who is not a transplant candidate should probably be considered ineligible for support in that any patient placed on ECMO may ultimately require cardiac transplantation for recovery (16).

However, a number of conditions previously thought to be unsalvageable or at risk for further complications with ECMO support have recently been treated with ECMO and should at most represent relative contraindications. Patients with shunted single ventricle physiology including patients with hypoplastic left heart syndrome after neonatal palliation were often denied support in the past due to difficulties in achieving balance between the pulmonary and systemic circulations in these patients. A number of recent studies have reported success with ECMO support of these patients (9,28,33). The blood flow through the shunt usually must be physically limited to ensure adequate systemic perfusion and to avoid "flooding" the lungs with excessive blood flow. We often perform this at the patient's bedside by placing a metallic clip to partially constrict the shunt, which is removed at the time of weaning. Completely occluding the shunt is not advisable due to the risk of extensive pulmonary infarction (28). In general, we have not developed rigid contraindications for mechanical support besides those features mentioned above but evaluate each case individually. In addition to shunted single ventricle patients we have successfully supported patients with presupport cardiac arrest, patients undergoing palliative cardiac operations, and cardiac patients with coexisting congenital diaphragmatic hernia. None of these represent absolute contraindications for ECMO support in our experience.

D. Outcome and Risk Factors for Death

Published series report variable survival statistics for pediatric cardiac ECMO. The latest cumulative survival rate for device weaning for neonatal and pediatric cardiac ECMO reported by the ELSO Registry is 42%, which has remained a relatively constant rate of survival (Fig. 3) (7). In our experience, two thirds of all patients placed on ECMO were successfully weaned from support, with 40%

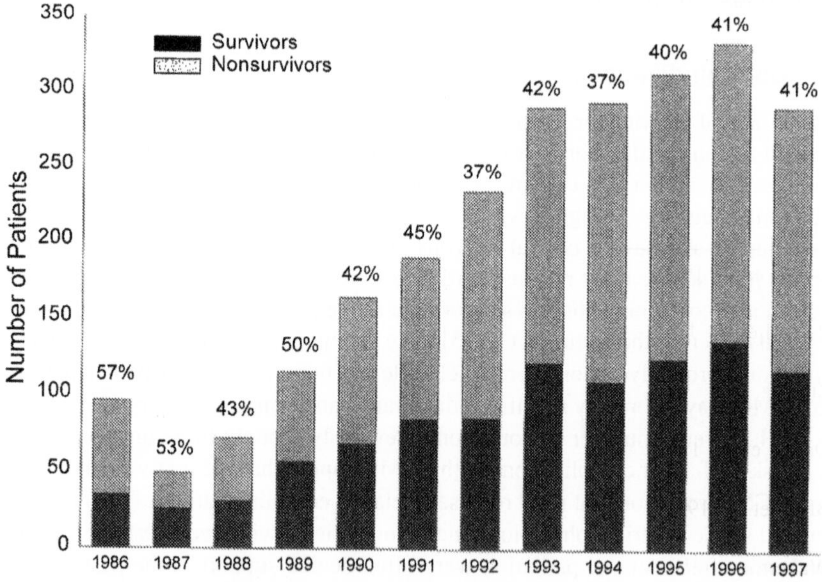

Fig. 3 ELSO data for annual percentage mortality for patients requiring ECMO for pediatric cardiac support.

of the original patients surviving to hospital discharge (9). This represents a fairly typical experience with other studies reporting a weaning rate of 45–80% and a hospital survival rate of 22–70% (12,15–18,20–22,28,33,36,37,41,42). Table 3 demonstrates the outcomes for several large series reported in the 1990s.

Reviewing risk factors for death from centers reporting a large experience with ECMO for pediatric cardiac cases reveals a number of unifying concepts. Several studies have identified the development of renal failure to have a significant adverse impact on survival (9,12,16,33,34). In addition to the development of overt renal failure as a risk factor, we found that survivors had a much greater urine output over the first 24 hours of support (9). Severe hemorrhage measured directly as the volume of blood lost or the need for excessive transfusion of blood products was a risk factor for death in a number of studies (9,18,33,34). In our experience nonsurvivors had a nearly twofold greater blood loss compared to survivors. The presence of residual cardiac lesions after cardiac surgery and the need for ECMO in cardiac surgical cases that fail to wean from cardiopulmonary bypass represent significant risk factors in some reports as discussed above (12,33). Other risk factors that have been identified in various reports include significant infectious complications, presupport cardiac arrest, and high inotropic dosages while on support.

Lack of return of ventricular function within 48–72 hours was an ominous sign in our experience. We examined the rate of return of ventricular function

Table 3 Summary of Reported Outcomes for ECMO Support of Pediatric Cardiac Patients

Study	Total no. patients	Weaned	Survivors	Ref.
Delius et al., 1992	25	13/25 (52%)	10/25 (40%)	21
Raithel et al., 1992	65	44/65 (68%)	23/65 (35%)	22
Ziomek et al., 1992	24	18/24 (75%)	13/24 (54%)	28
Dalton et al., 1993	29	18/29 (62%)	13/29 (45%)	16
Black et al., 1995	31	14/31 (45%)	13/31 (41%)	15
Walters et al., 1995	73	49/73 (67%)	42/73 (58%)	33
Duncan et al., 1999	67	45/67 (67%)	27/67 (40%)	9

for nontransplanted survivors compared with patients who were unable to be weaned from ECMO support (nonsurvivors and survivors who required cardiac transplantation) (Fig. 4) (9). Return of ventricular function was defined as the return of a pulsatile waveform on the peripheral arterial trace on maximal levels of support (80% of normal cardiac output provided by the device). Twenty-four of 25 nontransplanted ECMO survivors (96%) had return of a pulsatile waveform on the arterial line trace by 72 hours of support. We have used these data as additional prognostic information for these children. Postcardiotomy patients without return of ventricular function within 48–72 hours of support are currently considered for transplantation or termination of support if there are contraindications to transplantation. Delaying this decision while awaiting return of ventricular function beyond the first 48–72 hours of support is not justified based on these results. Due to the scarcity of organ donors in the pediatric population, early consideration for transplantation optimizes the chances of successful organ procurement.

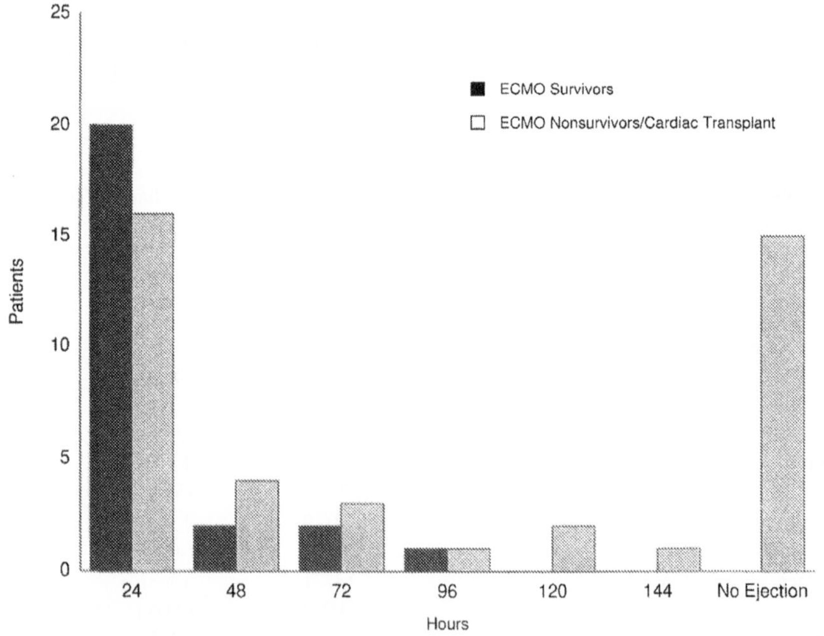

Fig. 4 Time to return of ventricular function versus survival for ECMO-supported patients.

E. Complications

Table 4 lists the complications by organ system that occurred in our experience at Children's Hospital, Boston (9). These same trends are also reflected in reports from other centers with hemorrhagic complications occurring in 10–70% of all patients (12,16–18,21,22,33,36,37). Most commonly in postoperative patients this takes the form of mediastinal bleeding, however, in all patients hemorrhage from the site of cannulation, the central nervous system, or gastrointestinal sources may occur. The negative impact of hemorrhagic complications on these patients' outcomes has been discussed in the previous section. Cardiovascular complications include arrhythmia or ongoing significant ventricular dysfunction. Neurological complications represent a source of considerable morbidity in these patients. We found intracranial hemorrhage, seizures, and cerebral infarction to be the three most common neurological complications comprising 36, 23, and 18% of all central nervous system complications, respectively. Neurological complications were more common in ECMO-supported patients as opposed to VAD-supported patients possibly due to ECMO support being instituted in a higher percentage of neonates with more coexisting disease. In our experience, neurological complications were independent of presupport cardiac arrest, the use of ca-

Table 4 Complication Rates and Survival

Complication	Incidence	Survival
Hemorrhage	28/70 (40%)	10/28 (36%)
Cardiovascular	26/70 (37%)	10/26 (38%)
Central nervous system	22/70 (31%)	10/22 (45%)
Any severe infection	19/70 (27%)	7/19 (37%)
Mechanical	18/70 (26%)	5/18 (28%)
Gastrointestinal	17/70 (24%)	6/17 (35%)
Renal failure (dialysis or serum creatinine ≥ 3.0)	15/70 (21%)	2/15 (13%)*
Pulmonary	15/70 (21%)	8/15 (53%)

* $p = 0.03$ for renal complications impact on survival.

rotid cannulation, or the performance of carotid reconstruction in patients who underwent neck cannulation (9).

Mechanical complications including tubing rupture, cannula dislodgment, or important thrombus formation in the circuit occurred in 26% of all cases that we analyzed. Our experience agrees with all other published reports in that mechanical complications did not represent a risk factor for death in these patients (17,21,28,34). Renal failure occurred in 21% of our patients and was a risk factor for death as it was in several other reports (22,33,34).

F. Causes of Mortality

Ongoing cardiac failure and multiple system organ failure were the most common causes of death for ECMO supported patients in our experience (9) (Table 5). Meliones' analysis of the ELSO registry listed ongoing cardiac failure (37% of the causes of death) and major central nervous system damage (15% of the causes of death) as the most common causes of mortality (31). Cardiac failure and complications arising from low cardiac output are likewise the most commonly reported causes of death in numerous other series (17,28,41). Attempts to improve the results achieved with pediatric cardiac ECMO should, therefore, address issues related to optimization of ventricular function and avoidance of extended periods of low cardiac output. Prompt institution of ECMO support achieves both of these goals by optimally preserving myocardial, central nervous system, and visceral perfusion. Allowing patients to continue in a low cardiac output state on increasing dosages of vasoconstrictive agents prior to ECMO may lead to established end-organ damage, which may not be reversible after circulatory support has been established. Once ECMO is initiated, meticulous patient management is required to limit infectious complications, which may contribute to an

Table 5 Causes of Death

Cause of death	Number	%
Ventricular failure	14	35
Multiple system organ failure	12	30
Respiratory failure	4	10
Anoxic brain injury	2	5
Intracranial hemorrhage	2	5
Arrhythmia	2	5
Inadequate flow rates due to poor venous drainage	2	5
Aortic cannula dislodgment	1	2.5
Hemorrhage (torn umbilical vein)	1	2.5
Total	40	100

ongoing clinical picture of sepsis that commonly progresses to multiple system organ failure. For salvage of continuing severe cardiac dysfunction, an early and aggressive approach to cardiac transplantation may be the only life-saving therapy available.

V. SUMMARY

The approach to children with increasingly complicated cardiac disease has required the development of innovative measures to help insure successful outcomes. The utilization of ECMO for cardiac support in children has arisen naturally in pediatric centers due to its widespread and highly successful treatment of respiratory failure in children. The ability to mechanically support the cardiorespiratory system in children with cardiac disease has been an important adjunct in the development of this field. It would not be overstating its importance to claim that a reliably successful surgical or medical approach to many of these cardiac lesions requires the availability of ECMO. However, a clear understanding of the differences between pediatric patients that require ECMO for cardiac conditions from those of respiratory origin must be appreciated. This chapter has attempted to highlight how these differences impact on the technical aspects of ECMO support for pediatric cardiac patients in terms of circuit design and management while on support. In addition, those clinical features that have been identified to be of importance in the treatment of these patients based on the increasingly large experience of many centers have also been presented. Finally, this chapter will provide background for important emerging areas of ECMO support that will be covered in later chapters such as the adjunctive treatment of cardiac transplantation patients, provision of support for severe cases of myocarditis and the use of ECMO for rapid resuscitation from cardiac arrest. All these topics of current importance should be appreciated in terms of their impact on the future of our field. Innovative approaches to mechanical circulatory support for children such as chronic implantable systems and small, pulsatile, cardiopulmonary support units will become a reality. The principles that we use in the application of ECMO to support these children today will serve as the foundation for developing these techniques in the future.

REFERENCES

1. Baffes TG, Fridman JL, Bicoff JP, Whitehill JL. Extracorporeal circulation for support of palliative cardiac surgery in infants. Ann Thorac Surg 1970; 10:354–363.
2. Soeter JR, Mamiya RT, Sprague AY, McNamara JJ. Prolonged extracorporeal oxy-

genation for cardiorespiratory failure after tetralogy correction. J Thorac Cardiovasc Surg 1973; 66:214–218.
3. Bartlett RH, Gazzaniga AB, Fong SW, Burns NE. Prolonged extracorporeal cardiopulmonary support in man. J Thorac Cardiovasc Surg 1974; 68:918–932.
4. Bartlett RH, Gazzaniga AB, Fong SW, Jefferies MR, Roohk HV, Haiduc N. Extracorporeal membrane oxygenator support for cardiopulmonary failure. J Thorac Cardiovasc Surg 1977; 73:375–386.
5. Hill JD, de Leval MR, Fallat RJ, Bramson ML, Eberhart RC, Schulte HD, Osborn JJ, Barber R, Gerbode F. Acute respiratory insufficiency treatment with prolonged extracorporeal oxygenation. J Thorac Cardiovasc Surg 1972; 64:551–562.
6. Tracy J, DeLosh T, Stolar CJH, The Registry of the Extracorporeal Life Support Organization, in ECMO, Zwischenberger JB, Bartlett RH, eds. Ann Arbor: Extracorporeal Life Support Organization, 1995:251–273.
7. ECMO Registry Report. Ann Arbor: Extracorporeal Life Support Organization, July 1998.
8. Trittenwein G, Furst G, Golej J, Frenzel K, Burda G, Hermon M, Marx M, Wollenek G, Pollak A. Preoperative ECMO in congenital cyanotic heart disease using the AREC system. Ann Thorac Surg 1997; 63:1298–1302.
9. Duncan BW, Hraska V, Jonas RA, Wessel DL, del Nido PJ, Laussen PC, Mayer JE, Lapierre RA, Wilson JM. Mechanical circulatory support in children with cardiac disease. J Thorac Cardiovasc Surg 1999; 117:529–542.
10. Chevalier JY, Couprie C, Larroquet M, Renolleau S, Durandy Y, Costil J. Venovenous single lumen cannula extracorporeal lung support in neonates. ASAIO J 1993; 39:M654–658.
11. del Nido PJ. Extracorporeal membrane oxygenation for cardiac support in children. Ann Thorac Surg 1996; 61:336–339.
12. Langley SM, Sheppard SB, Tsang VT, Monro JL, Lamb RK. When is extracorporeal life support worthwhile following repair of congenital heart disease in children? Eur J Cardiothorac Surg 1998; 13:520–525.
13. Saito A, Miyamura H, Kanazawa H, Ohzeki H, Eguchi S. Extracorporeal membrane oxygenation for severe heart failure after Fontan operation. Ann Thorac Surg 1993; 55:153–155.
14. Willms DC, Atkins PJ, Dembitsky WP, Jaski BE, Gocka I. Analysis of clinical trends in a program of emergent ECLS for cardiovascular collapse. ASAIO J 1997; 43: 65–68.
15. Black MD, Coles JG, Williams WG, Rebeyka IM, Trusler GA, Bohn D, Gruenwald C, Freedom R. Determinants of success in pediatric cardiac patients undergoing extracorporeal membrane oxygenation. Ann Thorac Surg 1995; 60:133–138.
16. Dalton HJ, Siewers RD, Fuhrman BP, del Nido PJ, Thompson AE, Shaver MG, Dowhy M. Extracorporeal membrane oxygenation for cardiac rescue in children with severe myocardial dysfunction. Crit Care Med 1993; 21:1020–1028.
17. Kanter KR, Pennington DG, Weber TR, Zambie MA, Braun P, Martychenko V. Extracorporeal membrane oxygenation for postoperative cardiac support in children. J Thorac Cardiovasc Surg 1987; 93:27–35.
18. Klein MD, Shaheen KW, Whittlesey GC, Pinsky WW, Arciniegas E. Extracorporeal

membrane oxygenation for the circulatory support of children after repair of congenital heart disease. J Thorac Cardiovasc Surg 1990; 100:498–505.
19. Hirschl RB. Devices, in ECMO: Extracorporeal Cardiopulmonary Support in Critical Care, Zwischenberger JB, Bartlett RH, eds. Ann Arbor: Extracorporeal Life Support Organization, 1995:150–190.
20. Anderson HL, Attori RJ, Custer JR, Chapman RA, Bartlett RH. Extracorporeal membrane oxygenation for pediatric cardiopulmonary failure. J Thorac Cardiovasc Surg 1990; 99:1011–1021.
21. Delius RE, Bove EL, Meliones JN, Custer JR, Moler FW, Crowley D, Amerikia A, Behrendt DM, Bartlett RH. Use of extracorporeal life support in patients with congenital heart disease. Crit Care Med 1992; 20:1216–1222.
22. Raithel RC, Pennington DG, Boegner E, Fiore A, Weber TR. Extracorporeal membrane oxygenation in children after cardiac surgery. Circulation 1992; 86(suppl II): II-305–II-310.
23. Wilson JM, Bower LK, Fackler JC, Beals DA, Berhus BO, Kevy SB. Aminocaproic acid decreases the incidence of intracranial hemorrhage and other hemorrhagic complications of ECMO. J Pediatr Surg 1993; 28:536–541.
24. Horwitz JR, Cofer BR, Warner BH, Cheu HW, Lally KP. A multi-center trial of 6-aminocaproic acid (Amicar) in the prevention of bleeding in infants on ECMO. J Pediatr Surg 1998; 33:1610–1613.
25. O'Connor TA, Downing GJ, Ewing LL, Gowdamarajan R. Echocardiographically guided balloon atrial septostomy during extracorporeal membrane oxygenation (ECMO). Pediatr Cardiol 1993; 14:167–168.
26. Koenig PR, Ralston MA, Kimball TR, Meyer RA, Daniels SR, Schwartz DC. Balloon atrial septostomy for left ventricular decompression in patients receiving extracorporeal membrane oxygenation for myocardial failure. J Pediatr 1993; 122:S95–99.
27. Kolobow T, Rossi F, Borelli M, Foti G. Long-term closed chest partial and total cardiopulmonary bypass by peripheral cannulation for severe right and/or left ventricular failure, including ventricular fibrillation. Trans ASAIO 1988; 34:485–489.
28. Ziomek S, Harrell JE, Fasules JW, Faulkner SC, Chipman CW, Moss M, Frazier E, Van Devanter SH. Extracorporeal membrane oxygenation for cardiac failure after congenital heart operation. Ann Thorac Surg 1992; 54:861–868.
29. Piena M, Albers MJ, Van Haard PM, Gischler S, Tibboel D. Introduction of enteral feeding in neonates on extracorporeal membrane oxygenation after evaluation of intestinal permeability changes. J Pediatr Surg 1998; 33:30–34.
30. Pettignano R, Heard M, Davis R, Labuz M, Hart M. Total enteral nutrition versus total parental nutrition during pediatric extracorporeal membrane oxygenation. Crit Care Med 1998; 26:358–363.
31. Kinsella JP, Gerstmann DR, Rosenberg AA. The effect of extracorporeal membrane oxygenation on coronary perfusion and regional blood flow distribution. Pediatr Res 1992; 31:80–84.
32. Secker-Walker JS, Edmonds JF, Spratt EH, Conn AW. The source of coronary perfusion during partial bypass for extracorporeal membrane oxygenation (ECMO). Ann Thorac Surg 1976; 21:138–143.
33. Walters HL, Hakimi M, Rice MD, Lyons JM, Whittlesey GC, Klein MD. Pediatric

cardiac surgical ECMO: Multivariate analysis of risk factors for hospital death. Ann Thorac Surg 1995; 60:329–337.

34. Meliones JN, Custer JR, Snedecor S, Moler FW, O'Rourke PP, Delius RE. Extracorporeal life support for cardiac assist in pediatric patients. Circulation 1991; 84(suppl III):III-168–III-172.
35. Hunkeler NM, Canter CE, Donze A, Spray TL. Extracorporeal life support in cyanotic congenital heart disease before cardiovascular operation. Am J Cardiol 1992; 69:790–793.
36. Rogers AJ, Trento A, Siewers RD, Griffith BP, Hardesty RL, Pahl E, Beerman LB, Fricker FJ, Fischer DR. Extracorporeal membrane oxygenation for postcardiotomy cardiogenic shock in children. Ann Thorac Surg 1989; 47:903–906.
37. Weinhaus L, Canter C, Noetzel M, McAlister W, Spray TL. Extracorporeal membrane oxygenation for circulatory support after repair of congenital heart defects. Ann Thorac Surg 1989; 48:206–212.
38. Goldman AP, Delius RE, Deanfield JE, de Leval MR, Sigston PE, Macrae DJ. Nitric oxide might reduce the need for extracorporeal support in children with critical postoperative pulmonary hypertension. Ann Thorac Surg 1996; 62:750–755.
39. Journois D, Pouard P, Mauriat P, Malhere T, Vouhe P, Safran D. Inhaled nitric oxide as a therapy for pulmonary hypertension after operations for congenital heart defects. J Thorac Cardiovasc Surg 1994; 107:1129–1135.
40. Kocis KC, Meliones JN, Dekeon MK, Callow LB, Lupinetti JM, Bove EL. High-frequency jet ventilation for respiratory failure after congenital heart surgery. Circulation 1992; 86(suppl II):II-127–II-132.
41. Ferrazzi P, Glauber M, DiDomenico A, Fiocchi R, Mamprin F, Gamba A, Crupi G, Cossolini M, Parenzan L. Assisted circulation for myocardial recovery after repair of congenital heart disease. Eur J Cardiothorac Surg 1991; 5:419–424.
42. Trento A, Thompson A, Siewers RD, Orr RA, Kochanek P, Fuhrman B, Frattallone J, Beerman LB, Fischer DR, Griffith BP, Hardesty RL. Extracorporeal membrane oxygenation in children. J Thorac Cardiovasc Surg 1988; 96:542–547.

2

Centrifugal Pump Ventricular Assist Device in Pediatric Cardiac Surgery

Tom R. Karl
Children's Hospital of Philadelphia, Philadelphia, Pennsylvania

Stephen B. Horton
Royal Children's Hospital, Melbourne, Australia

I. INTRODUCTION

Despite improvements in operative techniques, management of cardiopulmonary bypass, and myocardial protection, myocardial dysfunction is common after complex pediatric cardiac procedures. The impaired myocardium is characterized by decreased contractile force, abnormal diastolic relaxation, and a decreasing responsiveness to inotropic stimulation (1). A common feature of heart failure is that the disease either primarily involves or eventually produces excessive hemodynamic demands on the left ventricle. Thus, there is currently a great interest in and cumulative experience with ventricular assist devices (VAD) for circulatory support. The last decade has seen a plethora of new VAD systems placed into clinical use, many being suitable for patients down to the 20 kg range. However, the experience with VAD support of smaller children (<20 kg) remains limited to date. This is partly due to technical considerations and the fact that low flow rates may create a diathesis for thromboembolic complications when adult-sized systems are applied in the pediatric population (2). Moreover, there is also a longstanding perception that children with complex congenital heart disease will be unsuitable for univentricular support without an oxygenator. Many cardiac teams feel that extracorporeal membrane oxygenation (ECMO) is the best alternative, since implantable ventricular assist devices for small children are generally unavailable (3). Our own experience does not completely support this concept

(4–7). This chapter deals with our indications, technique, and outcome for short-term circulatory support in children, primarily employing a centrifugal pump VAD (4–9). We address the following issues:

1. Design characteristics of the centrifugal pump VAD circuit.
2. Indications and contraindications for support.
3. Intraoperative decision making for suitability for VAD support.
4. Cannulation and institution of VAD support.
5. Care of the patient and device during support.
6. Weaning patients from the device.
7. Outcome analysis.
8. The role of centrifugal pump VAD in relation to paracorporeal pulsatile devices and ECMO.

II. INDICATIONS AND CONTRAINDICATIONS

Postoperative support has been almost the exclusive indication for VAD in our own unit. The majority of patients so treated had undergone palliative or reparative open heart operations or cardiac transplantation and could not be weaned from cardiopulmonary bypass (CPB), despite optimization of blood volume, ventilation, acid-base status, and vasoactive/inotropic drug support. A small subset had refractory low cardiac output following (within 24 hours) satisfactory weaning from CPB. Rarely, low cardiac output not related to surgery (myocarditis, cardiomyopathy) was the primary indication.

Under what circumstances should VAD be used in a child? A great deal of judgment on the part of the surgeon, anesthetist, and perfusionist is required to decide exactly when extracorporeal support is justified in a given patient, since the devices themselves are not free of complications. In many published series, the strongest correlate of failure of extracorporeal support has been the presence of a residual cardiac defect. Our own experience supports the importance of this finding (10). Ideally, technical failure of the operation should have been ruled out prior to commencement of VAD, although in practice this may be quite difficult. Toward this end, there is a role for intraoperative assessment with transesophageal echocardiography, as well as direct cardiac chamber pressure and O_2 saturation measurements. An intraoperative review of preoperative data and imaging may also be helpful. One must ask whether there is a potential for recovery, and if not, whether or not transplantation is a realistic option. Family and social factors must also be weighed, including whether or not conversion of an intraoperative death to an ICU death several days later is a helpful or a punitive step for the particular family. Finally, one must consider which type of support is best for a given patient.

There are numerous *relative* contraindications to the use of VADs, which have been cited frequently in the surgical literature. Examples are multiorgan system failure, severe coagulopathy, intracranial hemorrhage, neurological impairment, uncontrolled sepsis, prolonged cardiac arrest, and the presence of a univentricular circulation. In practice, while all are relevant, most of these features are difficult or impossible to assess accurately in a child needing placement of a VAD, especially intraoperatively. Moreover, there is the ''problem'' of the improbable good outcome with this level of treatment in a highly compromised child. For example, addressing the sepsis issue, we have supported a patient with essentially untreated endocarditis (with evidence of cerebral embolism) following emergency aortic valve replacement with a prolonged but compete recovery. Every center involved with circulatory support in children could cite similar cases, and one might suggest that pediatric patients generally have a greater potential for recovery (without sequelae) than do adults. Therefore, in institutions capable of offering circulatory support, almost any child accepted for open heart surgery will also be a candidate for VAD should the need arise.

Is VAD appropriate for resuscitation following cardiac arrest? The main concern is neurological outcome, and the prearrest status is obviously a critical factor for both the brain and the heart. Recovery of cardiac function can occur well beyond the point of severe brain damage, but the upper limits are unknown. We have initiated both VAD and ECMO support during prolonged (1-hour) cardiac arrests with good quality survival. In the Pittsburgh experience 11 of 17 patients with cardiac arrest (6 of 11 who had greater than 15 minutes of cardiac massage) survived to discharge following ECMO support (11). Clearly we have been obliged to rethink the issue of acceptable resuscitation times for children in the era of circulatory support.

The general aim of postoperative centrifugal pump VAD support is recovery of the child within 5 days, although in selected cases there may be an option for a bridge to transplantation, with or without interim conversion to a pulsatile paracorporeal support system designed for longer-term use (see below) (11–15). For patients under 20 kg, 2 weeks would be considered the maximal realistic projected duration of support in our own unit.

Patients supported specifically for bridging (as opposed to recovery) must prospectively meet institutional criteria for transplantation (15). Issues such as size, blood group, and donor availability should be taken into consideration. Typically this group would include patients with acute myocarditis, cardiomyopathy, and inoperable end-stage congenital heart disease. Finally, there is a small subset of children with acute myocarditis who may recover (without transplantation) following prolonged VAD support (15). For a planned long-term support, centrifugal pump VAD is probably not the best choice of device, although in most units a better system is not yet available.

III. TECHNICAL DETAILS OF THE VAD CIRCUIT

Our VAD circuit consists of a centrifugal pump head (Bio-Medicus, Eden Prarie, MN) mounted on a flexible drive cable (Fig. 1). We employ inlet and outlet pressure monitoring and an in-line arterial flow probe. The tubing length is minimized by mounting the pump head directly onto the patient's bed. We have tended to employ heparin-bonded circuits in recent years, although this is not considered essential.

The centrifugal pump is preferred to a roller pump for VAD, as it is simple in concept and designed to run at constant (but operator determined) speed. There are no valves or diaphragms, since the device output is nonpulsatile. The constrained vortex pump design results in subatmospheric pressure at the tip of the cone, establishing suction in the venous cannula (Fig. 2). Care must be taken to keep this pressure above-20 mmHg, or excessive hemolysis can occur. In roller pumps, inlet obstruction results in a vacuum significant enough to cause collapse

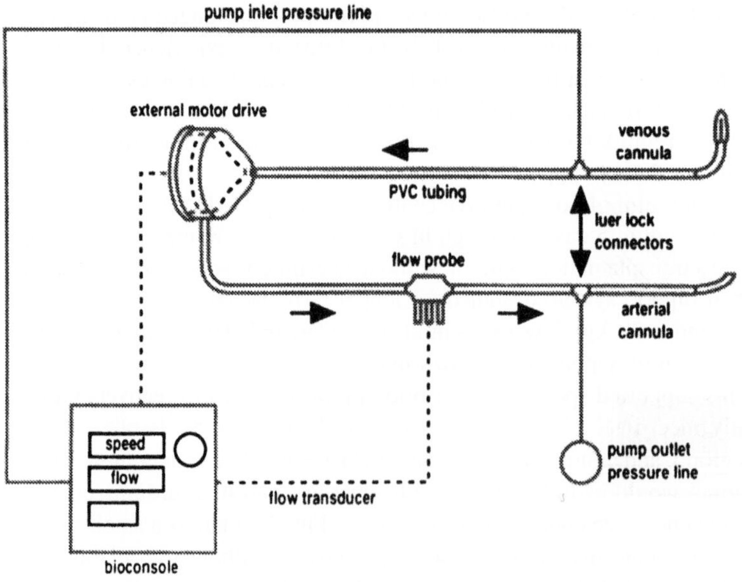

Fig. 1 Schematic of centrifugal pump.

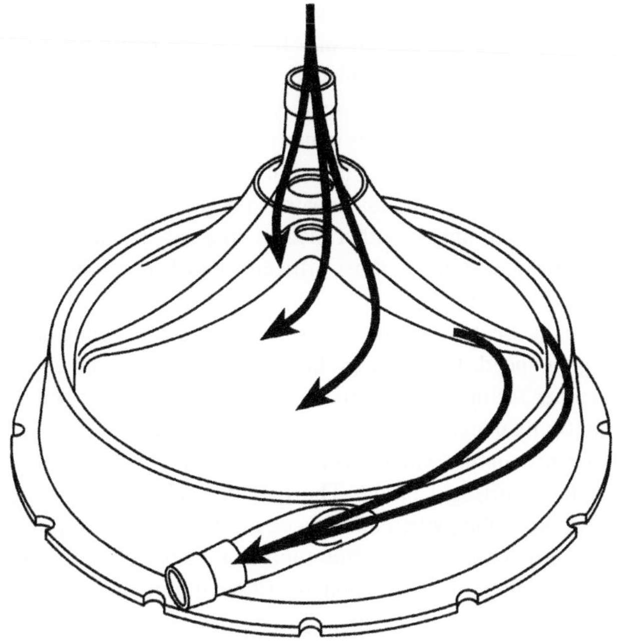

(a)

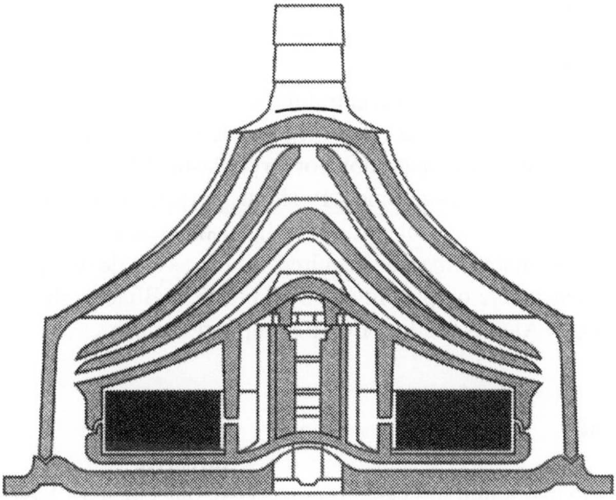

(b)

Fig. 2 BioMedicus centrifugal pump, intact (a) and cut away (b) views. Blood enters at the apex of the cone, and energy is implanted by the (constrained) vortex created by spinning cones along the vertical axis. Blood is ejected tangentially at the base of the cone. Mechanical energy is transferred to the cones by a spinning external magnet coupled to a second magnet inside the cone.

of the pump tubing. Roller pump ECMO circuits therefore usually employ a collapsible bladder that servo regulates the circuit. This system could be used for VAD, but pump support would stop if the bladder should collapse. With the centrifugal pump VAD system, a reduction in venous return will reduce pump output, with a reduction in inlet pressure. The operator must reduce the pump speed (rpm) at this point, which will not affect flow but will increase pump inlet pressure (i.e., render it less ''negative'' or less subatmospheric). The alternative is to increase venous return to the pump by other means, primarily by increasing vascular volume. The centrifugal pump is most efficient (and least hemolytic) when rpm are minimized for a given flow.

Although such problems are not encountered in roller pumps, which generate constant flow at a given speed, the latter probably have a greater potential for hemolysis relating to other factors. Studies in our own unit suggest that hemolysis is lower in the properly managed centrifugal pump circuit than in the roller pump circuit (16). Also, tubing rupture cannot occur, and the risk of air embolism is greatly reduced with the centrifugal pump. The battery back-up makes the pump convenient for transport of the patient and device during a period of assist. Most importantly, the centrifugal pump allows fine-tuning of the peripheral circulation prior to and during weaning, as it is responsive (flow at a given pressure) to the patients intravascular volume and resistance.

Biventricular assist is also possible with a centrifugal pump, and we have (rarely) employed right atrial/pulmonary arterial plus left atrial/aortic cannulation using two pump heads adjusted for approximately 100%/70% flow ratio. This set-up is technically cumbersome in a small child, however, and we would normally prefer ECMO in such a situation.

Is VAD possible in patients with a univentricular circulation? This is currently a point of controversy, but we (and others) have successfully supported patients with VAD after the Norwood operation for hypoplastic left heart syndrome as well as after bidirectional cavopulmonary shunts performed as part of the treatment of other complex univentricular variants. In such cases, higher than normal flows (~150% of calculated) may be required, as the assist device provides both pulmonary and systemic output. In our own practice, Blalock shunts have been left open during VAD (as well as ECMO) support in such cases.

IV. INSTITUTING VAD

The most common scenario in our unit has been intraoperative placement of VAD for patients who could not be weaned from CPB. In this circumstance, cannulation is usually transmediastinal, using the left atrial appendage or left atrial body (at the right superior pulmonary vein junction) for drainage and the ascending aorta for arterial return. For children with a univentricular circulation, the right atrial appendage and ascending aorta can be used. We employ standard or heparin-bonded CPB cannulas designed to carry 150 mL/kg/min flow. Cannulas are secured with pursestring sutures and tourniquets as for CPB. The tourniquets are held fast with vascular clips and left inside the mediastinum.

If VAD is instituted for a postoperative cardiac arrest (i.e., outside the operating theater), then CPB may be required initially, but in some cases we have been able to place asystolic postoperative patients undergoing open cardiac massage directly onto LVAD with a successful outcome.

VAD is commenced at minimum flow and quickly increased to 150 mL/kg/min. If the patient remains stable, flow is reduced to 70% of calculated output. We attempt to maintain a left atrial pressure of 3–4 mmHg, allowing for some cardiac ejection if possible. This may reduce the risk of stasis and thrombus formation. Heparin can be reversed with protamine, and hemostasis can then be secured as for other CPB cases. However, administration of protamine to patients supported with a heparin-bonded (Carmeda) circuit may neutralize some of the advantages of Carmeda coating and could result in a significantly greater heparin requirement or the potential for thrombus formation during VAD support (17). When hemostasis has been secured (often a prolonged exercise), the skin is closed, with cannulas exiting at either pole of the wound. Alternately, a PTFE membrane is sutured to the skin edges, leaving the sternum open in either case.

For some patients, it is not clear that univentricular support with a VAD will be adequate. For example, when global right ventricular (RV) and left ventricular (LV) failure are present, ECMO or biVAD probably will be required. The same could be said for patients with severe pulmonary hypertension or pulmonary dysfunction complicating their clinical picture. It should be borne in mind, however, that the decrease in left atrial pressure usually seen with LVAD may dramatically improve pulmonary hypertension and right ventricular dysfunction in borderline cases, especially with concurrent use of nitric oxide. Right ventricular function is sensitive to left ventricular function in a number of ways. By unloading the left ventricle with VAD, right ventricular filling is improved and the decrease in chamber size and septal shift may improve tricuspid valve function as well (17). Therefore, each case must be assessed on its own merits, and we prefer to employ the simplest effective level of support (i.e., VAD rather than ECMO) whenever possible.

In order to assess the prospects for VAD rather than ECMO intraoperatively, a venous cannula is placed in the left atrium, then the right atrial or caval cannula used for CPB is clamped. This system is used to assess the effect of partial left heart bypass. Right atrial and pulmonary artery pressure as well as right ventricular function are observed at 150 mL/kg/min pump flow. If all are satisfactory (right atrial pressure < 12 mmHg, pulmonary artery systolic pressure $< 1/2$ systemic, no right ventricular dilation), then the patient is ventilated normally while gas exchange in the oxygenator is temporarily interrupted. If pCO_2,

pO_2, acid-base status, and hemodynamics remain acceptable, the patient is recannulated for VAD. Otherwise, conversion to ECMO (or possibly biVAD) will probably be a better strategy. Once again a great deal of judgment will be required on the part of the entire surgical team, due to extreme patient variability.

V. MANAGEMENT OF THE PATIENT ON VAD

During VAD support, patients in our unit are sedated and fully ventilated. Inotropes are minimized to the level required to maintain optimal right heart function, based on central venous pressure, oxygenation, and echocardiographic assessment. Hourly records of arterial pressure, VAD inlet/outlet pressure, right and left atrial pressure, total flow, and activated clotting time (ACT) are recorded. When postoperative bleeding subsides, systemic heparin anticoagulation is begun (approximately 20 IU/kg/h), keeping the activated clotting time around 140–150 seconds.

Two different systems are commercially available for ACT measurement employing either diatomaceous earth (Hemochron, International Technidyne Corporation, Edison, NJ) or kaolin (Hemotec, Medtronic, Inc., Parker, CO). We have found the Hemotec method advantageous, as it requires only 0.2 mL of blood per sample to yield reproducible results. However, we have found that the Hemochron ACT was, on average, 1.1 times that obtained with Hemotec equipment.

With Carmeda heparin bonding, the system theoretically can be operated without heparin or at reduced doses in situations of high flow in larger patients. However, clots may form in heparin-bonded circuits with or without anticoagulation, and this risk of thrombosis must constantly be weighed against the risk of bleeding (18).

Inhaled nitric oxide is an effective and inexpensive treatment for pulmonary hypertension and is also useful for support of the right heart during low cardiac output states requiring support with a left ventricular assist device. Even if pulmonary artery pressure is normal, some patients may benefit haemodynamically, with improved left atrial filling. A secondary benefit may be an improvement in ventilation/perfusion mismatch in selected patients with pulmonary dysfunction. Methemoglobinaemia and NO_2 toxicity are rare in clinical practice, especially at doses less than 20 ppm.

Normothermia is maintained during VAD with a heating/cooling blanket and the heat generated by the centrifugal pump head itself. Peritoneal dialysis and/or venovenous hemofiltration are used as required for metabolic support and fluid removal. Vasodilators, parenteral nutrition, and antibiotics are also administered. In general, the measures used for metabolic support are much the same as those required for other critically ill cardiac patients not being supported with VAD.

Plasma free hemoglobin is monitored at least daily and should remain below 60 mg/dL. Elevated hemoglobin, especially in conjunction with noise or vibrations in the pump head, may be an indication that mechanical failure is imminent. In this case the pump head can be easily changed with only a very brief period off VAD. Generally, the pump head can be used for 7 days, after which we routinely change it. Occasionally we have replaced a pump head earlier in the presence of signs of imminent failure (see below). The median pump head life in our patients has been 71.5 hours (range 0.5–480).

VI. TROUBLESHOOTING THE VAD CIRCUIT

A number of technical problems relating to centrifugal pump VAD in children may be encountered. Some of the more common ones in our own practice are outlined in Table 1.

VII. WEANING THE PATIENT FROM VAD

In patients with improving ventricular function on VAD, one generally notes the appearance of a pulsatile systemic arterial pressure trace at full flow as the first sign. Transesophageal echo assessment is helpful at this point to further evaluate the ventricular contractility and the response to volume loading. A Starling response suggests that weaning can proceed. We employ gradual flow reduction as the left ventricle begins to eject, down to a minimum total flow of 150 mL/min. Temporary augmentation of heparin may be required at low flows, and the cannulas may be heparin flushed (5 IU/mL saline) to test the hemodynamics with pump support discontinued. Decannulation is generally performed in an operating theater, with concurrent sternal closure whenever possible.

VIII. OUTCOME OF VAD IN CHILDREN

From 1989 to 1998 we supported 53 infants and children with centrifugal pump VAD. This figure represents approximately 1.2% of our cardiopulmonary bypass cases during that time period. The median age was 3.5 months (2 days to 19 years) and the median weight was 4 kg (1.9–70). The diagnoses and operative procedures crossed the spectrum of congenital and acquired heart disease in chil-

Table 1 Common Problems Encountered with Centrifugal Pump VAD in Children and Possible Solutions

Problem	Comments and Possible Solutions
1. High arterial outlet pressure:	
Acute	
Cannula position has changed	Adjust cannula position
Thrombus partly obstructing cannula	Recannulate, adjust ACT as required
LV ejection above support provided by pump (equivalent of increased vascular resistance)	Considering weaning with flow reduction; vasodilator therapy
Chronic	
Flow too high for selected cannula	Recannulate with larger cannula
2. Low (subatmospheric) inlet pressure:	
Acute	
Cannula position has changed	Adjust cannula position
Thrombus partially obstructing cannula	Recannulate, adjust ACT as required
Atrial wall collapsed around cannula	Reduce flow temporarily (by decreasing rpm), then slowly return to normal flow
Hypovolemia	Infuse volume expander
Chronic	
Flow too high for selected cannula	Recannulate with larger cannula
Failing RV, poor LA filling	Pulmonary vasodilators, inotropes; consider RVAD or ECMO
3. Inability to achieve nominal flow:	
Any combination of circumstances outlined above	See Problems 1 and 2 above
Cardiac tamponade	

4. Excessive hemolysis:	
Low inlet pressure (< -20 mmHg)	See Problem 2 above
Thrombus in pump head (especially if pump head is noisy)	
Venous cannula too small (especially if inlet pressure is low)	
5. Inconsistent ACT readings:	
Incorrect preparation of kaolin suspension	Kaolin suspension should be mixed just prior to use
Incorrect preparation of cuvettes	Cuvettes should be stored at 2–25°C, and warmed to 37°C just before use
Sensor contaminated with blood	Clean sensor with H_2O_2; check to see that blood has actually clotted when ACT reading is made
Concurrent platelet infusion	Increase heparin dosage by 10% during platelet infusion
Ongoing variation in heparin metabolism	Adjust heparin dose
6. Air in VAD circuit:	
Air entrainment around insertion site (if inlet pressure is very low)	Reduce support to increase filling pressure in LA; infuse volume expander, revise cannulation suture to obtain a seal; positioning the outlet at 5 o'clock will create a bubble trap to sequester gross air, although small bubbles can still embolize
Open or faulty tap or connector in system	Change or close connectors or taps; Deair (venous side)
Crack in pump housing	Change pump head
Acute inlet obstruction with very low pressure	Under these circumstances, gas can be drawn out of solution in venous limb of circuit
7. Noisy pump head:	
Thrombus in pump head	Thrombus on wall of cone or bearing causes cone to spin eccentrically; hemolysis often occurs concurrently; pump head should be changed

dren Operations preceding VAD support included the Norwood procedure (10), mitral valve replacement (2), aortic root procedures (8), arterial switch (8), repair of supra-aortic stenosis (3), heart or heart lung transplant (3), ALCAPA repair (5), cavopulmonary connection (3), and others. Of the 53 children supported, 38 were weaned from VAD (0.72, CL = 0.57–0.83), and 24 were ultimately discharged from the hospital (0.46, CL = 0.31–0.61). Postweaning deaths generally reflected continued cardiac problems rather than morbidity specifically attributable to the VAD. Neither age, weight, timing of support (intra versus postoperative), cyanosis, nor presence of a mechanical valve was associated with incremental risk ($p > 0.05$ for all). The need for dialysis or ultrafiltration have been identified as risk factors for death in other published series (19). In our own unit however, both dialysis and ultrafiltration are used routinely (as needed) during both VAD and ECMO and have not emerged as independent risk factors. Taking initiation of VAD as day zero, Kaplan Meier survival at one year for all the VAD patients was 0.44 (CL = 0.31–0.58), suggesting a sharp decline in hazard function at the point of hospital discharge.

The median support time was 75 hours (range 19–428) for patients who could be weaned from VAD. For patients ultimately not weanable, it was 79.5 hours (range 2–114). For those discharged, the median support time was 71.5 hours (range 38–144), and for patients not discharged the median time was 88 hours (range 2–428). Thus, analyzed in various ways, VAD time was similar for survivors and non survivors ($p = 0.69$). The interpretation of support time data is confounded by the fact that VAD was electively terminated in some children who showed no signs of ventricular recovery after 72 hours, in the absence of a realistic transplant option.

The VAD group of particular interest to us consists of children under 6 kg, whose options for support are perhaps more limited and who have presented the greatest technical challenge. It has been suggested that many of these patients are suitable only for ECMO (9). We analyzed a subset of 34 of our patients, ages 2–258 days (median 60 days) and weight 1.9–5.9 kg (median 3.7 kg). Twenty-four were unweanable from cardiopulmonary bypass, and 10 required support in the intensive care unit for postoperative refractory low cardiac output. Weaning and decannulation were performed in 22 of 34 (0.63, CL = 0.45–0.78), similar to the patients above 6 kg ($p = 0.07$). One-year Kaplan-Meier survival was 0.31 (CL = 0.17–0.47), most deaths being due to irreversible cardiac disease. Within the 6 kg group, neither age, weight, VAD duration, cardiopulmonary bypass duration, cross clamp duration, nor the presence of univentricular anatomy proved useful in prediction of discharge from hospital ($p > 0.05$) (24). The smallest patient in our series was a 19-day-old, 1.9 kg baby with Taussig Bing anomaly and aortic arch obstruction, who was placed on VAD postoperatively, during a prolonged cardiac arrest, surviving with no neurological sequelae.

Complications were frequent in VAD patients of all ages, as has been the case in most reported series. Bleeding requiring exploration occurred in 15 patients. Three patients had sepsis with clinical signs and positive blood cultures, while positive blood cultures without clinical signs were found in another 5. Transient neurological defects were noted in 3 survivors, and 2 have had persistent mild neurological complications. There have been no permanent renal sequelae. Mechanical complications were also frequent (20 patients) but usually manageable with appropriate surveillance and action. Included were pump head failure, cracked connectors, kinked cannulas, and air or clots in the circuit. Only 4 patients required an emergency circuit change as the primary intervention. The true incidence of all complications is of course underestimated, as assessment was incomplete in the nonsurvivors.

Results of VAD and ECMO support have been remarkably similar across a number of published series (12,13,18,20–23). At least for postoperative support, a common feature in these series is that patients who are likely to recover tend to do so within the first few days. Beyond 2 weeks, complications of VAD such as sepsis and multiorgan system failure may supervene. A key question is whether or not *paracorporeal pulsatile systems* designed for longer-term support and patient mobilization will allow cardiac recovery to occur over a longer time span or allow more patients to survive in a good enough condition to undergo successful transplantation should a heart donor become available (see below).

Results with short-term VADs in our own unit and most others reflect a policy of expanding the indications to include nearly all cardiac surgical patients who are not expected to survive without support. Whether this strategy is appropriate or not is a decision to be taken by each team in the context of local resources and philosophy. To most of us, a 30–40% long-term survival probability would immediately justify the effort and expense, especially if the child might have minimal or no disability. Thus, improvements in the technical aspects, safety, and efficacy of centrifugal pump VAD may be obscured to a degree by the liberalization of indications for its use.

IX. CIRCUMSTANCES IN WHICH CENTRIFUGAL PUMP VAD MAY BE PARTICULARLY USEFUL

In our own unit and elsewhere, short-term circulatory support has been particularly effective for postoperative patients with anomalous origin of the left coronary artery from the pulmonary artery (ALCAPA), transposition of the great arteries (TGA) following arterial switch, and donor heart dysfunction following transplantation. Our patients with ALCAPA and TGA as a group had a 0.91 (CL = 0.59–1.0) overall survival probability ($p = 0.002$). The unifying thread in such cases is undoubtedly the presence of two anatomically normal ventricles with one being temporarily (but critically) impaired. Conversely, patients whose cardiac abnormalities bear a poor prognosis without VAD (left heart obstructive syndromes, complex univentricular hearts) also will do poorly after VAD support. Some of these situations deserve further commentary.

A. ALCAPA

In this rare congenital anomaly (about 10^{-5} of all infants), the entire left coronary system arises from the pulmonary artery. The basic pathophysiology is considered to be retrograde flow from the left coronary artery into the pulmonary artery, which may increase as the pulmonary vascular resistance drops postnatally (24,25). The result is a variable degree of myocardial ischemia, sometimes leading to extensive subendocardial or even transmural infarction. Despite its rarity, ALCAPA is the most common cause of myocardial infarction in children (24). There is a tendency to develop papillary muscle dysfunction, which causes mitral insufficiency, exacerbated further by LV dilation and loss of wall thickness (Fig. 3). The result may be severe low cardiac output syndrome, and the only effective treatment is surgery.

The preferred surgical option is direct implantation of the anomalous left coronary into the aorta (Fig. 4a) (22,26,28). An alternative is baffling the left coronary artery ostium within the PA to the aorta (Takeuchi operation) (29) (Fig. 4b). One may also connect the anomalous LCA to another systemic artery or ligate it to prevent run-off (least preferred option) (24).

The ischemic time required for most of these repairs exacerbates the compromised preoperative condition and may render some infants unweanable from CPB or cause severe postoperative low cardiac output. Such patients are usually good candidates for centrifugal pump LVAD support, as recovery can be expected within a few days.

The mechanism of recovery appears to be reperfusion of areas of dysfunctional but viable myocardium, as in salvage of "hibernating" myocardium after revascularization of ischemic myocardium in adults. Typically, there will be an early return of myocyte contractile function and augmented β-adenergic responsiveness during VAD support. Some extracardiac factors implicated in the progression of myocardial dysfunction such as cytokine-mediated toxicity, unfavorable neurohormonal stimulation, and excessive hemodynamic loading conditions are undoubtedly ameliorated as well. Because these mechanisms all have the

Fig. 3 Pathophysiology of ALCAPA: (a) sequence of events leading to severe low cardiac output; (b) anatomical changes that occur in the LV as a result of the above.

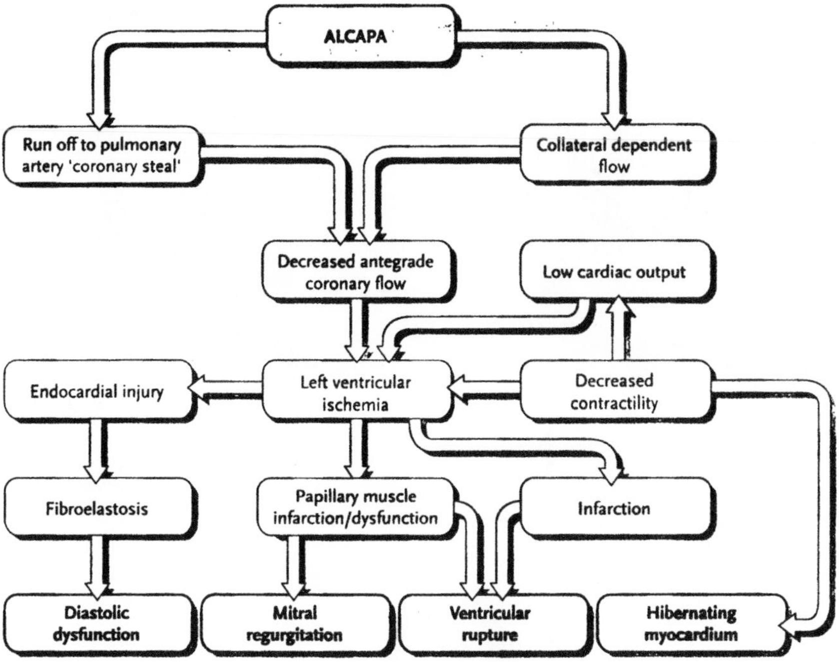
ALCAPA
Run off to pulmonary artery 'coronary steal'
Collateral dependent flow
Decreased antegrade coronary flow
Low cardiac output
Endocardial injury
Left ventricular ischemia
Decreased contractility
Fibroelastosis
Papillary muscle infarction/dysfunction
Infarction
Diastolic dysfunction
Mitral regurgitation
Ventricular rupture
Hibernating myocardium

(a)

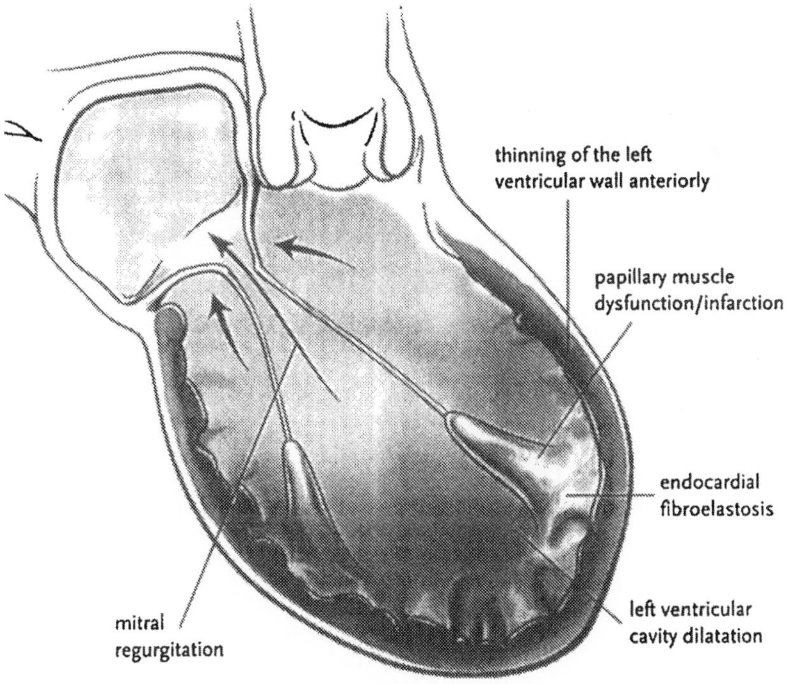
thinning of the left ventricular wall anteriorly
papillary muscle dysfunction/infarction
endocardial fibroelastosis
left ventricular cavity dilatation
mitral regurgitation

(b)

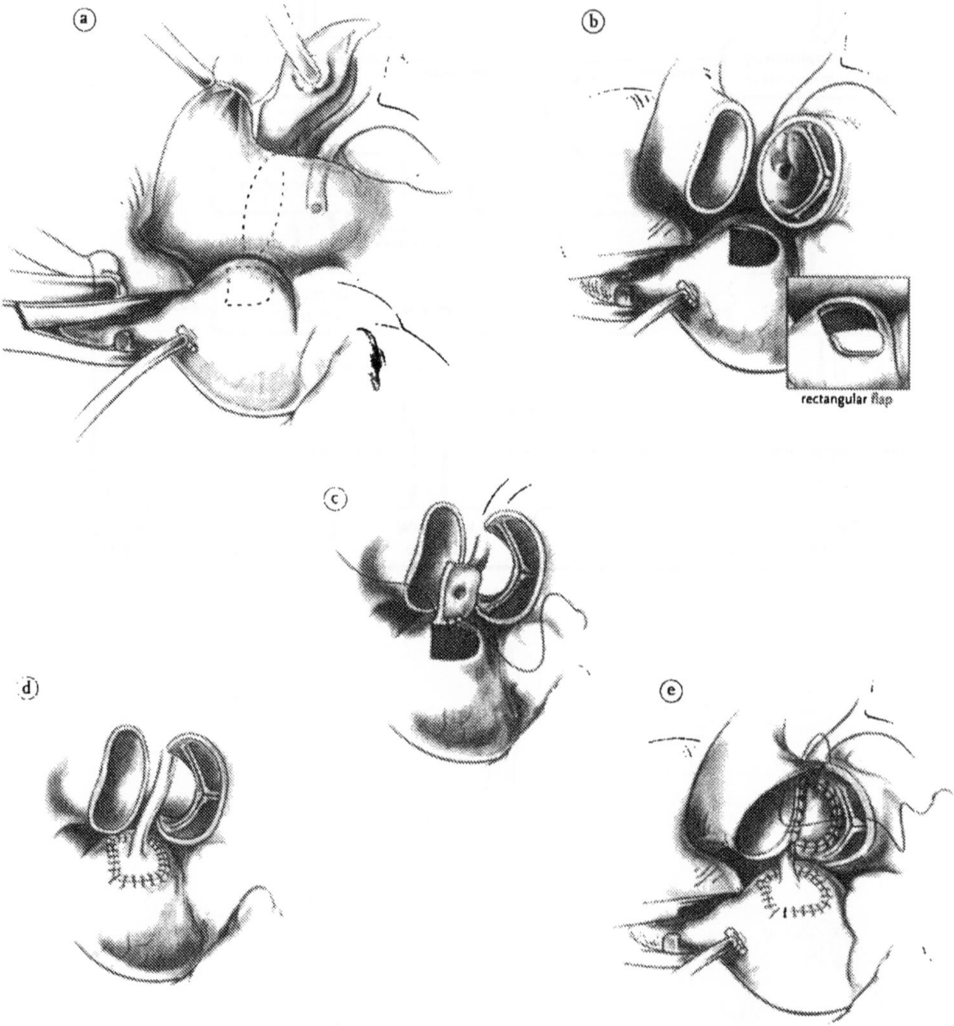

(a)

Fig. 4 Surgical options for ALCAPA: (a) Direct implantation of left coronary into aorta, using techniques of the ASO (b) The Takeuchi operation, employing a baffle within the pulmonary artery

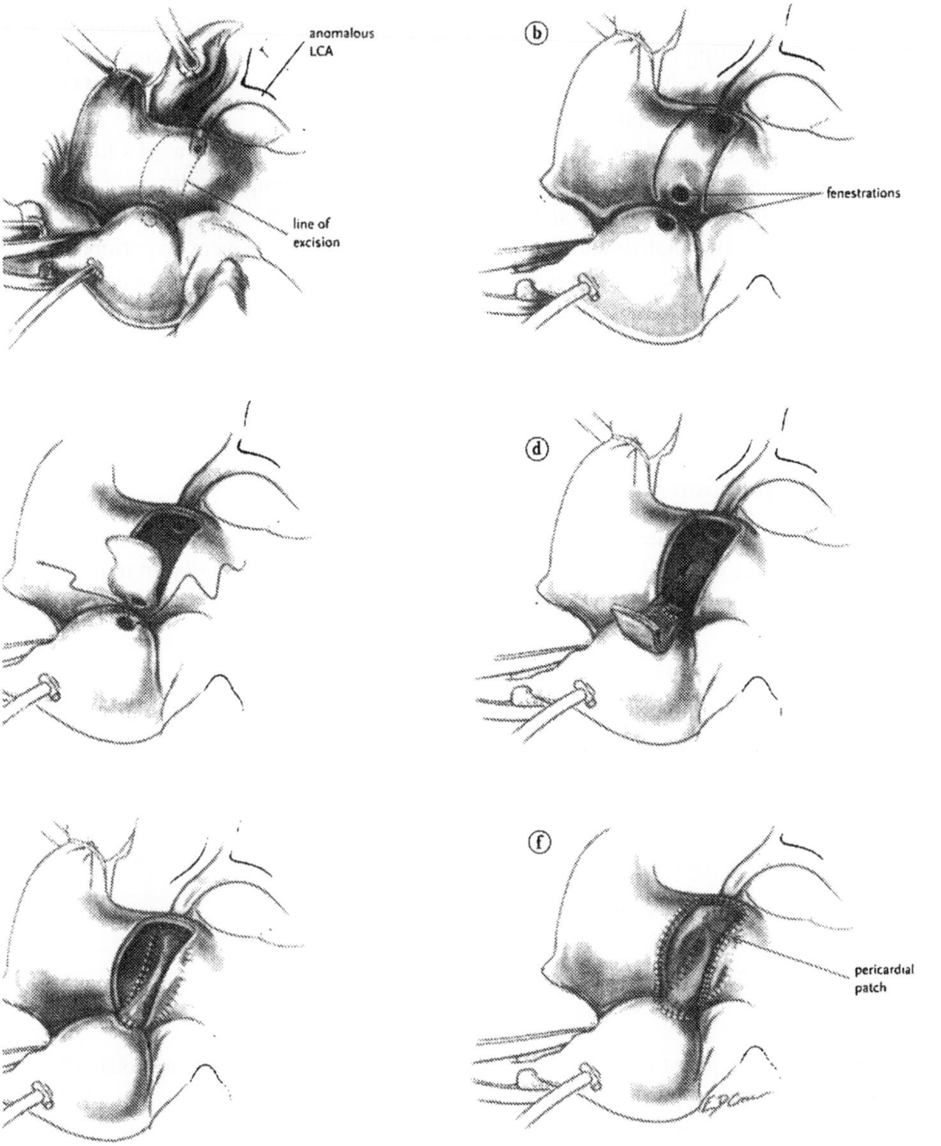
anomalous
LCA
line of
excision
b
fenestrations
d
f
pericardial
patch

(b)

potential to depress contractile function and promote myocyte loss through either ischemia or apoptosis, they also represent potential contributors to contractile improvement during and after VAD support (30). In ALCAPA patients, recovery of LV function in the long term is very good and the need for perioperative VAD does not predict a poor late functional status (25).

We have operated on 21 patients with ALCAPA, age range 6 weeks to 10 years (median = 9 months). The operative strategy was reimplantation in 7 and the Takeuchi procedure in 12. One patient had ligation of an isolated anomalous left circumflex, and another had an aortocoronary bypass. There were no perioperative deaths, but 5 patients required VAD support for 48–96 hours (median = 72). Long-term clinical outcome and LV function have been good, despite severe LV dysfunction at presentation. At late follow-up (Fig. 5) the VAD patients are virtually indistinguishable from the remainder of the cohort in terms of ventricular and mitral valve function as well as clinical status (24).

B. Transposition of the Great Arteries

Timing is critical for the safe conduct of the arterial switch operation (ASO) for TGA. In babies with TGA and intact ventricular septum, an involution in muscle mass of the LV takes place over the first month of postnatal life, as the pulmonary

LVEF resting: 66 ± 9% (range 50 - 73%)
exercise: 76 ± 8% (range 66 - 87%)

LVEF increased normally with exercise
(mean increase 10%, p = 0.001)

Wall motion defect was seen in one patient

RVEF first pass: 65 ± 6% (range 57 - 76%)

(a)

Fig. 5 Outcome for ALCAPA patients. Of 20 patients available for follow-up (total 147 patient years), 18 of 20 are in NYHA class and 2 of 20 are in class 2. Eight children had Bruce protocol exercise testing, and all scores were in the normal range (10th centile for age). (a) Summary of radionuclide studies of late LV function: 10 patients examined, 7 during exercise, 3 LVAD survivors; (b) recovery of LV function: LVEDD normal in 13, increased in 5 (3 with MR); (c) recovery of LV function: late fractional shortening = 34 (± 4%); (d) changes in mitral regurgitation; 56% improved at least one grade. The need for VAD could not be predicted with preoperative variables, nor did it influence the late outcome.

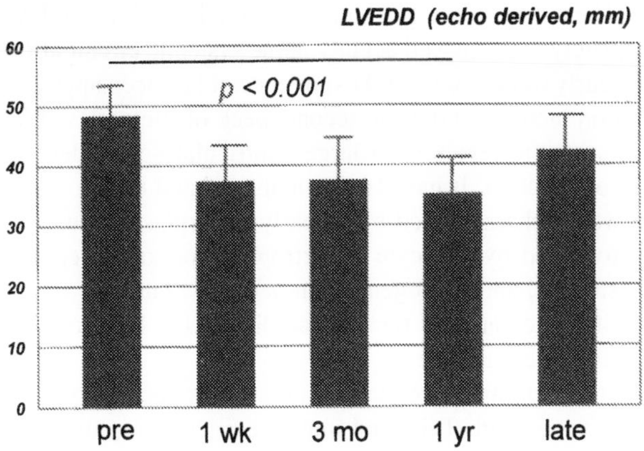
LVEDD (echo derived, mm)
60
50
40
30
20
10
0
p < 0.001
pre
1 wk
3 mo
1 yr
late

(b)

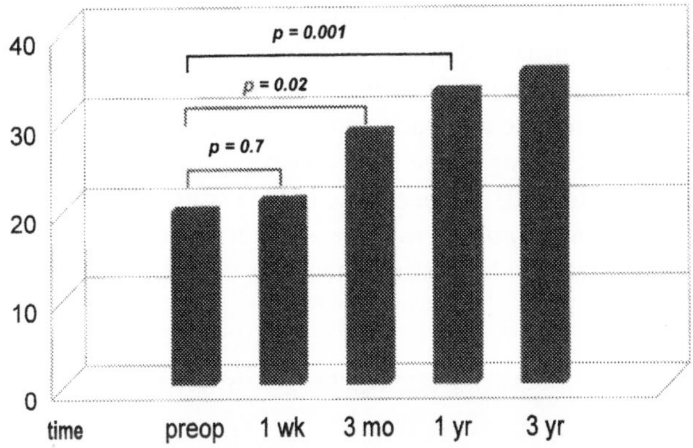
40
30
20
10
0
p = 0.001
p = 0.02
p = 0.7
time
preop
1 wk
3 mo
1 yr
3 yr

(c)

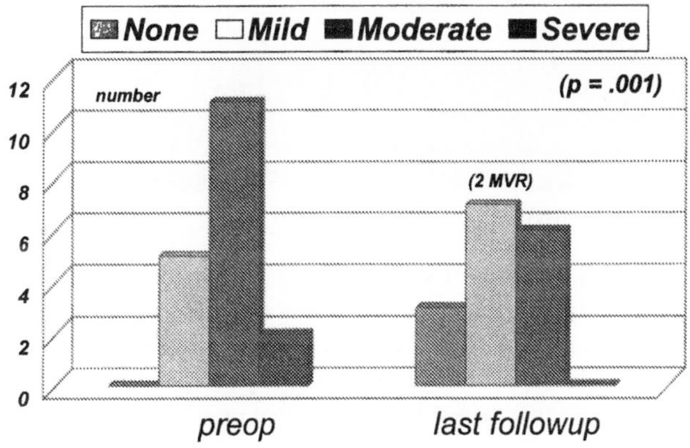
None
Mild
Moderate
Severe
12
10
8
6
4
2
0
number
(p = .001)
(2 MVR)
preop
last followup

(d)

vascular resistance drops. The consequence is a potential for a deconditioned LV that will not function adequately when placed acutely in the systemic circuit after an ASO (Fig. 6). Since the early days of the ASO experience, it has been appreciated that the risk of operation increases after the second week of life, unless LV pressure is maintained at systemic levels by a large ventricular septal defect, PDA, or LV outflow tract obstruction. It has also been appreciated that in postnatal life, myocardial growth is characterized by an early hyperplastic phase of myocyte and capillaries, followed by myocyte hypertrophy. Pressure overload induces hyperplasia, hypertrophy, and angiogenesis in neonates, but only myocyte hypertrophy later in life. The capacity for and rapidity of LV hypertrophy may therefore decrease with increasing age.

Based on the above information, a two-stage approach has been employed in many pediatric units for babies with TGA and intact ventricular septum presenting beyond 2–3 weeks of age (31). This approach consists of a primary pulmonary artery band plus modified Blalock Taussig shunt to induce LV hypertrophy while maintaining oxygenation. The ASO can be usually performed after a brief period of LV conditioning, usually 2 weeks or less. During this time, LV wall thickness and ventricular mass are seen to increase, based on echocardiographic studies. We prefer an alternate approach and have elected to perform a one-stage ASO for all babies presenting in the first 8 weeks of life, irrespective of LV mass, pressure, or geometry (32). If necessary, LVAD is used selectively as a means of rapid LV conditioning *postoperatively*, since it is clear that there is potential for a very rapid increase in LV mass in neonates up to this age. This

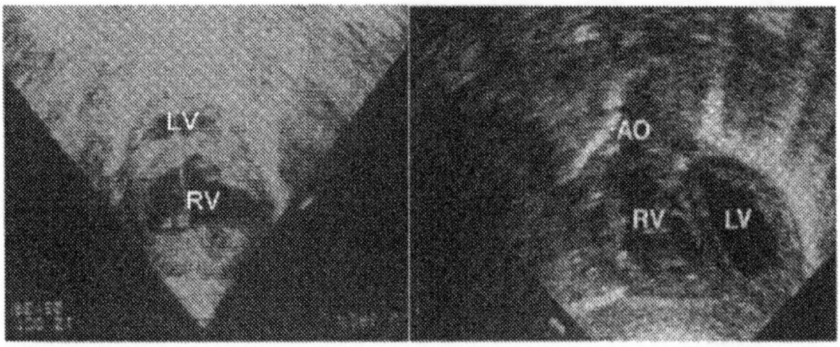

(a) **(b)**

Fig. 6 Echocardiographic assessment of the LV in TGA with intact septum: (a) The postnatal drop in pulmonary vascular resistance results in low (pulmonary) pressure in the LV. The interventricular septum bows into the LV due to the high (systemic) pressure in the RV. This patient is 4 weeks old. (b) A more normal geometry in a patient of similar age, but with a systemic LV pressure maintained by the presence of a VSD.

approach is less suitable for older children, who are likely to require a longer period of LV conditioning than can be safely provided with a centrifugal pump VAD.

Twenty-five children had a one-stage ASO (for TGA and IVS) after 3 weeks of age in our unit. Four required postoperative VAD support for rapid LV conditioning. Among the 25, there were 2 perioperative deaths, one related to a coronary artery technical problem, the other to extracardiac problems of prematurity. For this cohort, the results compare favourably with a two-stage ASO approach, even if VAD should be required.

We have also used VAD support in older patients undergoing a double switch (Senning plus ASO) for discordant TGA in the presence of a deconditioned LV, as well as in children with complex TGA whose main cause of LV dysfunction was a poor preoperative condition or a long ischemic time. The favorable results with VAD in ASO patients have been obtained in other units as well (33).

In any patient undergoing ASO, a technical problem with a coronary anastomosis must be ruled out as the primary cause of LV failure, otherwise VAD support will not be helpful. Appearance of the heart and ECG are useful in this regard, but once again a great deal of judgment is required in deciding whether to use VAD or revise the original repair, with the possibility of an additional ischemic insult.

C. Donor Heart Dysfunction

In the last decade, the proliferation of cardiac transplant candidates and transplant teams has led to a generalized shortage of donor organs. Likewise, the use of pretransplant mechanical support has increased the urgency in many cases, especially since the outcome in such patients is potentially as good as in those with less advanced cardiac failure. In most centers the magnitude of the problem increases inversely with the size of the patient. Consequently, the criteria for donor acceptability have been relaxed to the point that many units accept hearts with projected ischemic times greater than 6 hours or hearts with compromised ventricular function in the donor. Although reversibility of donor dysfunction is predicted in such cases, it may appear in delayed fashion, preventing weaning from CPB. Short-term centrifugal LVAD support is ideal in such cases, especially if pulmonary vascular resistance is low. The problem is greatly compounded in patients with elevated pulmonary vascular resistance. Although posttransplant right ventricular heart dysfunction may improve with nitric oxide therapy and time, it can become critical in the immediate posttransplant period. Right ventricular centrifugal assist (isolated or as biVAD) has been used successfully for right ventricular failure following cardiac transplantation in such cases (34).

X. VAD VERSUS ECMO FOR CHILDREN

Clearly, some patients are supportable only with ECMO, due to severe right heart failure, pulmonary problems, or complexity of the cardiac anatomy. However, in many children, even those with complex CHD, either type of system may be suitable. Previous institutional experience with neonatal ECMO for isolated pulmonary problems will have a strong influence on the choice of support systems due to availability of equipment and trained personnel. During the same time frame as our VAD experience, 40 children with cardiac or combined cardiopulmonary failure (not necessarily related to surgery) were supported with centrifugal pump ECMO (15). Of the ECMO patients, 19 were weaned, 3 bridged to transplant, and 19 eventually were discharged. The weaning probability was 0.48 ($p = 0.014$), and the discharge probability was similar 0.48 ($p = 1.0$). So although the weaning probability was better with VAD (0.71 vs 0.48, $p = 0.014$), the discharge probability was similar with VAD and ECMO (0.46 vs. 0.48, $p = 1.0$). In interpreting these results one must consider that most of the VAD patients could have been supported with ECMO, but the reverse would not generally apply.

One might consider the following points in decision making regarding centrifugal pump VAD versus ECMO.

A. Simplicity

VAD is straightforward in concept and design and requires little technical attention following insertion. Only a few minutes are required to set up and prime the circuit, providing an advantage in the cardiac arrest situation. ECMO is more complex to set up, prime, and debubble. On the other hand, with ECMO support can be established in some patients with peripheral closed chest cannulation, which is generally not possible with VAD in small children. The potential for complete left ventricular support with ECMO may be limited without the addition of a left ventricular vent, which complicates the system considerably.

B. Oxygenation

ECMO potentially provides pulmonary as well as cardiac support, although during periods of cardiac ejection the coronaries may be perfused with blood having a hemoglobin saturation closer to the left atrial level than to that of the oxygenator outlet. Therefore, there is a potential for myocardial ischemia if pulmonary function is severely impaired. The oxygenator itself may contribute to this problem. Patients supported with VAD are totally dependent on the lungs for gas exchange, but pO_2 tends to remain uniform throughout the arterial circulation, barring residual intracardiac shunts at ventricular level in patients with significant cardiac ejection. If an interatrial communication is present, significant right-to-left shunting (consequent to the low left atrial pressure) can cause uniform and significant arterial desaturation.

C. Anticoagulation and Blood Elements

LVAD requires little anticoagulation, especially at higher flows. Importantly, one can administer protamine and completely reverse anticoagulation before closure of the chest following intraoperative placement. By comparison, ECMO requires higher levels of anticoagulation, even with a heparin-bonded circuit. Also, the presence of the oxygenator results in more platelet damage, platelet consumption, and hemolysis, even when the centrifugal pump is used. The data from the pre-Carmeda era in our own institution suggest that there was a lower blood and platelet transfusion requirement for VAD than for ECMO ($p < 0.06$). The exact safe level of anticoagulation for either circuit may be difficult to establish, and an approach based on individual patient and circuit factors is required.

Carmeda-coated circuits may reduce the heparin requirement as well as the inflammatory response of both VAD and ECMO (35). In small children, the prospects for either type of support without heparin are still poor (36). The Carmeda bioactive surface covalently binds the polysaccharide containing the active sequence of heparin, through endpoint attachment, which is said to provide a uniform degree of thromboresistance. Limitations include difficulties in bonding heparin to certain surfaces required for the circuit and the need for continuous movement of blood over the surfaces of the circuit for the heparin bonding process to be effective. The blood/air interface should also be minimal. Theoretically, there is a risk of increased thrombogenecity in patients with antithrombin 3 deficiency.

Heparin-coated cardiopulmonary bypass circuits may offer clinical benefit in terms of reduction of release of inflammatory mediators, notably soluble selectins and β-thromboglobulins. Carmeda coating reduces complement activation during cardiopulmonary bypass (37,38). There is also a tendency toward thrombin activation (38,39) and granular release by neutrophils (38,40). The clinical significance of these findings has not been fully demonstrated, especially pertaining to VAD and ECMO.

D. Long-Term Support

Neither the centrifugal pump VAD nor ECMO system is eminently suitable for long-term support in children. The limiting factor for both systems is the development of sepsis. Our longest successful VAD and ECMO supports have been 144 and 120 hours, respectively, although good metabolic support has been provided for up to 428 and 384 hours, respectively, in eventual nonsurvivors. A major limitation has been our inability to wean most patients from ventilator support during centrifugal pump VAD and ECMO, mobilize them, and make then independent of ICU care. The experience compares unfavourably to that in adults, in whom patient extubation and mobilization can often be accomplished using a number of devices. Chronic support is possible in the latter group, either by way of recovery or bridge to transplant, and some patients can even be discharged from the hospital prior to (or as an alternative to) transplantation (15,41). To date, this degree of mobilization has not been possible with small children, even with implantable devices designed for chronic support. The usefulness of centrifugal pump VAD and ECMO as a bridge to transplant will therefore depend heavily on the immediate availability of suitable donor hearts, a major problem in many parts of the world.

E. Cost

In our institution LVAD adds $234 per day to the patients hospital costs versus $1050 per day for ECMO. We currently employ two nurses per patient (an ECMO specialist and the patient's regular ICU nurse) during ECMO support but only one for management of both the VAD system and the patient. In either case, a perfusionist, cardiac surgeon, and intensivist are available for assistance in troubleshooting the system and for patient-management problems.

XI. OTHER SUPPORT SYSTEMS

The future of centrifugal pump VAD might be considered uncertain in light of recent advancements with paracorporeal or totally implantable pulsatile systems. Examples of systems that may be suitable for children, or in some cases infants, include the following: Berlin Heart (15,42), the MEDOS/HIA assist (12,43) (both in clinical use in Europe), the Toyoba and Zeon pumps (44) (in clinical use in Japan), the Thoratec VAD (Thoratec Laboratories Corporation, Berkeley, CA) (in clinical use worldwide, included limited application in patients <20 kg), the University of Pittsburgh mini-centrifugal pump (not yet in clinical use) (45), the Pierce-Donachy pediatric system (not yet in clinical use) (46), the Jarvik 2000 (Symbion Incorporated, Salt Lake City, UT) and others (see subsequent chapters). Certainly these devices will play an important role in establishment of long-term support for recovery for bridging to transplantation. For short-term support, however, their role remains controversial. The costs involved at the time of this writing for the clinically available systems are substantially greater than for centrifugal pump VAD, both for the driving system and the disposable equipment required per ventricle per patient. We believe that for most cardiac surgical units, especially those not actively involved with transplantation, the simplicity, availability, cost-effectiveness, and good outcome (in selected cases) will ensure a place for centrifugal pump VAD in our surgical armamentarium for the foreseeable future.

REFERENCES

1. Kipla K, Mattiello JA, Jeevanandam V, Houser SR, Margulies KB. Myocyte recovery after mechanical circulatory support in humans with end-stage heart failure. Circulation 1998; 97:2316–2322.
2. Herwig V, Severin M, Waldenberger FR, Konertz W. MEDOS/HIA-assist system: first experiences with mechanical circulatory assist in infants and children. Int J Artif Organs 1997; 20:692–694.
3. Frazier EA, Faulkner SC, Seib PM, Harrell JE, Van Devanter SH, Fasules JW. Prolonged extracorporeal life support for bridging to transplant: technical and mechanical considerations. Perf 1997; 12:93–98.
4. Karl TR, Horton SB, Mee RBB. Left heart assist for ischaemic postoperative ventricular dysfunction in an infant with anomalous left coronary artery. J Cardiac Surg 1989; 4:352–354.
5. Karl TR, Horton SB, Sano S, Mee RBB. Centrifugal pump left heart assist in pediatric cardiac surgery: indications, technique and results. J Thorac Cardiovasc Surg 1991; 102:624–30.
6. Karl TR, Pennington GD. Extracorporeal circulatory support in infants and children. Semin Thorac Cardiovasc Surg 1994; 6:154–60.
7. Cochrane AD, Horton A, Butt W, Skillington P, Karl TR, Mee RBB. Neonatal and paediatric extracorporeal membrane oxygenation. Austr As J Cardiac Thorac Surg 1992; 1:17–22.
8. Karl TR. Circulatory support in children. In: Hetzer R, Hennig E, Loebe M, eds. Mechanical Circulatory Support. Berlin: Springer, 1997:7–20.
9. Thuys CA, Mullaly RJ, Horton SB, et al. Centrifugal ventricular assist in children under 6 kg. Eur J Cardio Thorac Surg 1998; 13:130–134.
10. Warnecke H, Berdjis F, Hennig E, et al. Mechanical left ventricular support as a bridge to cardiac transplantation in childhood. Eur J Cardio Thorac Surg 1991; 5: 330–333.
11. Del Nido PJ, Armitage JM, Fricker FJ, et al. Extracorporeal membrane oxygenation as a bridge to pediatric heart transplantation. Circulation 1994; 90:II66–69.
12. Konertz W, Reul H. Mechanical circulatory support in children. Int J Artif Organs 1997; 20:657–658.
13. Ashton RC Jr, Oz MC, Michler RE, et al. Left ventricular assist device options in pediatric patients. ASAIO 1995; 41:M277–M280.
14. Konertz W, Hotz H, Schneider M, Redlen M, Reul H. Clinical expertise with the MEDOS HIA-VAD system in infants and children: a preliminary report. Ann Thorac Surg 1997; 63:1138–1144.
15. Loebe M, Hennig E, Muller J, Spiegelsberger S, Weng Y, Hetzer R. Long-term mechanical circulatory support as a bridge to transplantation, for recovery from car-

diomyopathy, and for permanent replacement. Eur J Cardio Thorac Surg 1997; 11: S18–24.
16. Horton SB, Horton AM, Mullaly RJ, et al. Extracorporeal membrane oxygenation life support: a new approach. Perfusion 1993; 8:239–247.
17. Pavie A, Leger P. Physiology of univentricular versus biventricular support. Ann Thorac Surg 1996; 61:347–349.
18. Costa RJ, Chard RB, Nunn GR, Cartmill TB. Ventricular assist devices in pediatric cardiac surgery. Ann Thorac Surg 1995; 60:S536–538.
19. Pennington DG, Swartz MT. Circulatory support in infants and children. Ann Thorac Surg 1993; 55:233–237.
20. Duncan BW, Hraska V, Jonas RA, et al. Mechanical circulatory support in children with cardiac disease. J Thorac Cardiovas Surg 1999; 117(3):529–542.
21. Kanter KR, Pennington DG, Weber TR, Zambie MA, Braun P, Martychenko V. Extracorporeal membrane oxygenation for postoperative cardiac support in children. J Thorac Cardiovasc Surg 1987; 93:27–35.
22. Rogers AJ, Trento A, Siewers R, et al. Extracorporeal membrane oxygenation for postcardiotomy shock in children. Ann Thorac Surg 1989; 47:903–906.
23. Ziomek S, Harrell JE, Fasules JW, et al. Extracorporeal membrane oxygenation for cardiac failure after congenital heart operation. Ann Thorac Surg 1992; 54:861–886.
24. Karl TR, Cochrane AD, Brizard CP, Buxton B, Kitamura S, Frazier OH. Coronary anomalies in children. In: Buxton B, Frazier OH, Westaby S, eds. Surgery for Ischaemic Heart Disease Surgical Management. London: Mosby, 1997:261–287.
25. Cochrane AD, Coleman DM, Davis AD, Brizard CPR, Wolfe R, Karl TR. Excellent long term functional outcome after surgery for ALCAPA. J Thorac Cardiovasc Surg 1999; 117(2):332–342.
26. Neches WH, Mathews RA, Park SC, et al. Anomalous origin of the left coronary artery from the pulmonary artery. Circulation 1974; 50:582–587.
27. Grace RR, Angelini P, Cooley DA. Aortic implantation of anomalous left coronary artery arising from pulmonary artery. Am J Cardiol 1977; 39:608–613.
28. Laborde F, Marchand M, Leca F, Jarreau M, Dequirot A, Hazan E. Surgical treatment of anomalous origin of the left coronary artery in infancy and childhood. J Thorac Cardiovasc Surg 1981; 82:423–428.
29. Takeuchi S, Imamura H, Katsumoto K, et al. New surgical method for repair of anomalous left coronary artery from pulmonary artery. J Thorac Cardiovasc Surg 1979; 78:7–11.
30. Horton AM, Butt W. Pump-induced haemolysis: Is the constrained vortex pump better or worse than the roller pump? Perfusion 1992; 7:103–108.
31. Jonas RA, Giglia TM, Sanders SP, et al. Rapid two-stage arterial switch for transposition of the great arteries and intact ventricular septum beyond the neonatal period. Circulation 1989; 80:1203–1208.
32. Davis A, Wilkinson JL, Karl TR, Mee RBB. Arterial switch for TGA.IVS after 21 days of life. J Thorac Cardiovasc Surg 1993; 105:111–115.
33. Macha M, Litwak P, Yamazaki K, et al. In vivo evaluation of an extracorporeal pediatric centrifugal blood pump. ASAIO 1997; 43:284–288.
34. Barnard SP, Hasan A, Forty J, Hilton CJ, Dark JH. Mechanical ventricular assistance

for the failing right ventricle after cardiac transplantation. Eur J Cardio Thorac Surg 1995; 9:297–299.
35. Muehrcke DD, McCarthy PM, Stewart RW, et al. Extracorporeal membrane oxygenation for postcardiotomy cardiogenic shock. Ann Thorac Surg 1996; 61:684–691.
36. Schreurs HH, Wijers MJ, Gu YJ. Heparin-coated bypass circuits: effects on inflammatory response in pediatric cardiac operations. Ann Thorac Surg 1998; 66:166–171.
37. Mollnes TE, Videm V, Gotze O, Harboe M, Oppermann M. Formation of C5a during cardiopulmonary bypass: inhibition by precoating with heparin. Ann Thorac Surg 1991; 52(1):92–97.
38. Videm V, Mollnes TE, Garred P, Svennevig JL. Biocompatibility of extracorporeal circulation. In vitro comparison of heparin-coated and uncoated oxygenator circuits. J Thorac Cardiovasc Surg 1991; 101:654–660.
39. Larsson R, Larm O, Olsson P. The search for thromboresistance using immobilized heparin. Blood in contact with natural and artificial surfaces. Ann NY Acad Sci 1987; 516:102–115.
40. Borowiec J, Thelin S, Bagge L, et al. Heparin-coated circuits reduce activiation of granulocytes during cardiopulmonary bypass. A clinical study. J Thorac Cardiovasc Surg 1992; 104:642–647.
41. Fey O, El-Banayosy A, Arosuglu L, Posival H, Korfer R. Out-of-hospital experience in patients with implantable mechanical circulatory support: present and future trends. Eur J Cardio Thorac Surg 1997; 11:S51–S53.
42. Pasic M, Loebe M, Hummel M, et al. Heart transplantation: a single-center experience. Ann Thorac Surg 1996; 62:1685–1690.
43. Macha M, Litwak P, Yamazaki K, et al. In vivo evaluation of an extracorporeal pediatric centrifugal blood pump. ASAIO 1997; 43:284–288.
44. Takano H, Nakatani T. Ventricular assist systems: experience in Japan with Toyobo pump and Zeon pump. Ann Thorac Surg 1996; 61:317–322.
45. Litwak P, Butler KC, Thomas DC, et al. Development and initial testing of a pediatric centrifugal blood pump. Ann Thorac Surg 1996; 61:448–451.
46. Daily BB, Pettitt TW, Sutera SP, Pierce WS. Pierce-Donach pediatric VAD: progress in development. Ann Thorac Surg 1996; 61:437–434.

3
Intra-Aortic Balloon Counterpulsation for Children with Cardiac Disease

John A. Hawkins and L. LuAnn Minich
Primary Children's Medical Center, and University of Utah, Salt Lake City, Utah

1. INTRODUCTION

Intraaortic balloon pumping (IABP) is a standard therapeutic tool for managing acute left ventricular dysfunction after myocardial infarction or cardiac surgery in the adult patient. Its use in infants and children, however, remains limited for a variety of reasons, First, there is limited availability of the smaller-volume catheters needed for infants and small children. Second, the catheters are more difficult to insert than those in adults because children more commonly require a femoral arterial cut-down or aortic arch approach. Third, because infants and children are physiologically different from adults, many feel that IABP is inherently less effective in the more compliant pediatric vasculature.

This chapter reviews the past and present literature regarding the indications and results for IABP in children, including our own experience over the last 15 years. We will also include the technical aspects of insertion, timing of balloon inflation and deflation, care of the patient, as well as possible complications in the child undergoing IABP.

II. HISTORICAL ASPECTS

Moulopoulous and associates demonstrated the value of intra-aortic balloon counterpulsation in an animal model of left ventricular failure in 1962 (1). The first clinical application of the IABP was in 1967 by Kantrowitz and associates in Brooklyn, New York (2). They used the IABP in a 45-year-old female in cardiogenic shock, who surprisingly survived to hospital discharge. Although Kantrowitz's subsequent experience with other patients was not as favorable, the physiological principles were considered sound, and others persisted in exploring the clinical use of the IABP (3). The clinical efficacy of IABP was subsequently established in 1973 through a multicenter trial (4). The introduction of percutaneous placement in the late 1970s contributed to the widespread use of IABP in adults with left ventricular dysfunction. It is currently recognized as standard therapy in adults with moderate forms of left ventricular dysfunction.

Pollock and associates from Toronto reported the first series of IABP in children. They successfully pumped 6 of 14 children following cardiac operation (5). In 1983, Veasy and associates from Salt Lake City reported the use of small balloon catheters in a series of 15 children, including 4 infants (6). Despite the commercial availability of pediatric-sized balloon catheters in the early 1980s, IABP for children and infants has not become widespread.

III. PHYSIOLOGY OF IABP

The physiological benefits of intra-aortic balloon counterpulsation are dependent on precise balloon inflation at the onset of diastole with aortic value closure and deflation at the onset of systole with aortic value opening. The immediate and primary benefit of IABP is afterload reduction and diastolic augmentation. Inflation of the balloon results in displacement of a volume of blood equal to the volume of the balloon and augmentation of the diastolic pressure and coronary blood flow. Deflation of the balloon causes a drop in aortic afterload and aortic impedance to the failing ventricle and leads to a reduction in myocardial work and oxygen consumption and an increase in cardiac output. Other physiological benefits include a reduction in left atrial, left ventricular end-diastolic, and pulmonary artery pressures. Right ventricular function has also been show to improve with the IABP in adults with cardiogenic shock.

Although these physiological benefits should also be theoretically possible in children with a failing left ventricle, some investigators have suggested that the increased compliance and greater distensability of the immature aorta prohibits effective IABP in the pediatric population. Pollock and associates in 1980 reported IABP to be ineffective in children less than 5 years of age because of the greater compliance of the small aorta (5). They speculated that the pressure generated in diastole was less in the more compliant aorta, reducing both the afterload benefits as well as the diastolic augmentation. This speculation was supported by Lin and associates, who demonstrated greater augmentation in an adult canine model with significantly steeper aortic pressure-volume (compliance) curves than those in an immature calf model (7). They related balloon volume to aortic compliance and demonstrated comparable diastolic augmentation with half the balloon volume in the less compliant canine aorta.

Despite the fact that the pediatric aorta is more compliant, other investigators have been able to demonstrate clinical diastolic augmentation, even in infants (6). In an in vitro model of the pediatric circulation from our laboratory, we have been able to demonstrate that maximization of the balloon size will allow adequate diastolic augmentation, even in a very compliant aorta (8). Using a neonatal piglet model of acute left ventricular dysfunction, we were also able to demonstrate a significant increase in cardiac output, stroke volume, and mean aortic pressure, as well as a significant reduction in left atrial pressure with IABP (9). In a neonatal lamb model of acute left ventricular dysfunction using group B *Streptococcus*, IABP was demonstrated to improve cardiac output and decrease pulmonary artery pressure and pulmonary vascular resistance (10).

To achieve the maximal physiological benefits of IABP, balloon inflation and deflation must be properly synchronized to the cardiac cycle. In the neonatal piglet we compared timing the balloon using standard ECG and peripheral markers to echocardiographic timing using M-mode echocardiography (9). When the IABP was timed using standard ECG markers and peripheral arterial tracings, hemodynamic improvement could not be demonstrated. However, when accurate timing using M-mode echocardiography was used, cardiac output and mean aortic pressure increased and left atrial pressure decreased. M-mode echocardiography with alignment of the balloon and the aortic valve allows precise inflation of the balloon with aortic valve closure and balloon deflation with aortic valve opening (Fig. 1). Coronary blood flow in this model showed a trend towards an increase but was not statistically significant.

In summary, the physiological benefits of IABP have been demonstrated in pediatric and neonatal models provided balloon size is sufficient and timing is accurate. The physiological benefits in the clinical patient, however, have not been as well delineated because endpoints such as cardiac output, coronary blood flow, and afterload reduction are more difficult to measure. However, some indirect measures of cardiac output such as an increase in urine output have been demonstrated (11). Veasy and associates have also demonstrated a significant increase in the augmented diastolic pressure and a significant decrease in end-systolic and end-diastolic augmented pressures (12). The ultimate measure of IABP in infants and children is survival, of which detailed reports

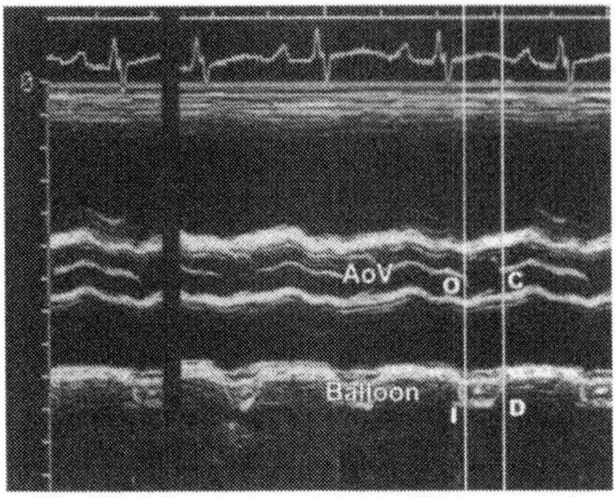

Fig. 1 M-mode echocardiogram from a parasternal transthoracic approach during IABP. Note that balloon inflation (I) occurs with aortic valve (AoV) opening (O) and balloon deflation (D) occurs with aortic valve closure (C).

are few. The specific reported results of IABP will be discussed in more detail later.

IV. INDICATIONS AND CONTRAINDICATIONS FOR PEDIATRIC IABP

The indications for IABP in adult patients have been well established. IABP equipment and procedures have been perfected and so well established in adult patients that percutaneous catheter placement is easily accomplished and therapy can be rapidly instituted. Balloon catheter insertion in children is a more invasive procedure, nearly alway requiring femoral arterial cutdown or insertion through the aortic arch. Therefore, careful consideration and more preparation is necessary before instituting IABP in children. As in adults, the general indication is low cardiac output that has become refractory to vigorous medical therapy. This exact point that IABP should be instituted becomes a clinical decision made by the surgeon and/or cardiologist and intensivist. Objective criteria include clinical signs of low cardiac output such as poor peripheral perfusion (low mean aortic pressure), persistent metabolic acidosis, mixed venous pO_2 persistently less than 25 torr, urine output less than 1 mL/kg/h and a left atrial pressure >20 mmHg. Additionally persistent malignant ventricular arrhythmias thought to be due to low coronary blood flow and catecholamine support at levels thought to be delete-

Table 1 Indications for Intra-Aortic Balloon Pumping in Children

Postoperative Left Ventricular Dysfunction	
	Failure to wean from cardiopulmonary bypass
	Refractory LV dysfunction in the intensive care unit
Preoperative Left Ventricular Support	
	Anomalous left coronary artery
	Pretransplant bridge
Medical Support	
	Myocarditis
	Kawasaki's disease
	Sepsis with ventricular dysfunction
	Persistent ventricular arrythmias

rious to the patient can be indications. The specific clinical situations where IABP should be considered are included in Table 1.

Contraindications to IABP in children include presence of a patent ductus arteriosus, recent coarctation or aortic arch repair, significant aortic valve insufficiency, and any situation where permanent recovery is not thought to be possible. If a postoperative patient has a significant residual lesion amenable to reoperation, then IABP should only be employed to permit the patient to be studied and reoperated.

V. TECHNIQUE FOR INTRAAORTIC BALLOON PUMPING

A. Catheter Selection

A variety of pediatric balloon sizes are available from Datascope Corporation (Paramus, NJ). The standard volume of balloons used in children are 2.5–20 mL in volume and are mounted on 4.5–7.0 Fr catheters. These catheters, unlike the adult-size balloons, do not contain an arterial pressure lumen for monitoring the central aortic pressure. The guidelines for choosing an appropriate size catheter have been previously published (12) and are included in Table 2. In general, we try to place a balloon that approximates 50% of the normal predicted stroke volume.

B. Technique of Insertion

While percutaneous techniques for balloon insertion have been perfected for adults, we have always inserted balloon catheters in infants and children by direct

Table 2 Guidelines for Sizing Intraaortic Balloons in Children

Age (yr)	Weight (kg)	Balloon volume (mL)	Catheter size (F)	Balloon length (cm)	Balloon diameter (mm)
<1	<8	2.5	4.5	10.7	6
1–2.5	8–13	5.0	5.5	12.8	8
2.5–5	13–18	7.0	5.5	14.2	9
5–12	18–40	12.0	7.0	17.8	10
>12	>40	20.0	7.0	19.4	19.4

exposure of the common femoral artery (Fig. 2). We make a small vertically oriented groin incision and expose the common femoral artery. After the child is heparinized, the artery is occluded proximally and distally to allow approximately a 2 cm section to be isolated. The appropriate sized balloon is premeasured and marked at the groin incision with a small silk suture while placing the tip at the suprasternal notch. This allows a good approximation for how far the catheter should be inserted. The balloon catheter is placed through a 3.5 or 4 mm

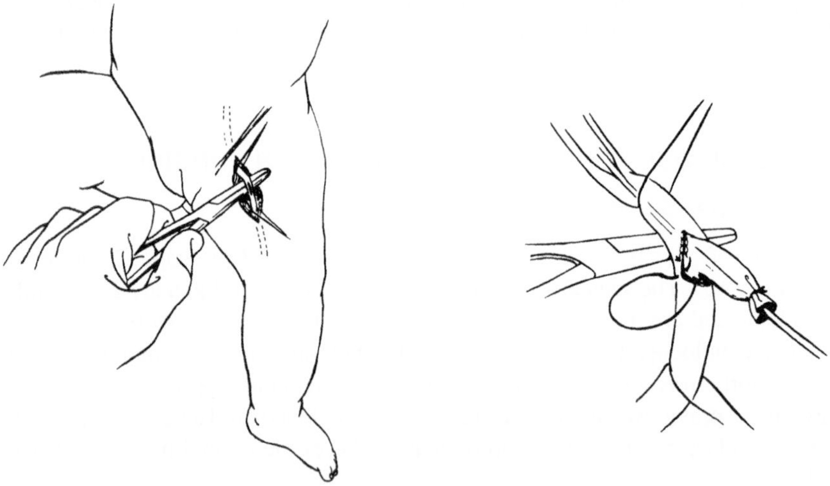

Fig. 2 Operative technique for femoral artery insertion of IABP catheter. The common femoral artery is isolated through a vertical groin incision. The balloon catheter is inserted through a sidearm graft of polytetraflouroethelyne. This graft is sewn to a longitudinal arteriotomy in the femoral artery.

diameter short section (1–2 cm) of expanded polytetrafluoroethylene graft material. A 4–5 mm longitudinal arteriotomy is made. The balloon is aspirated in order to remove all air (pediatric balloons do not come prewrapped) and lubricated with sterile mineral oil. The balloon can be manually "wrapped" by the surgeon to aid in insertion. The catheter is slowly advanced into position with a twisting motion using the previously placed suture mark as a guide for distance. The polytetrafluoroethylene graft is sewed to the arteriotomy using 6-0 polypropylene suture. IABP is started, and proper positioning of the tip of the balloon catheter just beyond the left subclavian origin is confirmed radiographically. While this is going on, the catheter is secured with a 2-0 or 3-0 tie around the graft to prevent bleeding. Hemostasis is achieved in the wound, and the skin incision is closed with a hemostatic continuous suture. When hemostasis seems secure, the patient is started on continuous heparin to maintain a partial thromboplastin time (PTT) of 40–60 seconds.

In some small infants or when femoral cannulation is not possible, other methods must be used. Some have reported success with aortic arch insertion through a purse string (13). This necessitates leaving the sternum open in the ICU, but most of these small children are ill and they would likely have an open chest anyway. An alternative, described by del Nido et al., uses an anterior flank incision and placement through a purse-string suture in the external iliac artery (14).

C. Timing of the Balloon Pump

Initial timing is done from the R wave of the ECG tracing while monitoring the arterial pressure waveform. The timing should be adjusted so that maximal diastolic augmentation and a maximal decrease in peak systolic pressure are obtained. The effectiveness of the augmented pulse can be assessed by obtaining a tracing with a 1:2 frequency comparing the assisted and nonassisted pulse (Fig. 3). Pulse contour timing from an arterial line is not desirable in our experience since there is a significant and unpredictable delay between the true central aortic pressure and a peripheral radial or even femoral arterial line (15).

We have found both experimentally and clinically that the best results can be obtained by triggering from the ECG and using M-mode echocardiography to accurately adjust the inflation and deflation points to aortic valve opening and closing (16). This can be done with a transthoracic, transesophageal, or epicardial approach. The transducer is positioned to obtain simultaneous images of both the aortic valve leaflets and the balloon in the same frame as seen in Fig. 1. While this image is obtained, the inflation and deflation points can be adjusted to perfectly coincide with aortic valve closure and opening.

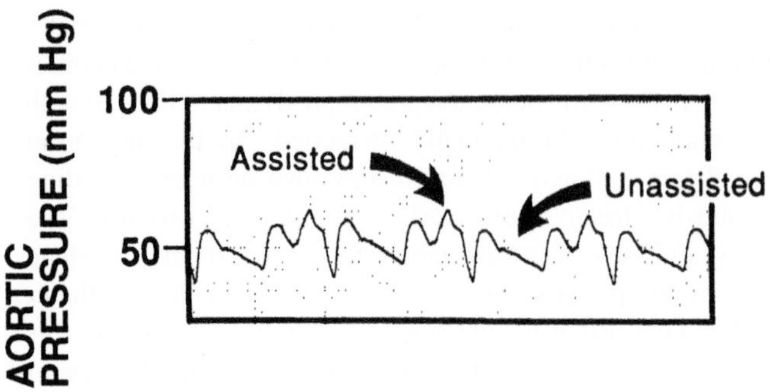

Fig. 3 Arterial tracing from a child on IABP at a 1:2 ratio. The assisted beat shows excellent diastolic augmentation.

D. Patient Care

Patients who undergo IABP are always in the intensive care unit with complete hemodynamic monitoring. Typically nursing care involves two nurses; one for care of the patient and one totally devoted to running the balloon pump. Besides the pump itself and general patient care, careful assessment of the involved lower extremity is important. The pulse in the foot of the involved extremity may disappear with balloon insertion, but viability is rarely, if ever, in question. Often the balloon improves systemic output enough that the capillary perfusion to the involved extremity is better than before balloon insertion, despite the fact that pulses may be diminished. Detailed specifics of nursing care for our IABP patients have been previously published (17).

E. Weaning from IABP

Weaning from IABP therapy should take place when pharmacological support has been substantially reduced and the overall patient condition warrants. We feel standard two-dimensional echocardiography provides good objective help in making the decision to wean the IABP. Echocardiography can document the return or improvement of ventricular function noninvasively while catecholamines are weaned. The left ventricular shortening fraction and ejection fraction should be showing some recovery before attempting to wean the IABP.

We typically go through a 24–48 weaning protocol depending on the patient's status. Prior to catheter removal, the pump is systematically taken from 1:1 to 1:2 and then 1:3 over the weaning period. Once the decision is made, the groin incision is reopened under sterile conditions. The ties around the polytetrafluoroethylene graft are then removed and the catheter is slowly removed after discontinuing the pump. We typically use an embolectomy catheter after removal of the balloon to remove any clot trapped in the common femoral artery. After confirming good arterial inflow and distal backflow, the graft is oversewn, leaving a small length of graft still attached to the femoral artery. This method of insertion through a side-arm graft allows removal without repair of the artery and preservation of arterial lumen size. Distal pulses are comfirmed prior to closing the incision so that further embolectomy can be performed if pulses are not present.

VI. RESULTS OF IABP IN INFANTS AND CHILDREN

The results of IABP in children to date have been limited because of the perceived ineffectiveness of IABP in pediatrics and the general lack of experience with large groups of children. We feel that IABP is effective in children as demonstrated experimentally, and it will take time and experience to demonstrate the real advantages in the clinical population. However, there are a few reports of pediatric IABP in the literature, and we have accumulated a moderate amount of experience over the last 15 years.

The first, and to date the largest published experience with IABP in children has come from the Toronto group as first reported by Pollock in 1980 (5) and later in limited form by del Nido (14). Pollock reported 14 children that underwent IABP following cardiac operation. Six children, or 43%, were long-term survivors. All 4 children in this group less than 5 years of age died, leading the authors to conclude that IABP was not effective for smaller infants. In a report from the same group, del Nido reported successful IABP in a 2 g infant and updated Toronto's total experience. In that report, there were 14 survivors out of 38 patients (37%), with the highest survival rate in the group where IABP was placed after valve surgery. Interestingly, the worst survival was in children undergoing the Fontan procedure, with only 1 survivor in 9 patients (11%). In this updated report from Toronto there was no correlation between patient age and survival.

In a report from Park and associates (11) of Columbia Presbyterian Medical Center in New York, 4 of 9 children survived (44%), almost identical to the survival rate in the Toronto series. In this group, 2 patients had IABP for medical reasons, with 1 survivor. Indications for IABP were expanded in this series to include its use as a bridge to transplantation. This group also documented a physiological benefit of IABP with a definite increase in urine output.

Our own experience with IABP in children has been previously reported (6,12,16–19) and has evolved over the years with respect to timing issues. Our total experience involves 43 infants and children accumulated over a 15-year period from 1983 to 1998. The patients ranged in age from 5 days to 18 years old (mean ± SD = 4.6 ± 5 years), and weights ranged from 4.2 to 40 kg (mean ± SD = 14.8 ± 12 kg). A total of 19 patients were less than 3 years old. During the entire 15-year experience, we were able to successfully wean 22 of the 43 patients from the IABP (51%), and 18 patients (42%) survived to be discharged from the hospital and became long-term survivors.

Because many children underwent IABP in our early years as a "last resort" application of support, our more recent experience is more indicative of the results that can be currently achieved with pediatric IABP. Over the last 10 years, 22 patients have undergone IABP at our institution (Table 3), with 13 patients (59%) successfully leaving the hospital and surviving long-term. Perhaps even more importantly, since we adopted echocardiographic timing in 1994, survival has been 78% (7/9) as compared to survival of 46% (6/13) with the more traditional ECG timing method. Survival has been 75% (6/8) in those children under 3 years of age as compared to 50% (7/14) for those 3 years of age and older. Survival for postsurgical patients was slightly better at 62% (8/13) than the survival of 56% (5/9) seen in the medical patients in the last decade. Three of the 4 deaths in the medical group were in patients listed for transplant who did not receive a donor heart.

Complications over the last decade have been relatively few. One patient had evidence of limb ischemia with loss of Doppler pulses in the involved leg but did not require early removal of the balloon pump. Another patient awaiting transplantation had evidence of sepsis while on the IABP, but again this did not require removal of the IABP. In this more recent 10-year experience, we have not seen any other complications reported with IABP such as balloon rupture, vessel perforation, hematoma, or wound infection.

There have been isolated reports of the use of IABP in children for specific cardiac problems including support for left ventricular dysfunction following repair of anomalous origin of the left coronary artery and the Fontan procedure.

Table 3 Results of IABP Placement in 22 Children, 1988–1998

Indication for IABP placement	Number	Survivors	Survival (%)
Postrepair of cardiac defect	13	8	62
Medical indications	9	5	55
Myocarditis	3	2	
Cardiomyopathy (bridge-to-transplant)	5	2	
Myocardial contusion	1	1	
Overall	22	13	59

Nawa and associates from Okayama, Japan, reported successful IABP in 1 out of 3 children following the Fontan operation (20). Similarly, del Nido reported only 1 survivor out of 9 children undergoing the Fontan procedure (14). We have had experience with only 2 children with IABP after the Fontan procedure, and both children survived. We would caution the use of IABP following the modified Fontan procedure and apply it only in specific circumstances when there seems to be primarily left ventricular dysfunction rather than the low cardiac output seen typically with an elevated right-sided pressures.

In contrast, however, we feel strongly that IABP is particularly helpful in those children with anomalous origin of the left coronary artery and left ventricular dysfunction. Pozzi and associates have recently pointed out the benefit of IABP in 2 infants who underwent successful IABP after repair of anomalous left coronary artery (13). We had a total of 5 children supported with IABP after repair of anomalous left coronary artery with 4 survivors. Ventricular dysfunction is common with anomalous origin of the left coronary artery, and IAB seems to be well suited since this is generally known preoperatively. As suggested by Pozzi preoperative or intraoperative placement of the IABP for this condition may allow better preservation of cardiac function and coronary flow before the onset of the low output state in the postoperative period.

VII. SUMMARY

Intra-aortic balloon pumping has not been widely applied in children over the years despite the fact its efficacy has been well established in adults. Even though IABP has not enjoyed widespread pediatric application, experimental and clinical data exist to show that the IABP is effective in children provided adequate sized balloons and accurate timing are used. We feel the most accurate timing for IABP utilizes triggering from the ECG and adjustments in timing made by using M-mode echocardiography. This accurately times inflation and deflation in relation to aortic valve opening and closure. Adopting this approach has allowed our group to achieve long-term survival and results that approach those seen routinely in adults. In addition, it appears that IABP is just as effective in the small infant as it is in larger children. It also appears to be equally effective for postcardiotomy and medical applications. IABP cannot be expected to be life-saving in those with severe LV dysfunction; formal ventricular assist device support will be needed in those children. However, IABP is well suited for children with more moderate forms of left ventricular dysfunction. Only more time and experience will show us if IABP will achieve the same widespread use in children as it has in adults with left ventricular dysfunction.

REFERENCES

1. Moulopoulos SD, Topaz S, Kolff WJ. Diastolic balloon pumping (with carbon dioxide) in aorta: mechanical assistance to failing circulation. Am Heart J 1962; 66:669–675.
2. Kantrowitz A, Akutsu T, Chaptal P-A, Krakauer J, Kantrowitz A, Jones RT. A clinical experience with an implanted mechanical auxiliary ventricle JAMA 1966; 197:525–529.
3. Kantrowitz A. Origins of intraaortic balloon pumping. Ann Thorac Surg 1990; 50: 672–674.
4. Scheidt S, Wilner G, Muyeller H, et al. Intra-aortic balloon counterpulsation in cardiogenic shock. Report of a cooperative clinical trial. N Engl J Med 1973; 288:979–984.
5. Pollock J, Charlton MC, Williams WG, Edmond J, Trusler GA. Intraaortic balloon pumping in children. Ann Thorac Surg 1980; 29:522–528.
6. Veasy LG, Blalock RC, Orth JL, Boucek MM. Intra-aortic balloon pumping in infants and children. Circulation 1983; 68:1095–1100.
7. Lin CY, Galysh FT, Ho KJ, Patel AS. Response to single-segment intraaortic balloon pumping as related to aortic compliance. Ann Thorac Surg 1972; 13:468–476.
8. Minich LL, Tani LY, Hawkins JA, Bartkowiak RR, Royall ML, Pantalos GM. In vitro evaluation of the effect of aortic compliance on pediatric intraaortic balloon pumping. Submitted.
9. Minich LL, Tani LY, Pantalos GM, Bolland BL, Knorr BK, Hawkins JA. Neonatal piglet model of intraaortic balloon pumping: improved efficacy using echocardiographic timing. Ann Thorac Surg 1998; 66:1527–1532.
10. Pribble CG, Shaddy RE. Intra-aortic balloon counterpulsation in newborn lambs infected with group B *Streptococcus*. ASAIO Trans 1991; 37:33–37.
11. Park JK, Hsu KT, Gersony WM. Intraaortic balloon pump management of refractory congestive heart failure in children. Pediatr Cardiol 1993; 14:19–22.
12. Veasy LG, Webster HF, McGough EC. Intra-aortic balloon pumping. adaptation for pediatric use. Crit Care Clin 1986; 2:237–249.
13. Pozzi M, Santoro G, Makundan S. Intraaortic balloon pump after treatment of anomalous origin of left coronary artery. Ann Thorac Surg 1998; 65:555–557.
14. Del Nido PJ, Swan PR, Benson LN, Bohn D, Charlton MC, Coles JG, Trusler GA, Williams WG. Successful use of intraaortic balloon pumping in a 2-kilogram infant. Ann Thorac Surg 1988; 46:574–576.
15. Cadwell CA, Quaal SJ. Intra-aortic balloon counterpulsation timing. Am J Crit Care 1996; 5:254–261.
16. Minich LL, Tani LY, McGough EC, Shaddy RE, Hawkins JA. A novel approach to pediatric intraaortic balloon pump timing using M-mode echocardiography. Am J Cardiol 1997; 80:367–369.
17. Geiger J, Hall T, Breeze E, Davey C, Jones A, Stackhouse D. Intra-aortic balloon pumps in children: a small-nursing-team approach. Crit Care Nurse 1997; 17:79–86.
18. Webster H, Veasy LG. Intra-aortic balloon pumping in children. Heart Lung 1985; 14:548–555.
19. Veasy LG, Webster H. Intra-aortic balloon pumping in infants and children. Cardiac Assists 1985; 2:1–6.
20. Nawa S, Sugawaqra E, Murakami T, Senoo Y, Teramoto S, Morita K. Efficacy of intra-aortic balloon pumping for failing Fontan circulation. Chest 1988; 93:599–603.

4

Extracorporeal Membrane Oxygenation Versus Ventricular Assist Device Support for Children with Cardiac Disease

Brian W. Duncan
Children's Hospital and Regional Medical Center and University of Washington School of Medicine, Seattle, Washington

I. INTRODUCTION

Utilization patterns for mechanical circulatory support devices differ for adult and pediatric patients due to a variety of factors. In adult patients, left ventricular failure due to coronary artery disease is successfully treated by intraaortic balloon counterpulsation (IABP) and left ventricular assist devices (LVAD). The success of long-term support with implantable LVAD systems has led to their increasing use in the management of adult patients with end-stage left ventricular failure. Extracorporeal membrane oxygenation (ECMO) has been used less frequently in adult patients but remains the most commonly used form of mechanical circulatory support in pediatric patients with cardiac disease. A major reason for this is the large experience possessed by most pediatric centers in utilizing ECMO support for neonatal respiratory failure. In addition, the development of pulsatile ventricular assist devices (VAD) for pediatric patients has been limited due to the need for availability of a number of different pump sizes to match the stroke volumes required over the range of patient sizes treated in the pediatric population. Both ECMO and VAD, however, may be used successfully to treat pediatric patients with cardiac disease. This chapter compares ECMO and VAD in the treatment of children with heart disease beginning with an analysis of experimental work that examines the effect of each modality on ventricular function. Following this is an examination of our clinical experience as well as that of other centers that specifically compare each of these modalities for the support of pediatric cardiac patients. From these analyses, we will demonstrate that both ECMO and VAD can be used effectively in the treatment of children with cardiac disease while identifying clinical settings where one modality may be a better choice than the other. This approach will hopefully show that both systems may be utilized in a complementary fashion in the treatment of this patient population.

II. EFFECT OF ECMO AND VAD ON VENTRICULAR FUNCTION—EXPERIMENTAL STUDIES

A. Animal Models

The ideal device for mechanical circulatory assistance must reliably support end-organ perfusion while providing optimal conditions for the recovery of myocardial contractile function. Both ECMO and VAD reliably support systemic perfusion to maintain end-organ function. Numerous studies, however, have raised questions regarding the possible deleterious effects of ECMO on ventricular function. If ECMO does not provide optimal chances for recovery of damaged myocardium, a strong argument could be made for the superiority of VAD in the treatment of children with cardiac disease. The validity of questions concerning the effect of ECMO on ventricular recovery can be assessed by a careful review of experimental studies that have addressed this issue.

With most cannula configurations employed for venoarterial ECMO, oxygenated blood from the arterial cannula fails to reach the coronary sinuses if there is any appreciable ventricular ejection. The source of coronary arterial blood flow is provided by the left ventricle in these cases (1–3). If there is significant pulmonary parenchymal damage or mechanical ventilation is withheld during ECMO support, hypoxic blood returning to the left ventricle may provide the sole source of coronary perfusion with deleterious effects on ventricular function and recovery. Other effects of ECMO with the potential to adversely impact recovery of impaired ventricular function relate to inadequate unloading of the left ventricle that may exist during ECMO support. Bavaria et al. demonstrated that although ECMO causes a small decrease in left ventricular end-diastolic volume, systolic wall stress increases substantially during ECMO support due to large increases in peak left ventricular pressure (4). These changes were most pronounced in hearts after an ischemic injury. Work by this same group demonstrated that LVAD caused a decrease in left ventricular end-diastolic volume with minimal effect on peak left ventricular pressure leading to an overall decrease in systolic wall stress (5). Decreased wall stress in LVAD-supported hearts was also observed after a previous ischemic injury to the myocardium.

Despite these findings, experimental evidence also exists that ECMO, when properly conducted, can provide ample opportunity for recovery of ventricular function. Eugene et al. demonstrated that venting the left ventricle during ECMO resulted in identical hemodynamics compared to LVAD in supporting a model of left ventricular ischemia (6). These same investigators also found good preservation of myocardial function in a biventricular failure model supported with vented ECMO (7). One report found ECMO to provide superior hemodynamic effects over LVAD in supporting a model of biventricular ischemia (8). These results were probably due to ECMO providing true biventricular support during episodes of severe, recurrent ventricular dysrhythmia that occurred in this model.

B. Clinical Studies

Several studies have examined the effects of ECMO on myocardial function in neonates that require support for respiratory failure. Echocardiographic monitoring has demonstrated a decrease in systolic phase indices of myocardial performance such as ejection fraction and aortic flow velocity during ECMO support (9,10). These changes were transient in all cases and returned to normal after ECMO was discontinued. However, an elegant study performed by Berdjis et al. demonstrated that systolic phase indices of myocardial performance are inaccurate during ECMO due to extreme variations in preload and afterload imposed by extracorporeal circulation (11). These authors used the velocity of circumferential fiber shortening corrected for heart rate/end-systolic wall stress relation (VCFc/ESS) as a load-independent measure of myocardial performance. The VCFc/ESS was maintained in the normal range for patients during ECMO support.

C. Summary of Animal and Clinical Experimental Studies Comparing ECMO to VAD

There is a pervasive opinion that VAD is superior to ECMO in terms of creating a physiological milieu conducive to recovery of ventricular function after myocardial injury. Based on the above studies and our clinical experience, however, we have found that ECMO not only provides reliable perfusion for preservation of end-organ function but also optimizes conditions for recovery of damaged myocardium. Appropriate management of ECMO support is crucial to its success in treating patients who have suffered cardiac injury. The most important aspects of ECMO management that will encourage myocardial healing include adequate decompression of the left ventricle and provision of oxygenated blood perfusing the coronary arteries. Our clinical experience agrees with experimental evidence that ECMO can mechanically unload the left ventricle if decompression of the left side of the circulation is performed (6,7). This may be accomplished by direct venting of the left atrium with a drainage catheter that is "Y-ed" into the systemic venous drainage limb of the circuit in patients that have ECMO instituted transthoracically. For patients who have had support instituted by neck cannulation, creation of an atrial septostomy under echocardiographic guidance or in the cardiac catheterization laboratory also provides reliable left sided decompression (12,13). Provision of oxygenated blood flow to the coronary arteries is also vitally important and is easily accomplished by continuing to provide moderate levels of ventilation for all patients that require ECMO support for cardiac disease. This ensures that fully oxygenated pulmonary venous blood returns to the left atrium and serves as the source of coronary perfusion (1–3). With these modifications of the conduct of ECMO support, we have observed recovery of ventricular function even in patients demonstrating profound myocardial dysfunction (14,15). Based on our experience both ECMO and VAD reliably provide optimal conditions for recovery of ventricular function. Choosing which modality provides the greatest chance of successful support in a given patient, therefore, depends on a number of other considerations that will be discussed in the next section.

III. CLINICAL EXPERIENCE WITH ECMO AND VAD IN PEDIATRIC PATIENTS WITH CARDIAC DISEASE

A. Patient Characteristics and Outcome

We reviewed all patients with a primary diagnosis of cardiac disease supported with ECMO (67 patients) or VAD (29 patients) at Children's Hospital, Boston (14). This report served as a summary of our experience and an attempt to provide a comparison of the clinical use of these two modalities. The patients who were supported constituted a diverse group including cardiac surgical patients who required support in the preoperative or postoperative period, as well as cardiac medical patients who did not require other surgical intervention. The median age of the ECMO-supported patients [2.6 months (range 1 day to 243 months)] was considerably younger than the median age of the VAD supported patients [20.2 months (range 2 days to 280 months)]. This was also reflected in the median weights for the two groups [ECMO 4.3 kg (range 2.4–82 kg) vs. VAD 9.0 kg (range 2.7–71 kg)]. However, both modes of support were successfully utilized in patients over the entire spectrum of sizes encountered in our practice, from newborns to young adults. The median duration of support was longer for the ECMO-supported patients [4.8 days (range 0–29 days)] than for the VAD-supported patients [1.8 days, (range 0–7.8 days)].

Three ECMO-supported patients required two periods of support (runs) for a total of 70 ECMO runs. One VAD-supported patient required support with two runs, while one patient required three runs for a total of 32 VAD runs. Sixty-four of the 70 ECMO runs employed venoarterial support, while six of the runs employed venovenous support. For the 32 VAD runs there were 24 LVAD runs,

6 right ventricular assist device (RVAD) runs, and 2 bi-ventricular assist device (BVAD) runs. Four VAD patients required conversion to ECMO for oxygenator support with one (25%) survivor. No ECMO patients were converted to VAD after satisfactory institution of support. One patient was initially supported with intraaortic balloon counterpulsation prior to the institution of ECMO and did not survive. The proportion of these patients successfully weaned from support [ECMO 45/67 (67.2%); VAD 19/29 (65.5%)] and those that survived to hospital discharge [ECMO 27/67 (40.3%); VAD 12/29 (41.4%)] was nearly identical for the two modes of support (Fig. 1).

B. Cardiac Diagnoses and Indications for Support

The survival according to cardiac diagnoses and the indications for support are listed in Tables 1 and 2, respectively. Examining the underlying diagnoses of these patients demonstrates that the appropriate utilization of ECMO or VAD is based on considerations regarding the specific anatomy and physiology present in a given case. Complex, cyanotic heart disease was present in more than half of the children supported with ECMO. The most common diagnoses in the VAD-supported patients were cases with predominant univentricular failure such as

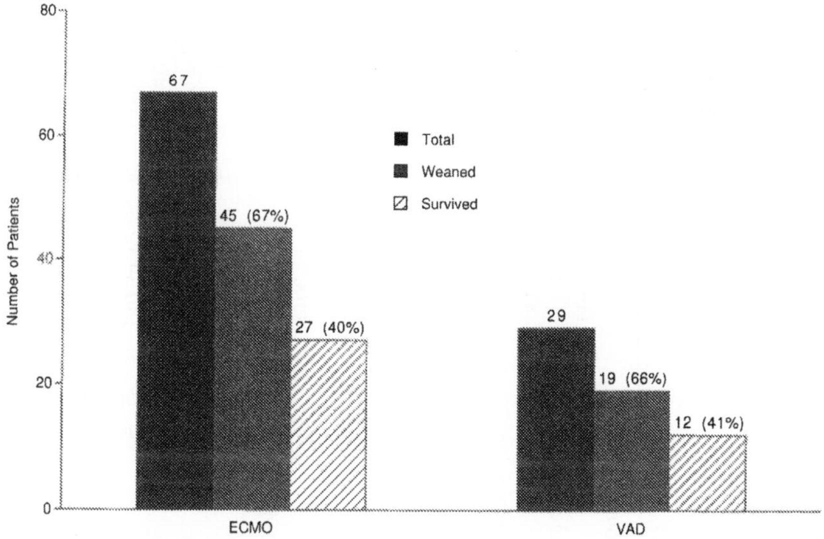

Fig. 1 Total patients supported, patients weaned from support, and hospital survivors for ECMO and VAD patients. (From Ref. 14.)

Table 1 ECMO and VAD Diagnostic Groups and Survival

	ECMO			VAD		
Diagnosis	Survivors	Nonsurvivors	Total	Survivors	Nonsurvivors	Total
L-to-R shunt	1 (14.3%)	6 (85.7%)	7	0	1 (100%)	1
L-sided obstruction	5 (41.7%)	7 (58.3%)	12	1 (25%)	3 (75%)	4
R-sided obstruction	1 (100%)	0	1	0	2 (100%)	2
Cyanosis, ↑ PBF	8 (36.4%)	14 (63.6%)	22	1 (25%)	3 (75%)	4
Cyanosis, ↓ PBF	7 (41.2%)	10 (58.8%)	17	1 (50%)	1 (50%)	2
ALCAPA	1 (100%)	0	1	5 (71.4%)	2 (28.6%)	7
Cardiomyopathy	3 (75%)	1 (25%)	4	3 (60%)	2 (40%)	5
Other	1 (33.3%)	2 (66.7%)	3	1 (25%)	3 (75%)	4
Total	27 (40.3%)	40 (59.7%)	67	12 (41.4%)	17 (58.6%)	29

ALCAPA = Anomalous left coronary artery from pulmonary artery; PBF = pulmonary blood flow. *Source*: Ref. 14.

Table 2 ECMO and VAD Indications for Support and Survival

	ECMO			VAD		
Indication	Survivors	Nonsurvivors	Total	Survivors	Nonsurvivors	Total
Hypoxia	11 (44%)	14 (56%)	25	—	—	—
Preop cardiac failure	1 (100%)	0	1	—	—	—
Postop cardiac failure	2 (28.6%)	5 (71.4%)	7	0	2 (100%)	2
Cardiac arrest	7 (41.2%)	10 (58.8%)	17	2 (40%)	3 (60%)	5
Bridge to transplant	2 (67%)	1 (33%)	3	2 (50%)	2 (50%)	4
Failure to wean from CPB	1 (10%)	9 (90%)	10	7 (36.8%)	12 (63.2%)	19
PHT	1 (25%)	3 (75%)	4	—	—	—
Failure no operation	2 (67%)	1 (33%)	3	1 (50%)	1 (50%)	2
Total	27 (38.6%)	43 (61.4%)	70	12 (37.5%)	20 (62.5%)	32

CPB = Cardiopulmonary bypass; PHT = pulmonary hypertension.
Source: Ref. 14.

anomalous left coronary artery from the pulmonary artery (ALCAPA) or cardiomyopathy. We feel that ECMO is superior to VAD for the support of most children with complex congenital heart disease such as cyanotic lesions where hypoxia, pulmonary hypertension, and bi-ventricular failure contribute to the pathophysiology necessitating mechanical circulatory support. ECMO provides greater flexibility than VAD in these instances. In lesions where univentricular failure predominates such as ALCAPA, VAD provides an effective approach.

Examination of the indications for support demonstrates the high incidence of hypoxia and pulmonary hypertension in ECMO patients. ECMO was required in several of these patients despite the use of high-frequency ventilation, nitric oxide, and liquid ventilation. These measures have been reported to decrease the need for ECMO when used to treat neonatal and pediatric respiratory failure (16–18). Our experience indicates that these adjunctive respiratory measures may fail when severe hypoxia occurs in the setting of congenital heart disease, with many of these children still ultimately requiring ECMO support. In cases of respiratory failure and unrelenting pulmonary hypertension, the presence of an oxygenator in the ECMO circuit makes it the modality of choice for these patients.

Both modalities of support demonstrated equivalent results for the indications of cardiac arrest and bridge to transplantation. Patients requiring ECMO support for failure to wean from cardiopulmonary bypass demonstrated 90% mortality (Table 2). Although not a statistically significant improvement in outcome, VAD supported patients who failed to wean from cardiopulmonary bypass fared somewhat better with 7 survivors out of 19 total patients (37%). A major difference in these two groups was due to the influence of the LVAD-supported ALCAPA patients, many of whom fail to wean from cardiopulmonary bypass yet have an overall good outlook with mechanical circulatory support. The predominance of younger patients with complex cyanotic lesions was largely responsible for the poorer outcome of patients with ECMO support instituted in the operating room. Failure to wean from cardiopulmonary bypass is not a contraindication for ECMO support, but its use in younger patients with complex anatomy should be selective in this setting due to an appreciation of the poor outlook for this group.

C. Complications

Table 3 compares the relative complication rates by organ system for ECMO and VAD. For this analysis, the occurrence of a given complication was determined for each individual ECMO (N = 70) or VAD run (N = 32). No complications were more frequent for the VAD-supported patients. While hemorrhagic complications were the most common complication in both groups, excessive blood loss was a statistically significant risk factor for death only in the ECMO-supported patients. Risk factors for excessive bleeding in our patients included

Table 3 Comparison of Complication Rates for ECMO and VAD Runs

Complication	ECMO incidence	VAD incidence	*p*-value
Hemorrhage	28/70 (40.0%)	14/32 (43.8%)	0.72
Central nervous system	22/70 (31.4%)	4/32 (12.5%)	0.042
Cardiovascular	26/70 (37.1%)	13/32 (40.6%)	0.74
Pulmonary	15/70 (21.4%)	4/32 (12.5%)	0.28
Gastrointestinal	17/70 (24.3%)	1/32 (3.1%)	0.009
Mechanical	18/70 (25.7%)	3/32 (9.4%)	0.058
Renal failure (dialysis or serum creatinine ≥ 3.0)	15/70 (21.4%)	3/32 (9.4%)	0.14
Any severe infection	19/70 (27.1%)	10/32 (31.3%)	0.67
Mediastinitis	3/70 (4.3%)	2/32 (6.3%)	0.67
Pneumonia	10/70 (14.3%)	1/32 (3.1%)	0.092
Positive blood cultures	9/70 (12.9%)	4/32 (12.5%)	0.96

Source: Ref. 14.

chest cannulation and the need for support in the operating room (data not shown). Renal failure in ECMO-supported patients also had a negative impact on survival.

Neurological complications were more common during ECMO support as opposed to VAD support. Neurological complications were not associated with higher mortality in these patients but obviously represent a source of great morbidity. Table 4 lists the neurological complications in these children. Much of the increased incidence of neurological complications in the ECMO patients can be attributed to higher rates of intracranial hemorrhage, which reflects the younger age of the ECMO-supported patients (including a large number of newborns) in addition to the higher levels of anticoagulation required for the ECMO circuit. Anoxic encephalopathy was seen in three of the four neurological complications occurring in VAD-supported children. The higher incidence of central nervous system complications was independent of carotid cannulation or reconstruction in ECMO-supported patients.

Table 4 Type and Number of Neurological Complications Occurring During ECMO and VAD Runs

Central nervous system complication	Number of runs (% of total CNS complications)
ECMO	
Cerebral infarction	4 (18.2%)
Intracranial hemorrhage	8 (36.4%)
Seizures	5 (22.7%)
Developmental delay	1 (4.6%)
Horner's syndrome	1 (4.6%)
Abnormal EEG	1 (4.6%)
Anoxic encephalopathy	2 (9.2%)
Total	22
VAD	
Anoxic encephalopathy	3 (75%)
Prolonged muscle weakness	1 (25%)
Total	4

Source: Ref. 14.

The relatively higher rate of mechanical complications in the ECMO group is due to the increased complexity of the circuit. The presence of the oxygenator itself is a significant source of morbidity resulting in trauma to blood elements and activation of systemic inflammatory and coagulation cascades. In addition, multiple connector sites required in the ECMO circuit increase the risk of air and particulate embolism while oxygenator failure requires interruption of flow and replacement. Complications related to the circuit were not associated with a significantly higher mortality.

D. Causes of Death

Cardiac failure and multiple system organ failure were the major causes of death in both ECMO- and VAD-supported patients (Table 5). For both of these

Table 5 ECMO and VAD Causes of Death

	ECMO		VAD	
Cause of death	Number	%	Number	%
Ventricular failure	14	35	9	53
Multiple system organ failure	12	30	4	23
Respiratory failure	4	10	—	—
Anoxic brain injury	2	5	2	12
Intracranial hemorrhage	2	5	—	—
Arrhythmia	2	5	1	6
Inadequate flow rates due to poor venous drainage	2	5	—	—
Aortic cannula dislodgement	1	2.5	—	—
Hemorrhage (torn umbilical vein)	1	2.5	—	—
Hemorrhage (mediastinal)	—	—	1	6
Total	40	100	17	100

Source: Ref. 14.

conditions, early and aggressive consideration for transplantation may lead to higher salvage rates. We have maintained patients for as long as 4 weeks with mechanical circulatory support, however, the development of infectious complications and multiple system organ failure eventually supervenes. The use of pulsatile circulatory perfusion devices for chronic support in children may delay the development of this process. Although no pulsatile flow systems are currently available in the United States for chronic pediatric circulatory support, the development of such devices will be a welcome addition to the therapeutic options for these critically ill children.

E. Other Studies

There are few other reports that compare the use of ECMO and VAD in the treatment of children with cardiac disease. Karl reported the use of ECMO and/or VAD in 51 pediatric cardiac patients with similar results to ours. The survival to hospital discharge of ECMO- and VAD-supported patients did not demonstrate a statistically significant difference (33% vs. 48%, respectively; $p = 0.37$) (19). Important features of this report include a description of the meticulous management and decision making employed by the authors in determining the suitability of ECMO or VAD support for patients that are unable to wean from cardiopulmonary bypass. Karl also found that VAD was most useful for postoperative support of patients with ALCAPA. Khan and Gazzaniga reported the use of ECMO, VAD, and IABP in 15 pediatric cardiac patients with an excellent overall survival of 74% (20). These authors found that the preoperative use of ECMO was frequently useful in conditions that demonstrated refractory pulmonary hypertension and hypoxia prior to operation. In addition, they reported that ECMO was most often useful in neonates and infants, while VAD was technically easier and more likely to be successful in older children and young adults (20).

IV. SELECTION OF THE APPROPRIATE MODALITY OF SUPPORT—ECMO VERSUS VAD

Table 6 is a ''scorecard'' based on the above experimental and clinical experience that demonstrates the advantages and disadvantages of ECMO and VAD relative to each other in the treatment of pediatric cardiac patients. These general points may aid in selecting the appropriate mode of support in a given clinical setting. Pediatric centers have extensive experience with ECMO for the treatment of neonatal respiratory failure where expansion of its use to include pediatric cardiac patients is often easily accomplished. As opposed to adult cardiac units, however, the experience of pediatric centers with VAD may be limited. Due to the absence of an oxygenator, VAD circuits are simpler, requiring less anticoagulation and resulting in less blood trauma than is the case for ECMO. ECMO may be instituted peripherally with neck or groin cannulation, while VAD requires a sternotomy. Left ventricular decompression is more effectively performed by LVAD or BVAD, while the occurrence of left ventricular distension requires aggressive monitoring and prompt treatment with left atrial venting or balloon atrial septostomy in patients supported with ECMO. ALCAPA results in a relatively pure form of left ventricular dysfunction and represents the paradigm lesion for successful LVAD support. ECMO, on the other hand, provides greater flexibility in dealing with forms of complex congenital heart disease where pulmonary hyper-

Table 6 Scorecard for Appropriate Modality of Support—ECMO versus VAD

	ECMO	VAD
Experience in pediatric centers	√	
Simplicity of circuit		√
Peripheral cannulation	√	
Left ventricular decompression		√
Anomalous left coronary artery from the pulmonary artery		√
Treatment of pulmonary hypertension and hypoxia	√	
Biventricular support in neonates	√	

Source: Ref. 14.

tension and hypoxia contribute significantly to the pathophysiology. Finally, biventricular support is easier to institute with ECMO, which requires only two cannulation sites compared to four cannulation sites required for BVAD. This may not be a problem in older patients but is an important consideration when biventricular support is required in neonates.

REFERENCES

1. Secker-Walker JS, Edmonds JF, Spratt EH, Conn AW. The source of coronary perfusion during partial bypass for extracorporeal membrane oxygenation (ECMO). Ann Thorac Surg 1976; 21:138–143.
2. Nowlen TT, Salley SO, Whittlesey GC, et al. Regional blood flow distribution during extracorporeal membrane oxygenation in rabbits. J Thorac Cardiovasc Surg 1989; 98:1138–1143.
3. Kato J, Seo T, Ando H, Takagi H, Ito T. Coronary arterial perfusion during venoarterial extracorporeal membrane oxygenation. J Thorac Cardiovasc Surg 1996; 111: 630–636.
4. Bavaria JE, Ratcliffe MB, Gupta KB, Wenger RK, Bogen DK, Edmunds LH. Changes in left ventricular systolic wall stress during biventricular circulatory assistance. Ann Thorac Surg 1988; 45:526–532.
5. Ratcliffe MB, Bavaria JE, Wenger RK, Bogen DK, Edmunds LH. Left ventricular mechanics of ejecting, postischemic hearts during left ventricular circulatory assistance. J Thorac Cardiovasc Surg 1991; 101:245–255.
6. Eugene J, Ott RA, McColgan SJ, Roohk RV. Vented cardiac assistance: ECMO versus left heart bypass for acute left ventricular failure. Trans ASAIO 1986; 32: 538–541.
7. Eugene J, McColgan SJ, Roohk HV, Ott RA. Vented ECMO for biventricular failure. Trans ASAIO 1987; 33:579–583.
8. Zobel G, Dacar D, Kuttnig M, Rodl S, Rigler B. Mechanical support of the left ventricle in ischemia induced left ventricular failure: an experimental study. Int J Artif Organs 1992; 15:114–119.
9. Kimball TR, Daniels SR, Weiss RG, et al. Changes in cardiac function during extracorporeal membrane oxygenation for persistent pulmonary hypertension in the newborn infant. J Pediatr 1991; 118:431–436.
10. Martin GR, Short BL. Doppler echocardiographic evaluation of cardiac performance in infants on prolonged extracorporeal membrane oxygenation. Am J Cardiol 1988; 62:929–934.
11. Berdjis F, Takahashi M, Lewis AB. Left ventricular performance in neonates on extracorporeal membrane oxygenation. Pediatr Cardiol 1992; 13:141–145.
12. Koenig PR, Ralston MA, Kimball TR, Meyer RA, Daniels SR, Schwartz DC. Balloon atrial septostomy for left ventricular decompression in patients receiving extracorporeal membrane oxygenation for myocardial failure. J Pediatr 1993; 122:S95–S99.

13. O'Connor TA, Downing GJ, Ewing LL, Gowdamarajan R. Echocardiographically guided balloon atrial septostomy during extracorporeal membrane oxygenation (ECMO). Pediatr Cardiol 1993; 14:167–168.
14. Duncan BW, Hraska V, Jonas RA, et al. Mechanical circulatory support in children with cardiac disease. J Thorac Cardiovasc Surg 1999; 117:529–542.
15. Duncan BW, Ibrahim AE, Hraska V, et al. Use of rapid-deployment extracorporeal membrane oxygenation for the resuscitation of pediatric patients with heart disease after cardiac arrest. J Thorac Cardiovasc Surg 1998; 116:305–311.
16. Goldman AP, Delius RE, Deanfield JE, de Leval MR, Sigston PE, Macrae DJ. Nitric oxide might reduce the need for extracorporeal support in children with critical post-operative pulmonary hypertension. Ann Thorac Surg 1996; 62:750–755.
17. Journois D, Pouard P, Mauriat P, Malhere T, Voune P, Safran D. Inhaled nitric oxide as a therapy for pulmonary hypertension after operations for congenital heart defects. J Thorac Cardiovasc Surg 1994; 107:1129–1135.
18. Kocis KC, Meliones JN, Dekeon MK, Callow LB, Lupinetti JM, Bove EL. High-frequency jet ventilation for respiratory failure after congenital heart surgery. Circulation 1992; 86(suppl II):II-127–II-132.
19. Karl TR. Extracorporeal circulatory support in infants and children. Semin Thorac Cardiovasc Surg 1994; 6:154–160.
20. Khan A, Gazzaniga AB. Mechanical circulatory assistance in paediatric patients with cardiac failure. Cardiovasc Surg 1996; 4:43–49.

5

Intensive Care Management of Cardiac Patients on Extracorporeal Membrane Oxygenation

David L. Wessel, Melvin C. Almodovar, and Peter C. Laussen
Children's Hospital and Harvard Medical School,
Boston, Massachusetts

Mechanical support of the failing circulation in children has much of its origins in cardiovascular surgery. Adaptation of heart-lung machines to support patients in cardiogenic shock has been attempted by clinicians since the 1950s. Support of children with postoperative pulmonary hypertension associated with repair of congenital heart disease was reported as early as 1963. However, it was not until the important contributions of Bartlett and colleagues (1) that technological advances permitted prolonged mechanical support of children with cardiorespiratory failure to become a routine aspect of intensive care life.

I. IMPACT OF MECHANICAL SUPPORT

The availability of extracorporeal cardiorespiratory support for children with congenital heart disease has had a dramatic impact on a broad range of issues in the intensive care unit (ICU) (1–11). Prolonging intraoperative cardiopulmonary bypass (CPB) for cardiac surgical patients returning to the ICU was an early and obvious extension of CPB technology. The effect on hospital mortality is unequivocal and even more obvious when used as rescue therapy during cardiopulmonary resuscitation (12,13). But the impact is felt across many disciplines, including medicine, surgery, nursing, pharmacy, and respiratory therapy, and involves cardiovascular surgeons, cardiologists, intensivists, anesthesiologists, neonatologists, and extracorporeal membrane oxygenation (ECMO) specialists. Extracorporeal cardiorespiratory support has expanded our options for supporting reversible heart failure and utilizing organ transplantation (14,15). It has enabled us to perform difficult catheter interventions in unstable patients and allowed treatment of life-threatening arrhythmias with catheter ablation techniques. It has altered the way intensive care physicians select patients for intervention and conduct cardiopulmonary resuscitation, and it has made clinicians confront practical issues of informed consent for starting and stopping potentially life-saving treatment. This in turn has challenged medical ethicists to opine on study designs involving ECMO and the important issues of parental input and consent. The technology has confused the clergy by introducing ambiguities about the temporal domains of life and death in the ICU. It has put extraordinary demands on administrators and ECMO specialists to provide more time and personnel during an era of cost reduction. The care of these patients provides intellectual challenges in understanding unique pathophysiology and requires expertise that physicians and other healthcare professionals seek to obtain. The intensity and experience associated with using the ultimate resuscitative tool to achieve sudden shifts from near certain death to dramatic recovery is highly motivating and enormously gratifying.

Tables 1 and 2 show the cumulative activity through 1999 in the Extracorporeal Life Support Organization (ELSO) registry with survival by diagnostic category. Figure 1 shows the number of ECMO cases for neonatal respiratory failure in over 120 centers, predominantly in the United States (ELSO registry). With the advent of high-frequency oscillatory ventilation, use of surfactant, inhaled nitric oxide, and other advances in critical care of the newborn, the need for ECMO for hypoxemic respiratory failure has declined since its peak in 1992. Cardiac ECMO (including adults) seems to have declined more recently as adult

Table 1 Cumulative ELSO Registry Data Through 1999

	Total patients	Survived ECMO (%)	Survived to discharge (%)
Neonatal			
Respiratory	14,543	84	79
Cardiac	1,085	55	40
Pediatric			
Respiratory	1,711	62	55
Cardiac	1,642	52	39
Adult			
Respiratory	483	52	49
Cardiac	244	36	32

Table 2 Cumulative ELSO Registry Data Through 1999 for Neonatal Respiratory Failure by Diagnostic Category

	Total runs	Avg. run time (hr)	Percent survived
MAS	5177	127	94
CD hernia	3132	216	55
Sepsis	2088	138	76
PPHN/PFC	2065	137	80
RDS	1268	132	80
Pneumonia	151	216	55
Other	740	164	68

use of ventricular assist devices (VADs) (including implantable) has gained acceptance (Fig. 2). In contrast, Fig. 3 shows that the proportion of children who received ECMO support for congenital or acquired heart disease at Children's Hospital, Boston, has steadily increased; this is typical of the pediatric experience in many large cardiac centers. More than half of all ECMO runs in our institution are now for cardiovascular support rather than respiratory support. Survival for patients on ECMO after cardiac surgery has also steadily improved but has not

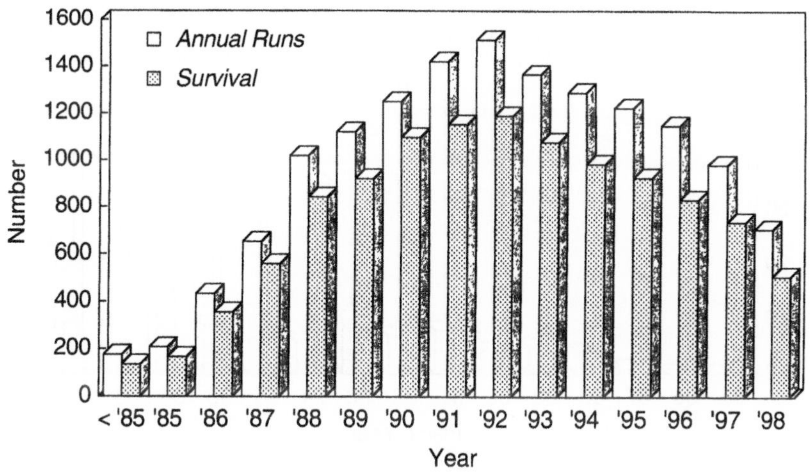

Fig. 1 ELSO Registry data for neonatal respiratory failure. Open bars show total number of ECMO cases per year. Shaded bars show total number of survivors per year.

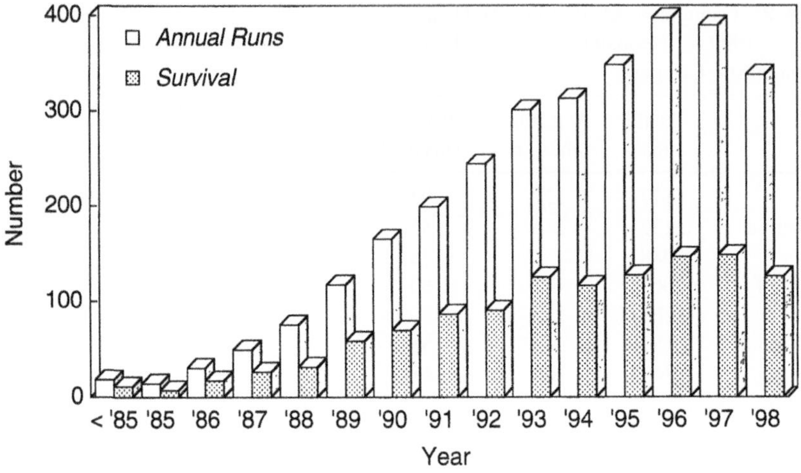

Fig. 2 ELSO Registry data for adult and pediatric cardiac support. Open bars show total number of ECMO cases per year. Shaded bars show total number of survivors per year.

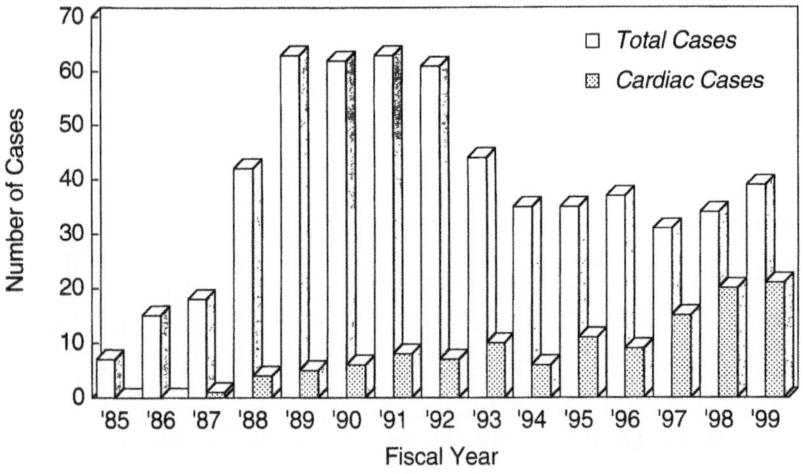

Fig. 3 ECMO activity at Children's Hospital, Boston. Open bars show total number of ECMO cases per year. Shaded bars show total number of ECMO cases used for cardiac support per year. Approximately half of all ECMO cases are now for cardiac support rather than respiratory failure.

reached the survival rates of neonates on ECMO for respiratory failure (Table 1; Fig. 1). Substantial institutional variability in patient selection for ECMO makes comparison of published experience difficult. Even within institutions, practice has substantially evolved, and this confounds the interpretation of trends over time. Overall, one can propose that the use of ECMO for cardiovascular support is increasing, results are improving, but there is room for further progress (16). Refinement of ECMO personnel and organization to include an in-hospital team for rapid resuscitation may improve outcome (13) (see Chapter 9). During 1999 at Children's Hospital, Boston, more than 20 patients were cannulated for cardiovascular support during resuscitation for cardiac arrest; hospital survival exceeds 60%. Survivors among neonates has dramatically improved to 70%, including those patients with hypoplastic left heart syndrome who have undergone a Norwood operation.

II. INDICATIONS FOR ECMO

General indications for use of mechanical support in patients with heart disease include inadequate oxygen delivery or a requirement for temporary support during cardiac catheterization interventions. Inadequate oxygen delivery is caused most commonly by either low cardiac output, profound cyanosis with intracardiac shunting and cardiovascular collapse, or profound hypoxemia from associate lung disease (Table 3).

The most common cause of inadequate oxygen delivery in a pediatric cardiac ICU stems from low cardiac output, which is usually a result of myocardial dysfunction. Ventricular dysfunction may occur as a component of chronic cardiomyopathy or from other causes of congestive heart failure. It may occur more dramatically with acute decompensation typified by acute fulminant viral myocarditis.

Patients who fail to wean from cardiopulmonary bypass may be converted to an ECMO circuit in the operating room and brought to the ICU in hopes of recovering myocardial function (17). These children typically have poorer survival rates for multifactorial reasons, including severity and complexity of disease, as well as increased bleeding. Other children have progressive myocardial failure after successful weaning from CPB. This typically occurs during the first 24 hours after cardiac surgery, and subsequent survival may be better in this group of patients following a period of myocardial rest and decompression.

Pulmonary hypertensive crises after CPB may be refractory to therapy and necessitate mechanical support of the right heart. These patients are notoriously difficult to resuscitate after cardiac arrest if they have advanced pulmonary vascular obstructive disease. Resuscitation is facilitated if a small right-to-left communication is created or left in place at the time of surgical intervention.

Table 3 Indications and Relative Contraindications for ECMO

	Typical Indications for ECMO
I.	Inadequate oxygen delivery
	A. Low cardiac output
	1. Chronic (cardiomyopathy)
	2. Acute (myocarditis)
	3. Weaning from CPB
	4. Progressive postoperative failure
	5. Pulmonary hypertension
	6. Refractory arrhythmias
	7. Cardiac arrest
	B. Profound cyanosis
	1. Intracardiac shunting and cardiovascular collapse
	C. Profound hypoxemia
	1. Child
	a) pneumonia or acute respiratory failure exaggerated by underlying heart disease
	2. Newborn
	b) CHD, complicated by other newborn indications for ECMO such as meconium aspiration syndrome, PPHN, pneumonia, sepsis, respiratory distress syndrome, etc.
II.	Support for intervention during cardiac catheterization
	A. Ablation
	B. Dilation
	C. Device closure
	Relative Contraindications for ECMO
I.	End-stage, irreversible, or inoperable disease
II.	Family, patient directives to limit resuscitation
III.	Significant neurological impairment
IV.	Uncontrolled bleeding within major organs
V.	Extremes of size and weight
VI.	Inaccessible vessels during CPR
VII.	Residual, operable, anatomical lesion (reoperation rather than ECMO)

Refractory arrhythmias are occasionally controlled only after the heart has been decompressed on ECMO and sufficient time has been gained to achieve adequate pharmacological control of the arrhythmia (9).

Cardiac arrest may occur suddenly in the postoperative period without substantial warning. It may also occur as the culmination of progressive postoperative myocardial dysfunction, resistant to therapy. Although anticipation of this event with timely preparation for ECMO is preferable, cannulation during CPR is not uncommon (13,16).

III. RELATIVE CONTRAINDICATIONS TO ECMO

Although there may be few structural heart defects that preclude the use of ECMO, there are some potentially important contraindications that should be considered (Table 3). Obviously if the underlying disease is felt to be irreversible or inoperable, common sense may dictate that mechanical support of the circulation merely prolongs a terminal illness, which is destined to have a fatal outcome in the near future. However, perspective on the term ''inoperable'' may vary among healthcare professionals and is closely tied to the parents' perception of the likelihood of survival and the quality of life during survival.

Significant central nervous system disease or injury may also preclude the use of ECMO. Chromosomal abnormalities associated with central nervous system impairment may complicate the assessment of patients and affect predictions about quality of life. Generally speaking, the presence of trisomy 21 has not been considered recently to be a contraindication to ECMO after cardiac surgery. However, most families and practitioners believe that the severe limitation in cognitive function and predicted life span associated with trisomy 13 or 18 would not be consistent with the guideline that the underlying disease or diseases must be reversible in order to merit consideration for ECMO.

Active bleeding from relatively inaccessible locations such as the brain or abdominal structures prior to initiation of ECMO may also present a relative contraindication since heparinization would in all likelihood aggravate previously existing disease. Extremes of size and weight may pose limitations on ECMO technology, but those limits expand each year.

Unattainable vascular access may deter ECMO cannulation during CPR. Occasionally, a child with congenital heart disease will have had surgery many weeks or months prior to an in-hospital cardiopulmonary arrest, which would otherwise prompt consideration for ECMO as part of the resuscitative maneuvers. However if the jugular veins or superior vena cava are known to be obstructed from previous interventions and there are anatomical limitations (size or previous procedures) to cannulating through the groin, then the notion of continuing CPR through a prolonged procedure to reopen the sternum through extensive scar tissue may be inadvisable.

Finally, if progressive myocardial dysfunction characterizes the postoperative course of a patient who is identified as having significant residual anatomical disease, then the temptation to support the child with ECMO must be balanced against the more prudent need to return to the operating room and directly address the residual anatomical lesion.

IV. IDENTIFYING RESIDUAL DISEASE

The importance of identifying residual or previously undiagnosed anatomical disease in the postoperative patient with progressive myocardial dysfunction and low cardiac output cannot be underestimated. This is one of the prime responsibilities of those who participate in postoperative management (18,19). Intracardiac catheters to measure pressure and sample blood for oxygen saturation will help assess the adequacy of diagnosis and repair. Transthoracic and transesophageal echocardiography are valuable in the postoperative evaluation of the child with low cardiac output. When acoustic windows are limited with echocardiography, the patient may benefit from cardiac catheterization, including physiological assessment and angiographic imaging. Aggressive diagnostic intervention is a critical component in the assessment of low cardiac output in the postoperative patient. This is especially appealing if suspected residual lesions can be addressed with interventional catheterization techniques.

V. CAUSES OF LOW CARDIAC OUTPUT BEFORE ECMO

Although some causes of low cardiac output after cardiopulmonary bypass are attributable to residual or undiagnosed structural lesions, progressive low cardiac output states do occur. A number of factors have been implicated in the development of myocardial dysfunction following cardiopulmonary bypass, including (a) the inflammatory response associated with cardiopulmonary bypass, (b) the effects of myocardial ischemia from aortic cross clamping, (c) hypothermia, (d) reperfusion injury, (e) inadequate myocardial protection, and (f) ventriculotomy (when performed). The expression and prevention of reperfusion injury after aortic cross clamping on cardiopulmonary bypass is currently the subject of intense investigation. Figure 4 shows the decrease in cardiac index in newborns following an arterial switch operation. In this group of 122 newborns, the median maximal decrease in cardiac index that occurred typically 6–12 hours after separation from cardiopulmonary bypass was 32% (20). A quarter of all of these newborns reached a nadir of cardiac index of <2 L/min/m^2 on the first postoperative night. Low cardiac output states do occur in the postoperative patient, but appropriate anticipation and intervention can do much to avert the need for mechanical support.

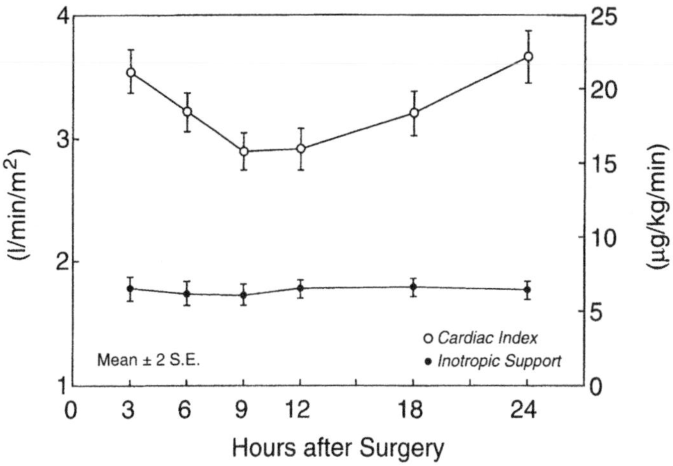

Fig. 4 Cardiac index (left axis) and inotropic drug score (right axis) in 122 newborns following cardiopulmonary bypass for an arterial switch operation. The decline and recovery of cardiac index is thought to be attributable in part to the inflammatory response and ischemia-reperfusion injury after bypass. (From Ref. 20.)

VI. OPTIMIZING CARDIAC OUTPUT BEFORE AND AFTER MECHANICAL SUPPORT

Physicians in the ICU bear the responsibility of anticipating changes in cardiac output after cardiac surgery, excluding residual disease as a causative factor, and optimizing physiological conditions that will achieve optimal cardiac output. The need for mechanical support of the circulation can often be averted by an experienced appreciation of therapeutic modalities to support oxygen delivery short of ECMO (18,21). But even if these therapies are inadequate to sustain the patient prior to invoking ECMO, they must again be thoughtfully applied in the effort to wean the patient from mechanical support as soon as possible after myocardial function has returned and adequate organ perfusion can be guaranteed. Table 4 summarizes various considerations and treatment strategies available to the child with low cardiac output.

VII. INSTITUTION OF MECHANICAL CIRCULATORY SUPPORT

Initiation of ECMO requires the prompt and coordinated efforts of the entire mechanical support team. Algorithms for action to proceed will vary among insti-

Table 4 Supporting the Failing Myocardium in the ICU

I. Extent of the Problem
- A. One quarter of newborns will decrease their cardiac index to <2.0 L/min/m^2 after CPB

II. Exclude Residual Disease
- A. Tranesophageal echocardiography and intracardiac catheters provide important anatomical and physiological data for planning the need for reintervention.

III. Optimize Preload
- A. Monitor filling pressure and interpret values in light of underlying cardiac disease.

IV. Enable R → L Shunting for Right Heart Failure
- A. Newborn after right ventriculotomy (TOF and truncus arteriosus).
- B. Baffle fenestration in patients undergoing a Fontan operation helps preserve cardiac output and oxygen delivery and reduces right atrial pressure.
- C. Preserving a R → L shunt in patients with known elevation in pulmonary vascular resistance may preserve cardiac output during postoperative pulmonary hypertensive crises or during CPR.

V. Pharmacological Support
- A. Catecholamines
  1. Dopamine (5–15 μg/kg/min) supports cardiac output and preserves aortic perfusion pressure during weaning from cardiopulmonary bypass. Dobutamine may reduce afterload.
  2. Prolonged high dose epinephrine after cardiopulmonary bypass in neonates is associated with myocardial necrosis and marked diastolic dysfunction and is increasingly avoided.
- B. Afterload reduction
  1. Milrinone, a phosphodiesterase inhibitor, increases cardiac output and lowers filling pressures. Nitrates are commonly employed as vasodilators.
  2. Phenoxybenzamine is a potent alpha blocker and has been advocated as part of the postoperative management of patients with hypoplastic left heart syndrome but has a long duration of action.
  3. Nitric oxide is a selective pulmonary vasodilator, which will reduce the afterload on the right heart.

VI. Rhythm
- A. A-V sequential pacing is important for arrhythmias such as JET or complete heart block.
- B. Atrio-biventricular pacing may improve hemodynamics substantially in patients with complete right or left bundle branch block.

VII. Ventilation/Cardio-respiratory Interactions
- A. Positive pressure ventilation reduces left ventricular afterload, but decreases preload and may raise pulmonary vascular resistance and RV afterload.
- B. Negative pressure ventilation (Hayek oscillator) may augment R heart function.

VIII. Hypothermia
- A. There is renewed interest in lowering core body temperature to 34°–35°C for patients in low cardiac output states in an effort to reduce oxygen consumption and optimize oxygen delivery.

IX. Ischemia Reperfusion Injury
- A. Anti-inflammatory agents including monoclonal antibodies, competitive receptor blockers, inhibitors of compliment activation and preoperative preparation with steroids are being actively investigated in an effort to prevent and protect major organs from ischemic injury imposed by cardiopulmonary bypass and the reperfusion injury associated with the recovery period.

tutions. In the authors' experience, the decision to proceed with ECMO is usually made at the bedside by those attending the patient: cardiac surgeon, cardiac intensivist, bedside nurse, and nurse in charge. Cross-trained personnel such as ECMO specialists who are also respiratory therapy staff facilitate communication and streamline personnel requirements. As the ECMO specialist is notified, the transfusion service is contacted and a blood prime is planned. The operating room nursing staff are called and a scrub nurse is made available whenever possible. The precise moment of the procedure start time may vary according to the availability of personnel and necessary components when resuscitation is not impending or underway.

VIII. RAPID-DEPLOYMENT ECMO FOR RESUSCITATION

When ECMO is utilized during an ongoing resuscitation, our goal is to have a circuit ready in 15 minutes and cannulation complete in less than 30 minutes after cardiac arrest. Since 1996 we have utilized an in-hospital rapid deployment team to respond to an emergency need for ECMO cannulation during cardiopulmonary arrest and resuscitation at a variety of locations throughout the hospital (13) (see Chapter 9). These include the ICU, cardiac catheterization laboratory, emergency department, inpatient wards (rarely), and noncardiac operating rooms. In our hospital, the senior physician at the resuscitation initiates the rapid deployment call by contacting the ICU secretary or nurse-in-charge, who executes a rapid series of urgent telephone pages from a predefined contact list. This includes all personnel noted above and an ECMO specialist, who carries a "priming pager" and is in-hospital at all times. The transfusion service can respond to the urgent page in less than 45 minutes, but the ECMO rapid resuscitation circuit, which stands ready and CO_2-vacuum primed at all times in the ICU, is immediately crystalloid-primed and ready for use in 15 minutes. Blood products are added when they are available (typically after cannulation), and crystalloid is removed by direct withdrawal from the circuit into a syringe or by a volume-matched amount of ultrafiltration. Cardiac surgeons who are trained in cannulation techniques for open chest, groin, or neck routes are based in the ICU, along with cardiac ICU fellows 24 hours per day. At night, these are senior trainees who have been oriented to the rapid resuscitation protocol and have attending physician backup immediately available.

Hospital survival of pulseless patients resuscitated with ECMO now exceeds 60%. Obviously the effectiveness of ECMO as a tool to achieve successful resuscitation of cardiac patients will depend on the nature of the underlying disease and the efficiency of the technique. Typically we now wait only 5 minutes (or one round of medication administration) before determining that return of cardiovascular stability during CPR is unlikely and the ECMO circuit should be primed. A circuit prepared and primed with crystalloid but unused can be maintained in readiness for 24 hours but will usually be discarded after that time. Delay in cannulation during CPR is rarely the result of prolonged circuit preparation time.

A parallel consideration involves the decision process for determining suitability for ECMO. This must occur *prior* to cardiac arrest whenever possible. Institutions may adopt general philosophies about rapid resuscitation ECMO for broad categories of patients in the ICU. For example, infants with two ventricles and uncomplicated repair of CHD who have no other underlying disease may all be candidates for ECMO should they have a sudden, unexpected cardiac arrest in the early postoperative period. In contrast, it may be generally inadvisable to impose ECMO on an older patient with end-stage heart disease or severe neurological disease who declines or is not otherwise a candidate for transplantation but has an acute decompensation and cardiac arrest. In between these extremes is an area that requires discussion and individualization of care plans that must be accomplished prior to any anticipated or unanticipated decompensation. Thus, daily patient rounds in the intensive care unit must now incorporate a dialogue among physicians, nurses, family, and support staff that addresses the patient's suitability for ECMO. The moment after cardiac arrest is not the time to initiate discussions about the appropriateness of invasive, potentially life-prolonging technology. Addressing these issues during rounds and fully discussing the appropriate limitation of technology is an important new responsibility.

IX. BASIC PHYSIOLOGY OF ECMO

The primary physiological goal of ECMO is to maintain adequate oxygen delivery while minimizing oxygen consumption. A normal ratio of oxygen delivery to oxygen consumption is sought to avoid metabolic acidosis and cellular injury during recovery from the primary physiological insult. Oxygen consumption can be minimized by use of sedation, muscle relaxation, avoidance of catecholamine infusion (if possible), infection, and fever. Active cooling of patients during and after resuscitation with ECMO may be protective against further neurological injury during reperfusion. In patients with cardiac disease, acceptable oxygen delivery is achieved almost exclusively with the use of venoarterial extracorporeal support. Oxygen delivery is proportional to blood flow and oxygen content of arterial blood, which is largely influenced by the hemoglobin concentration and, to a lesser degree, dissolved oxygen. Additional contributions from native cardiac output and pulmonary function may be beneficial.

In many centers, blood flow is driven by a roller pump using a servoregulatory mechanism. This system permits high flow rates with minimal hemolysis and protects against entrainment of air. Flow is preserved at the expense of pressure if impedance to flow is encountered in the membrane or the patient. Systemic venous blood drains by gravity from the right atrium or large systemic vein using one or more large-bore cannulae and passes through the pump to a membrane oxygenator or artificial lung where oxygen is introduced and carbon dioxide eliminated (see Chapter 1). Blood is returned to the body via the "arterial" limb of the circuit directly into the aorta, common carotid, or common iliac arteries. The rate of blood flow is limited by the size of the venous and arterial catheters, tubing, membrane oxygenator, and patient factors such as size intravascular volume status, and systemic vascular resistance. Central venous, intracardiac, and peripheral arterial blood pressure catheters are connected to standard transducers and allow continuous pressure monitoring with intermittent blood sampling as a means of frequently assessing the adequacy of the circulation and oxygen delivery. Additional important factors are closely monitored and include the following: physical examination, pulse oximetry if the heart is ejecting and flow is pulsatile, and indices of renal (serum blood urea nitrogen and creatinine, hourly urine output) and hepatic (serum transaminases, coagulation profile, and serum albumin) function. Persistent or new-onset metabolic acidosis, a rising lactate, and diminishing urine output argue strongly for inadequate oxygen delivery. This triad merits aggressive diagnostic evaluation. Pump flow should be increased to 150 mL/min or even higher if there is an anatomical lesion with runoff of systemic flow to the lungs.

X. EQUIPMENT AND SUPPLIES

A standard mobile ECMO cart in our center consists of a roller pump with control dial, tubing, volume- or pressure-sensitive bladder-transducer system for flow servoregulation, membrane oxygenator/heat exchanger, in-line premembrane and postmembrane pressure monitors, and a backup battery pack with a charger. In addition, a well-organized, readily accessible supply of arterial and venous cannulae of different sizes and shapes (Table 5), mediastinal tray with appropriate surgical instruments, drapes, and antiseptic solutions are stocked in the cardiac ICU. A vacuum-primed rapid-resuscitation circuit is maintained for emergency ECMO cannulation and initiation of support within 15 minutes.

XI. PRECANNULATION PREPARATION

After blood group typing with antibody screening has been performed and baseline complete blood count, prothrombin time, partial thromboplastin time, and fibrinogen level have been measured, blood products are ordered for the initial circuit prime. Blood product components are ordered as neonatal, pediatric, adult,

Table 5 ECMO Cannula Characteristics

Manufacturer	Features	Connector	Size (Fr)	Length (cm)	Maximum drainage (L/min)	Maximum infusion (L/min)	Radiographic appearance
Kendall	Double-lumen	1/4″	14	10	—	0.5	Opaque throughout
Origen Biomedical	Double-lumen	1/4″	12	9	—	0.5	Opaque throughout
			15	9		0.6	
			18	9		1.0	
Biomedicus							
96820	Arterial	1/4″	8	19	—	—	Coil ends 0.5 cm from tip
			10	19			
			12	19			
96830	Venous	1/4″	8	19	—	—	Radiopaque dot at tip
			10	19			Coil ends 4 cm from tip
			12	19			
			14	19			
96350	Percutaneous kit with side holes; arterial or venous	3/8″	15	18	2.0	2.8	Coil ends 4 cm from tip
			17	18	3.0	4.0	
			19	18	3.5	5.4	
			21	18	4.5	6.8	
96540	Percutaneous kit with side holes; arterial or venous	1/2″	23	25	6.5	—	Coil ends 4 cm from tip

96600	Percutaneous kit (femoral vein)	3/8″	17	50	1.5	2.5	Coil ends 4 cm from tip
			19	50	2.5	3.5	
			21	50	3.2	4.5	
96370	Femoral venous kit with introducer	1/2″	23	50	4.5	6.7	Coil ends 4 cm from tip
			25	50	5.2	8.2	
			27	50	6.5	9.5	
Medtronic DLP	Venous right angle	1/4″	12	37	—	—	Metal tip
			14	37			
			16	37			
			18	37			
			20	38			
	Venous right angle	3/8″	20	37	—	—	Metal tip
			22	37			
			24	37			
			28	38			
	Arterial straight tip	1/4″	8	18	—	—	Radiopaque line ends 2 cm from tip
			10	18			
			12	18			
			14	18			
	Arterial straight tip	3/8″	16	18	—	—	Radiopaque line ends 3 cm from tip
			18	18			
			20	18			

Table 6 Circuit Priming Components

ECMO Circuit/ blood "packs"[a]	Weight (kg)	Membrane (m^2)	PRBC (ml)	FFP (ml)	Cryoprecipitate (units)	Platelets (units)	"Keep ahead" (PRBC-ml)
Neonates/Infants	<15	0.8–1.5	500[b]	200	2	2[Conc]	1000[c]
Pediatric	16–35	2.5–3.5	1000[c]	400	3	4	1000[c]
Adult	>35	4.5	1500[c]	500	4	6	1000[c]
Rapid resuscitation[d]	<25	0.8–1.5	200[d]	100	2	2–4	—

PRBC = Packed red blood cells; FFP = fresh frozen plasma; Conc = concentrated platelets.
[a] Blood products ordered in packages according to patient size (i.e., neonatal, pediatric, adult).
[b] Leukopore filtered, <7 days old.
[c] <7 days old.
[d] Leukopore filtered, <21 days old.
[e] Normosol® primed with addition of 50 cc 5% albumin; blood products added when available.

Table 7 ECMO Circuit Characteristics

	Neonatal	Pediatric	Adult	Rapid resuscitation	
Patient weight (kg)	2–15	16–35	>36	>25	<25
Membrane (m^2)	0.8–1.5	2.5–3.5	4.5 (1–2)	hollow fiber	0.8–1.5
Membrane volume (cc)	174	455–575	665–1330	260	174
Circuit volume (cc)	580	1500–1600	2500–3200	1000	580
Prime					
5% Albumin (cc)	50	100	100	100	50
PRBC (cc)	500[a]	1000[b]	1500[b]	1000[c]	200[c]
FFP (cc)	200	400	500	400	100
Cryoprecipitate (units)	2	3	4	3	2
Platelets (units)	2	4	6	6	2–4
Normosol®	—	—	—	—	Yes
Other					
Heparin (Units)	500	500	800	500	100
THAM® (cc)	100	200	300	200	100
Ca^+ gluconate (mg)	1500	3000	4000	3000	1500
Na^+ bicarbonate (meq)	20	40	60	40	20
Minimum blood flow (ml/min)	100	200–250	300–600	500	100–200
Maximum blood flow (L/min)	1.8	4.5–5.5	6.5–13	8	1.8
Sweep gas range (L/min)	1–4.5	2–11	2–13	0.5–20	1–4.5

PRBC = packed red blood cells; FFP = fresh frozen plasma; THAM® = tris-hydroxymethyl aminomethane; Normosol® = isotonic crystalloid solution (Na-140 meq/L, Cl-90 meq/L, K-5 meq/L, Mg-3 meq/L).

[a] Leukopore filtered red cells, <7 days old.

[b] <7 days old.

[c] Leukopore filtered red cells, <21 days old.

or emergency "packs" according to patient size. Priming volumes are determined by the surface area of the oxygenator membrane and range from approximately 350 mL in neonates to nearly 2.5 L in adults.

The ECMO specialist primes the fully assembled circuit as follows: first, the circuit is filled with carbon dioxide to eliminate nitrogen, which would lead to bubble formation after introduction of the saline priming solution; second, normal saline or Normosol® solution (Abbott Laboratories, Abbott Park, IL) is used to displace the carbon dioxide; third, the system is debubbled followed by the addition of 5% albumin to decrease adsorption of fibrinogen to the circuit components during the subsequent blood priming. Guidelines for blood product priming components, equipment, and operational characteristics of the ECMO circuit according to patient size are displayed in Tables 6 and 7.

XII. CANNULATION AND INITIAL STABILIZATION

Depending on the circumstances of hemodynamic decompensation (impending or actual cardiac arrest; nonoperated or postoperative cardiac patient) and surgeon preference, vascular access is obtained either by transthoracic approach with direct cannulation of the right atrium and aorta or peripherally through the neck or femoral vessels. The size (internal diameter and length) of the arterial and venous cannulae are chosen according to the size of the vascular structures, patient, and desired circuit flow rate. Table 8 shows guidelines for cannulae size with respect to patient weight.

Medical support and resuscitation (i.e., airway stabilization with hand ventilation, intravascular volume replacement, catecholamine infusions, correction of electrolyte imbalance, sodium bicarbonate administration, arrhythmia suppres-

Table 8 Guidelines for Cannula Size According to Patient Weight

Weight (kg)	Venous cannula I.D.	Arterial cannula I.D.
2–4	8–14	8–10
5–15	15–19	12–15
16–20	19–21	15–17
21–35	21–23	17–19
35–60	23	19–21
>60	23	21

I.D. = internal diameter (French scale).

sion, cardiac pacing, core temperature cooling, and cardiac massage, etc.) are continued throughout the cannulation procedure and commencement of veno-arterial extracorporeal support until a stable circulation is achieved. Prior to skin incision or chest exploration the patient is anesthetized (fentanyl infusion 5–20 μg/kg) and paralyzed (pancuronium 0.1–0.3 mg/kg or cisatracurium 0.2–0.4 mg/kg). Following cannulation, the patient is connected to the ECMO circuit and the roller pump dial is adjusted to gradually achieve the desired flow rates of 100–150 ml/kg depending on the underlying cardiopulmonary physiology. Intracardiac and arterial blood pressures including waveform characteristics are noted. Usually, inotropic infusions are weaned to maintain mean arterial blood pressure of >45 mmHg in neonates and >60–70 mmHg in children and adults. A chest x-ray is obtained to check cannulae and line position as well as endotracheal tube and lung parenchymal status.

Assessing the adequacy of flow soon after initiation of ECMO is of paramount importance. Answering a checklist of questions facilitates this assessment:

1. Is the ventricle adequately decompressed?
   a. If not, should one place a vent in the left atrium, augment ventricular ejection, or increase ECMO flow?
2. Is systemic perfusion adequate?
   a. Is there hypo- or (rarely) hypertension?
   b. What is the clinical appearance of the patient?
   c. Is acidosis clearing and lactate decreasing?
   d. Are any intracardiac shunts (e.g., aorto-pulmonary) adequately controlled?
   e. Are the cannulae appropriately sized and positioned?
3. Is hemostasis achieved?
   a. Is there surgical bleeding?
   b. Is there a coagulopathy?
   c. Is there a need for coagulation factors, antifibrinolytics, cell saver?

If the answers to questions 1, 2, and 3 are yes, then one can reasonably proceed with routine monitoring and maintenance. If a need for increased systemic perfusion is warranted but more flow cannot be achieved with the existing circuit and physiological conditions, then further analysis should be undertaken as outlined in Table 9. Note that actions taken during this period may entail assessment with echocardiography or reexploration of the mediastinum.

Venting the left atrium with a small left atrial cannula or transcatheter atrial septal defect creation in patients with two ventricles may lower left atrial pressures, decrease left ventricular wall stress and contractility, and minimize ongoing myocardial injury. Left atrial decompression also serves to limit the development of pulmonary edema and the length of time on ECMO.

Table 9 Assessment of Low Flow States During ECMO

Problem	Observations	Treatment options
Inadequate oxygen delivery and organ perfusion	Tachycardia, mottled skin, cool extremities, poor capillary refill, hypotension, oliguria, metabolic acidosis, hyperlactatemia, rising serum creatinine and liver function tests	Increase ECMO flow Increase native cardiac output
Attempts to increase ECMO flow fail: circuit chatters, bladder collapses, inadequate venous return or high post-membrane pressures	If atrial pressures are not extremely high or low consider:	
	1. Venous cannula malposition	1. Reposition venous cannula
	2. Venous cannula too small	2. Replace or add second venous cannula
	3. Venous thrombus formation	3. Surgical removal of thrombus or thrombolysis
	4. Excessive runoff through aorto-pulmonary shunt	4. Narrow shunt, embolize collaterals
	If atrial pressures unusually low consider:	
	5. Bleeding	5. Surgical exploration, administer coagulation factors and blood, antifibrinolytics, reduce heparin
	6. Severe vasodilation	6. Treat sepsis, administer vasoconstrictors
	If atrial pressures unusually high consider:	
	7. Tamponade	7. Surgical exploration, evacuation of blood and clot
	8. Left ventricular over distension	8. Place vent in left atrium, support ejection with catecholamine
	9. Aortic regurgitation	9. Reposition aortic cannula, asses need for aortic valve replacement
	If high membrane pressure, consider:	
	10. Arterial cannula malposition	10. Reposition cannula
	11. Arterial cannula too small	11. Replace or add second arterial cannula (bifemoral arterial cannulation)

Note: Atrial pressures measured with intracardiac catheters during ECMO are not a reliable measure of the functional status of the heart, especially when flow exceeds minimal support. Therefore, all of the observations and treatment options must also be considered independently from the measured atrial pressures.

Hypotension with mean arterial blood pressure of <30 mmHg in neonates or <50 mmHg in larger children and adults requires prompt evaluation and treatment. Colloid or blood products can be given empirically for volume expansion in the setting of low central venous pressure, continuous bleeding from chest drains (postcardiotomy patients), or other sites, especially if there is frequent pump shutdown triggered by bladder deflation. The latter suggests either hypovolemia or impaired venous return to the circuit. If increased circuit flow, fluid administration, bed height adjustment to optimize venous drainage, and cannula repositioning do not improve blood pressure, then inotropic infusions should be started or increased. Under these circumstances, plasma ultrafiltration should be suspended until hemodynamic variables are stabilized. With unexplained hypotension, a possible source of surgical or occult intracranial (neonates and infants) or intra-abdominal bleeding should be considered. A thorough evaluation for septicemia should be undertaken with the addition or modification of broad-spectrum antibiotics if abnormal findings on exam, complete blood count, urinalysis, or in the absence of other probable causes of sustained hypotension. Whole blood plasma exchange may be useful in treating severe cases of sepsis with profound coagulopathy and hemodynamic instability.

Immediately following cannulation, especially after the use of a rapid resuscitation circuit, hematocrit concentration, fibrinogen levels, and platelet count, are usually below acceptable values. Packed red blood cell transfusion (up to 20 cc/kg at a time) is given to maintain hematocrit of greater than 35%. Cryoprecipitate is given to keep serum fibrinogen >150 mg/dL, and concentrated platelet transfusions are given to maintain platelet count >100,000/mm^3. A delicate balance between the natural tendency for thrombogenesis and deliberate anticoagulation is required for proper circuit function while avoiding spontaneous and potentially catastrophic bleeding within the body. A heparin bolus (30 units/kg) is usually given at the authors' institution at the time of cannulation followed by infusion (20–30 units/kg/hr) adjusted to maintain activated clotting time of 180–200 seconds. A coagulation profile should be checked if there is persistent bleeding and abnormalities corrected by the replacement of clotting factors, platelets, red blood cells, and modification of heparin infusion rate to maintain activated clotting time of 160–180 seconds. In patients with active bleeding or significant risk factors for bleeding (see below), aminocaproic acid bolus (100 mg/kg) followed by infusion (30 mg/kg/hr) is started immediately after cannulation and is continued for up to approximately 72 hours following the initiation of ECMO or until nonsurgical bleeding ceases (22). Due to the potential for circuit thrombosis, the circuit is changed after approximately 120 hours during aminocaproic acid infusion or sooner if clots are found anywhere within the circuit. An alternative for persistent postcardiotomy bleeding may be aprotinin 30,000 IU/kg bolus and 10,000 IU/kg/hour for 6 hours.

Risk factors for bleeding complications on ECMO are as follows:

Post–cardiac surgery (<12 hours post-op)
Prematurity (gestational age < 37 weeks)
Preexisting intraventricular hemorrhage
Sepsis
Prolonged cardiopulmonary arrest (pH < 7.1)

Systemic hypertension following cannulation for ECMO is unusual unless patients with cardiac disease and good function are placed on ECMO for respiratory support. Generally hypertension is avoided to minimize risk of myocardial impairment imposed by increased afterload. Hypertension also drives excessive blood across a systemic-to-pulmonary artery shunt in patients with single ventricle physiology. This is generally deleterious and further volume loads the single ventricle. Avoidance of hypertension also helps to minimize arterial bleeding at suture sites in all patients following cardiac surgery and intracranial hemorrhage in neonates and infants. Control of hypertension is, therefore, extremely important and is achieved by controlling patient and circuit factors after ensuring adequate analgesia. ECMO flows can be reduced and modified ultrafiltration (Amicon filter) can be initiated if excessive volume is a contributing factor. Peripheral vasoconstriction resulting in elevated systemic vascular resistance can be manipulated with continuous nitroprusside, nitroglycerin, or intermittent doses of hydralazine, the latter two being less effective as antihypertensive agents than nitroprusside. Control of a hyperdynamic state can be addressed by weaning inotropes, providing adequate sedation and analgesia, and controlling fever or infection. Beta-blockade is also useful in controlling heart rate and hypercontractility due to a heightened adrenergic state. This occurs more commonly during ECMO for respiratory failure when myocardial performance is good. In our experience,

Table 10 Common Agents for Blood Pressure Control and Afterload Reduction

	Dose	Potential disadvantage(s)
Nitroprusside	0.5–5 μg/kg/min	Cyanide and thiocyanate toxicity, reflex tachycardia, tachyphylaxis
Esmolol	100–500 μg/kg bolus, 50–300 μg/kg/min	Myocardial depression, arrhythmia, bradycardia
Hydralazine	0.1–0.3 mg/kg q 4–6 hrs	Agranulocytosis, hypersensitivity, tachycardia
Milrinone	50 μg/kg bolus (20 min) 0.25–1.0 μg/kg/min	Hypotension
Labetolol	0.25–1 mg/kg/dose q 4 hrs 0.25–1.0 mg/kg/hr	Bronchospasm
Nitroglycerin	0.5–5 μg/kg/min	Tachycardia, tachyphylaxis

combination therapy using nitroprusside/esmolol or nitroprusside/milrinone has been effective in reducing afterload without associated excessive tachycardia. Common agents used for blood pressure control and afterload reduction are shown in Table 10. Notably, altered pharmacokinetics in fluid-overloaded ECMO-supported patients with a large volume of distribution and abnormal hepatic and/or renal function may require dosing modification to achieve the desired effect and avoid toxicity. In some instances, a larger initial or loading dose followed by a lower infusion rate is necessary.

XIII. DAILY MANAGEMENT ON ECMO

Successful daily management of a patient on ECMO or other forms of extracorporeal life support requires meticulous attention to patient care and technical factors by all members of the ECMO team.

A. Circuit Maintenance

Frequent inspection of the circuit with appropriate maintenance is performed during every shift. Alarms, pressure monitors, and integrity of the tubing and membrane are checked regularly. Continuous inspection for visible thrombi is important, especially if there are sudden changes in arterial blood gas values. Inability to eliminate carbon dioxide despite maximal sweep gas flow rate may necessitate replacement of the oxygenator. Elevated premembrane pressures (i.e., >350 mmHg) at normal flows without change in postmembrane pressure or evidence of blood-to-gas leak constitute membrane oxygenator dysfunction and may dictate oxygenator replacement. Extensive thrombus or consumptive coagulopathy with hypofribrinogenemia and thrombocytopenia constitute other indications for circuit replacement.

B. Hemodynamic Monitoring and Myocardial Conditioning

Hemodynamic variables including arterial and intracardiac pressures are monitored continuously in cardiac patients on ECMO. If the heart is ejecting, changes in pressure and waveform may provide important information about the adequacy of circulatory support and potential cardiac function. They often provide clues to changes in underlying heart rhythm, ventricular ejection, atrio-ventricular valve regurgitation, aortic regurgitation from arterial cannula malposition, inadequate venous cannula drainage, tamponade with impaired venous return and arterial flow, or development of intracardiac thrombus. When ECMO flow appears inadequate to meet the needs of the patient and limited venous drainage restricts additional flow, proper interpretation of arterial and atrial pressures may aid the formulation of a differential diagnosis (Table 9). Low flow states and/or significant hypotension require immediate analysis and intervention.

Following cannulation and resuscitation of vital organs, the need is often felt to run "full flow" and "rest" the heart. Decompressing an overdistended heart is likely to benefit the failing myocardium. However, the heart must eventually be retrained to accommodate a normal workload. For this reason inotropic support, although dramatically reduced after cannulation, is reintroduced earlier in cardiac patients compared to those on ECMO purely for respiratory support. Optimizing preload without overdistending the heart, establishing atrio-ventricular synchrony, and pharmacologically stimulating the heart to eject some blood, may have multiple merits, including:

1. Ventricular ejection facilitates decompression of the left heart, thereby avoiding the need in most cases for left atrial cannulation and venting.
2. By definition, total cardiopulmonary bypass excludes antegrade flow from entering the pulmonary circulation from the right heart. The bronchial circulation and alveolar ventilation will usually sustain the lung parenchyma, but there may be inadequate blood flow to the pulmonary vascular endothelium. Transient endothelial dysfunction is a common sequela of cardiopulmonary bypass, leading to elevated pulmonary vascular resistance and ventilation-perfusion abnormalities (23). Permitting or promoting the heart to eject some blood into the pulmonary circulation while on ECMO will oppose this effect and guard against pulmonary hypertension when ECMO is weaned off. However, pulmonary blood flow on ECMO necessitates adequate alveolar ventilation with oxygen so that pulmonary venous blood entering the left ventricle and ejected into the coronary circulation is not markedly desaturated.
3. Pulsatile flow contributed by the ejecting ventricle may contribute to more effective systemic perfusion as compared to nonpulsatile flow generated by the circuit alone.
4. Myocardial conditioning of the failing ventricle may be achieved by encouraging native cardiac output, especially after 24–48 hours of hemodynamic support. Gradual escalation of nonmechanical support during a graded reduction in ECMO flow during the final hours of ECMO may facilitate a timely separation from ECMO.
5. Risks of intracardiac thrombosis and thromboemboli may be reduced in ejecting versus nonejecting ventricles on ECMO.

Blood gas analysis including measurement of mixed venous O_2 saturation (sampled from the venous limb of the circuit in patients without atrial level mixing or indwelling SVC or IVC catheters) is used to assess the adequacy of the circulation on a given level of support. Serum lactate levels may be useful indicators for tissue oxygen delivery and perfusion in unstable patients on ECMO

(24,25). Transthoracic or transesophageal echocardiography is useful in assessing ventricular systolic function, right ventricular and pulmonary artery pressures, residual anatomical lesions, cannula position relative to intracardiac structures, and the presence of mediastinal or pericardial fluid collection that might preclude successful weaning or indicate the need for surgical or transcatheter intervention.

C. Fluid Retention and Management

Fluid retention is inevitable in cardiac patients on ECMO because of:

1. Endothelial dysfunction and capillary leak associated with reperfusion injury and inflammatory cascade activation after cardiopulmonary bypass and ECMO itself
2. Shifts in oncotic pressure from a large crystalloid burden and volume administration during priming
3. Renal dysfunction and decreased urine flow, which occur normally after cardiopulmonary bypass as a result of endocrine disturbances in antidiuretic hormone, renin-angiotensin, and atrial natriuretic factor production
4. Impaired renal function from low cardiac output, possibly nonpulsatile blood flow, and use of nephrotoxic drugs
5. Chronic renal insufficiency from long-standing cyanotic disease or acyanotic heart failure

Following cannulation, intravenous fluids are administered in the form of blood products plus maintenance dextrose in ½ normal saline. Diuretic therapy is started soon after cannulation in order to optimize fluid balance as soon as possible. Furosemide bolus (1 mg/kg) followed by continuous infusion (0.2–0.3 mg/kg/hr) is usually sufficient to induce diuresis and hourly urine output of 3–5 cc/kg/hr or more. Chlorothiazide (10 mg/kg per dose every 12 hours) is added if the response to furosemide is suboptimal. Careful surveillance and replacement of electrolytes is necessary with this diuretic regimen until contents of intravenous fluid and parenteral nutrition can be adjusted. Modified ultrafiltration using an Amicon filter (W.R. Grace and Co., Beverly, MA) is utilized in the setting of excessive fluid retention despite maximal diuretic therapy and circulatory support (26). Plasma is filtered continuously or intermittently with a goal to achieve slightly negative fluid balance over a 24-hour period depending on the size of the patient and the total body water overload. Ultrafiltration is discontinued after resolution of pulmonary and peripheral edema or if hourly urine output falls below 1 cc/kg or if blood urea nitrogen and creatinine rise precipitously. Suspension of ultrafiltration is advisable in the setting of low atrial pressures with hypotension and frequent circuit shutdown due to low volume or pressure sensing within the bladder, at least until hemodynamics stabilize. Daily laboratory investigation includes routine chemistries, liver and renal function tests, blood and coagulation analysis, and blood lactate levels.

D. Respiratory Support and Management

On venoarterial ECMO, native heart and lung function is completely or partially circumvented by the ECMO circuit depending on respiratory and circulatory needs of the patient. Normal gas exchange is achieved through manipulation of both the circuit and ventilator parameters. On full bypass, oxygen uptake and carbon dioxide elimination occur within the membrane oxygenator. Ventilating gas, consisting of oxygen alone or in combination with carbon dioxide, is delivered to the membrane at a constant rate (sweep gas flow in L/min) where oxygen diffuses into the blood and carbon dioxide is transferred from the blood to the efferent limb of the gas tubing. Unlike oxygen uptake and delivery to the tissues, carbon dioxide elimination is less dependent on blood flow through the circuit, but is highly dependent on the surface area of the membrane, the sweep gas flow rate, and the CO_2 content of the venous blood. In patients with minimal lung disease and some pulmonary blood flow resulting from native cardiac output, gas exchange occurs within the lungs as well as the membrane oxygenator. Excessive carbon dioxide elimination may result and is treated by adding carbon dioxide to the sweep gas or decreasing sweep gas flow rate. Optimal arterial blood gas values are as follows: pH, 7.35–7.45; P_aCO_2, 35–45 mmHg; P_aO_2, >60–100 mmHg.

Following cannulation, ventilator settings are adjusted primarily according to lung compliance, which may reflect the degree of preexisting cardiac-related or new-onset lung disease. Tidal volumes of 7–9 mL/kg with peak inspiratory pressures not exceeding 25–28 cmH_2O and FiO_2 of 0.3–0.4 are usually maintained in patients with normal lung compliance. However, lung parenchymal abnormalities resulting from pneumonia, pulmonary edema, pulmonary hemorrhage, or acute respiratory distress syndrome require increased airway pressures to maintain alveolar recruitment and pulmonary venous oxygenation. Changes in ventilator settings are infrequent and are guided by physical examination and the appearance of the lung fields on daily chest radiographs. Likewise, endotracheal tube and cannulae positions are assessed daily by chest radiograph or when sudden changes in lung compliance or ECMO flow are encountered provided the patient can tolerate the procedure. To assist with the maintenance of pulmonary toilet as well as to minimize the risk of secondary pulmonary infection, intermittent endotracheal tube suctioning is conducted while on ECMO depending on the presence or severity of underlying lung disease.

E. Neurological Surveillance

Neurological assessment, although difficult in patients on ECMO, must be regularly and carefully performed. Physical examination, including pupillary response to light, spontaneous movements, and purposeful movements to tactile or auditory stimuli, is performed frequently. A high index of suspicion for seizure activity is maintained in paralyzed patients with abrupt changes in heart rate, blood pressure, skin perfusion, and pupillary size. Concerning findings are promptly evaluated by cranial ultrasound or head CT scan, as evidence of irreversible injury including massive hemorrhage, will dictate discontinuing further ECMO therapy. In patients with an open fontanel, cranial ultrasonography is routinely performed prior to or immediately following cannulation when possible to evaluate for new intracranial hemorrhage or extension of previously known lesions. Follow-up studies are obtained after 24 hours and then every 48 hours while on ECMO. Electroencephalography is performed to diagnose seizures and assess background cerebral cortical activity, which may impact the decision ultimately leading to discontinuing ECMO support.

F. Sedation, Analgesia, and Muscle Relaxation

Continuous sedation and analgesia is maintained with fentanyl (3–10 μg/kg/hr) or morphine sulfate (0.05–0.15 mg/kg/hr) and midazolam (0.05–0.1 mg/kg/hr) infusions with intermittent doses for agitation and painful procedures or unexplained hypertension. Long-term fentanyl infusion is less commonly used by some groups as drug levels vary widely and unpredictably, or tolerance may develop (27,28). Others have shown good analgesia with relatively low doses of fentanyl (29). Additional agents used for analgesia include lidocaine (2 mg/kg via the tracheal tube) prior to tracheal tube suctioning and ketamine (1–2 mg/kg/dose) for some painful procedures. Propofol may be useful as an anesthetic for procedures or for short periods of adjunctive analgesia or hypnosis but is generally avoided for prolonged (days) treatment as the primary sedative. Muscle relaxation is advisable in unstable patients on mechanical support but can be used intermittently as needed when the patient stabilizes. Pancuronium (0.1 mg/kg/dose) is effective, but undesired tachycardia or propensity for other arrhythmias may preclude its use. Cis-atracurium (infused at 0.2–0.4 mg/kg/hr) is more expensive but boasts a safe hemodynamic profile and offers considerable advantage in patients with hepatic and renal dysfunction since it is metabolized by Hoffman degradation. When possible, the use of muscle relaxants is minimized to allow restrained spontaneous movement for frequent neurological assessment.

G. Nutritional Support

Parenteral nutritional support is often initiated within 24–48 hours after cannulation. Daily protein, carbohydrate, and lipid intake is adjusted according to the nutritional needs of the individual patient. Lipid intake should not exceed 1 g/kg/day to prevent accumulation and embolism within the circuit. Baseline measurements of serum electrolytes, blood urea nitrogen and creatinine, and indicators of hepatic synthetic function are performed prior to starting parenteral nutrition and with significant changes in nutritional intake.

H. Prevention and Management of Infection

Patients receiving mechanical support are at high risk for nosocomial infection, especially from skin flora with a direct portal of entry through catheters, chest sites, and open or closed sternotomy wounds. Likewise, indwelling urinary catheters and tracheal tubes can lead to local infection followed by bacteremia in these potentially immunocompromised hosts. Recommended antibiotics at our institution while on ECMO for respiratory failure (including pneumonia) are: ampicillin (100 mg/kg/day every 6 hours; if <7 days of age, then 50–100 mg/kg/day every 12 hours); oxacillin (150–200 mg/kg/day every 4 hours; if <7 days of age, then 100 mg/kg/day every 12 hours); cefotaxime (150 mg/kg/day every 8 hours; if <7 days of age, then 100 mg/kg/day every 12 hours). Cardiac patients on ECMO for hemodynamic support have fewer ''routine'' indications for prophylactic broad-spectrum antibiotic use. Commonly, cefazolin, used routinely in the perioperative patient, is continued while the child is on ECMO. Postoperative cardiac patients who suffer cardiac arrest and are resuscitated and cannulated through an open chest may be at greater risk for mediastinitis with associated high mortality. Therefore, a second- or third-generation cephalosporin in combination with a course of vancomycin or oxacillin is used in these patients. Patients with unexplained hemodyamic instability, coagulopathy, and elevated white blood cell count or fever are aggressively treated for septicemia, which may require replacement of the circuit itself.

XIV. WEANING AND DECANNULATING FROM ECMO

A. Individualized Weaning Protocols

Given the high risk of complications and substantial mortality in cardiac patients associated with the duration of mechanical circulatory support beyond 1 week, consideration as to when and how to wean cardiac patients from ECMO should begin soon after cannulation once circulatory stability has been established. The disease process and circumstances resulting in hemodynamic failure or cardiac arrest may influence the expected duration of mechanical support. For example, patients who fail to separate from cardiopulmonary bypass after cardiac surgery due to severe pulmonary hypertension usually respond to a period of 24–48 hours on ECMO with inhaled NO therapy and inotropic support of the right heart. Similarly, patients who suffer cardiac arrest after cardiac surgery may have residual or newly discovered repairable defects that allow rapid weaning and decannulation soon after reoperation. ECMO instituted for catheter intervention or arrhythmia ablation procedures may be discontinued within hours of patient cannulation. In contrast, patients with severe cardiomyopathies or those awaiting heart transplantation may require mechanical assistance for days or weeks. Patients with severe bronchiolitis due to respiratory syncytial virus complicating repair of congenital heart disease on cardiopulmonary bypass typically require 2–3 weeks of ECMO support for respiratory failure. Still, return of stable cardiopulmonary function must be carefully evaluated as the criteria necessary for successful weaning from ECMO are multifactorial and require understanding of the underlying disease-specific cardiac physiology. The likelihood of recovery of ventricular function should be decided within the first 48–72 hours so that cardiac transplantation status can be ascertained.

B. Weaning for Respiratory Failure

Prior experience in the management of neonates with structurally normal hearts who require ECMO support for respiratory failure has shaped our parameters for gas exchange required for decannulation. In such cases, the ability to wean is dependent on resolution of the primary pulmonary process with little need for support of the myocardium beyond moderate inotropic support, fluid and electrolyte management, and nutritional support. Once lung compliance and gas exchange have normalized, marked improvement of the lungs on chest radiograph is apparent, and a stable circulation with sufficient negative fluid balance has been achieved, the patient is sedated, paralyzed, and fully ventilated and the ECMO circuit clamped. Blood continues to flow through the circuit via a bridge of tubing. Arterial blood gases are sampled at 15 and 90 minutes. At the Children's Hospital, Boston, criteria for decannulation of patients without heart disease on ECMO for neonatal respiratory failure include: stable hemodynamics; $P_aO_2 > 60$ mmHg and $P_aCO_2 < 45$ mmHg with pH > 7.35 and < 7.50 on an FiO_2 of 0.35; ventilator set to peak inspiratory pressure $= 30$ mmHg, positive end-expiratory pressure $= 5$ mmHg, and ventilator rate $= 25$ breaths/min for 2 hours.

C. Weaning for Cardiac Failure

Patients requiring cardiovascular support with ECMO are partially weaned within the first 48 hours in order to assess myocardial function by echocardiography and hemodynamic evaluation. This provides prognostic information, assists in planning the method and timing of subsequent weaning attempts and trials off ECMO, and may prompt a discussion with the family about transplantation considerations. ECMO flow may be partially or fully reinstituted after this evaluation.

Table 11 Expected P_aO_2 During Successful Weaning from ECMO in Selected Cardiac Diseases

Examples of cardiac disease	Typical reasons for ECMO	Acceptable P_aO_2 (during weaning)
Acquired heart disease		
Cardiomyopathy (chronic)	Biventricular failure	>60 mmHg
Cardiomyopathy (acute)	Hypotension	
	Intractable arrhythmias	
Heart transplant	Graft dysfunction	
Kawasaki disease	Myocardial infarction from giant aneurysms	
Repaired congenital heart disease		
TGA s/p arterial switch	Coronary ischemia with right or left heart failure	>60 mmHg
	Unprepared LV in infants	
ALCAPA	Myocardial infarction	
	LV failure, MR	
TAPVR	Pulmonary hypertension	
	Small left heart	
TOF	Right heart failure	>45 mmHg (if R → L intracardiac shunt)
	Pulmonary hemorrhage after angioplasty	
Truncus arteriosus	Pulmonary hypertension	
Palliated single-ventricle physiology		
S/P systemic-to-pulmonary artery shunt		
HLHS	Ventricular dysfunction and excessive pulmonary blood flow	~30–40 mmHg

Tricuspid atresia/PS	Decreased PBF, Hypoxia	
Pulmonary atresia/IVS	Intractable arrhythmia (VF)	
S/P shunt or PA band		
Other single ventricle	RSV, sepsis, unexplained hypotension	
S/P bidirectional Glenn shunt		
Single ventricle	Decreased PBF, Hypoxia	>30–50 mmHg
	Ventricular failure	
	Pneumonia	
S/P Fontan procedure (fenestrated)		
Single ventricle	Ventricular dysfunction (pretransplant)	>45–50 mmHg
	Arrhythmia	
Unrepaired congenital heart disease		
TGA	Hypoxia, acidosis, PPHN s/p BAS	>30 mmHg
TOF/PA/APCs	Pneumonia/sepsis	>40 mmHg
Neonatal Ebstein's anomaly	Bridge to surgery	>40 mmHg
	Catheter ablation of arrhythmia	
TAPVR (obstructed)	Unrecognized congenital heart disease	>45 mmHg

TGA = Transposition of the great arteries; ALCAPA = anomalous left coronary artery from the pulmonary artery; TOF = tetralogy of Fallot; TAPVR = total anomalous pulmonary venous return; HLHS = hypoplastic left heart syndrome; IVS = intact ventricular septum; VF = ventricular fibrillation; RSV = respiratory syncitial virus; PBF = pulmonary blood flow; PA = pulmonary valve atresia; PPHN = persistent pulmonary hypertension of the newborn; BAS = balloon atrial septostomy; APCs = aortopulmonary collaterals.

Compared to respiratory failure patients, basic differences in underlying cardiac anatomy and physiology dictate the important weaning variables and indicators of cardiac function while gradually weaning from full cardiopulmonary support. For example, an acceptable P_aO_2 obtained while the ECMO circuit is clamped will vary substantially according to the underlying anatomy and pathophysiology (Table 11).

If transthoracic cannulation was used and problems with bleeding were encountered during the ECMO run, the mediastinum may require exploration for removal of thrombi, gel foam packing, and other debris prior to or during the weaning process. If only a short reconditioning period is anticipated, the patient is frequently sedated and paralyzed, dopamine infusion is increased to 5–10 μg/kg/min, intravascular volume status is optimized, and ventilator settings are adjusted according to lung compliance and expected arterial O_2 saturation. ECMO flow is decreased by 25–50% over a period of several hours until the circuit is clamped. The clinical evaluation used to wean and separate cardiac patients from ECMO includes:

1. Physical examination (skin perfusion, peripheral edema, direct mediastinal observations)
2. Mean arterial blood pressure, pulse pressure and waveform, intracardiac pressures, assessment of intravascular volume and inotropic need
3. Electrocardiogram (i.e., rhythm, strain pattern, ST-T wave changes)
4. Lung compliance and gas exchange; radiographic appearance of the lungs (pulmonary edema, atelectasis, pneumothorax, etc.)
5. Estimate of pulmonary vascular resistance and performance of the right heart and pulmonary circulation
6. Echocardiographic assessment of ventricular systolic function, valvar function, systemic and pulmonary outflow obstruction, and location and direction of intracardiac shunts (This often occurs after the designated period of myocardial conditioning and just as the reduced flow is stopped when the cannulae are clamped.)
7. pH, P_aO_2, P_aCO_2, and end-tidal CO_2
8. Serum lactate levels, systemic (mixed) venous saturation

The cardiac surgeon performs decannulation only if the patient has maintained stable hemodynamics and acceptable gas exchange for a period of 1–2 hours without contribution from the circuit. Cardiac output should be optimally supported just before and during this time (Table 4). Mechanical support is resumed if the patient is marginal during this time with continued conditioning, partial ECMO support, and repeat attempts within 24 hours. Further testing may be indicated (i.e., diagnostic or interventional catheterization), depending on the reasons for failure.

XV. SPECIAL CONSIDERATIONS

The management of patients after Norwood palliation for hypoplastic left heart syndrome (HLHS) can be especially challenging. Blood is ejected from the single right ventricle through the reconstructed outflow tract (Stansel anastomosis) and is directed to the upper body via the brachiocephalic vessels and the lower body through the reconstructed aortic arch. In a parallel fashion, blood flow to the lungs is supplied from the aorta through a surgically created Blalock-Taussig shunt between the inominate or right subclavian artery and the right pulmonary artery. Thus, blood flows to the body and lungs in parallel with the total cardiac output (Q_T) resulting from the sum of systemic blood flow (Q_S) plus pulmonary blood flow (Q_P). Due to complete mixing of systemic and pulmonary venous blood, the arterial oxygen saturation is ~80% when Q_P and Q_S are equal and pulmonary vein saturation and systemic cardiac output are normal. Importantly, the ratio of pulmonary flow to systemic flow (Q_P/Q_S) is determined by the driving pressure across the shunt and the relative resistances of the systemic and pulmonary circuits. Given that the resistance of blood vessels in the lung is normally only a fraction (~10%) of the systemic vascular resistance, Q_P/Q_S typically exceeds 1 (0.5–>4), with the primary restriction to pulmonary blood flow offered by the 3.5 mm shunt.

Inadequate systemic blood flow and secondary end organ injury may result from impaired right ventricular function in the setting of ventricular volume loading due to excessive run-off of blood into the lungs or other perioperative myocardial insults in patients undergoing a Norwood operation. On ECMO, circuit flows up to 150 mL/kg/min or more are usually necessary to maintain adequate systemic perfusion while accounting for run-off into the pulmonary circulation through the shunt. Although partial temporary narrowing of the shunt may be advisable in some circumstances, it is unwise to completely occlude the only source of pulmonary blood flow to the pulmonary endothelium. Anecdotal reports of lung infarction after clipping the modified Blalock-Taussig shunt while on ECMO have emerged and are consistent with predictions based on other studies. On full cardiopulmonary support, target indicators of systemic perfusion are no different than other mechanically supported patients. It is possible to bypass the membrane oxygenator in Norwood patients without lung disease if higher flows are maintained and the shunt is patent. This maneuver simplifies the circuit and may permit less use of heparin. ECMO thus effectively becomes a ventricular assist device.

Weaning and decannulation criteria also require modification in patients with single-ventricle physiology. P_aO_2 should range from 35 to 45 mmHg on an FiO_2 of 0.3 with a clear chest radiograph and low inotropic requirement. P_aO_2 in the range of 50 mmHg or higher with marginal hemodynamics suggests excessive pulmonary blood flow, which may preclude discontinuing ECMO. In this case, resizing the shunt to restrict pulmonary blood flow and allow successful weaning and decannulation.

Patients with single-ventricle physiology and complex venous anatomy related either to abnormal visceral situs or multiple prior catheterizations, etc., need forethought and understanding as to the patency of large vessels prior to ECMO cannulation. In addition, the size of the patient and sites of available unoccluded vessels as well as physiological requirements for effective cardiopulmonary bypass might influence the number of venous cannulae used. Patients with a superior cavopulmonary anastomosis (bidirectional Glenn shunt) as the primary source of pulmonary blood flow require separate venous drainage of the SVC and IVC unless congenital interruption of the infrahepatic IVC with drainage of lower body blood to the azygous vein exists. In the latter case a single venous cannula in the SVC might be sufficient. To complicate matters further in patients with a bidirectional Glenn shunt is the potentially reduced drainage of venous blood from the brain by cannula placement in the SVC. This may lead to diminished cerebral perfusion and CNS injury—a scenario that concerns all patients with single-ventricle anatomy and Glenn or even Fontan physiology. Additional considerations pertaining to ECMO support of patients with single ventricle disease and arterial blood gas parameters during weaning are included in Table 11.

XVI. VENTRICULAR ASSIST DEVICES IN THE ICU

Mechanical assist devices most commonly employed in the intensive care unit are not limited to ECMO but include ventricular assist devices (VAD). Utilization of VAD for pediatric patients varies among centers but has gained a definite niche for certain applications. Practically speaking, however, their use is limited compared to the experience in adults because of size disparities between young patients and implantable or easily portable devices. The most conventional VAD is the external centrifugal-type pump, which has a set of rotating cones that impart kinetic energy to the circulating blood. A VAD may be used to support either ventricle. VAD support of the left ventricle (LVAD) requires cannulae to be inserted in the left atrium (usually through the atrial appendage), with the arterial return from the VAD into the ascending aorta or femoral artery. Adequate function of the right ventricle is crucial for successful use of LVAD; the right ventricle must be able to support a full cardiac output into the lungs in order for there to be adequate left atrial filling/pulmonary venous return to the pump without causing cavitation and air embolus. Continuous monitoring of right and left atrial filling pressures is necessary. A low left atrial pressure in the face of a rising right atrial pressure is indicative of right heart failure; low left atrial pressure with a low right atrial pressure may signify hypovolemia. Similarly, VAD support of the

Table 12 Comparison of Mechanical Support Technology in the ICU

VAD—Advantages over ECMO	
	Simplicity of circuit
	Less anticoagulation
	Less blood trauma at low flow rates
	Less priming volume
	Better unloading of ventricle
	Possibly implantable
	Possibly pulsatile
ECMO—Advantages over VAD	
	Biventricular support
	Blood flow support during lethal arrhythmias
	Support gas exchange
	Servoregulation less affected by afterload
	Substantial experience in newborns
	In-hospital respiratory therapists dually trained

right ventricle (RVAD) requires right atrial cannulation with RVAD return to the pulmonary artery, and left ventricular function must be adequate for RVAD to be effective. Biventricular assist using two separate VAD may be technically feasible in larger pediatric patients but is significantly more complicated if there are dynamic changes in hemodynamics. Compared to ECMO, VAD requires less anticoagulation but is unable to overcome coexisting pulmonary disease. Hospital survival may exceed 40%. Use of VAD is now usually confined to patients with isolated left ventricular dysfunction (ALCAPA) or single ventricle lesions. At the current time more than 90% of devices to support the circulation in pediatric ICUs involve ECMO. Comparative features of VAD and ECMO in the ICU are shown in Table 12.

XVII. CONCLUSION

Extracorporeal cardiorespiratory support is a complex, labor-intensive tool that is life-saving in the ICU. Few areas in medicine and surgery require more integrated, multidisciplinary support. Virtually every healthcare worker can contribute positively to this evolving technology where continued improvements will be needed to achieve the success that has been realized elsewhere in pediatric cardiovascular critical care.

REFERENCES

1. Bartlett RH, Roloff DW, Custer JR, Younger JG, Hirschl RB. Extracorporeal life support. The University of Michigan experience. JAMA 2000; 283:904–908.
2. Delius RE, Bove EL, Meliones JN. Use of extracorporeal life support in patients with congenital heart disease. Crit Care Med 1992; 20:1216–1222.
3. Marx M, Salzer-Muhar U, Wimmer M. Extracorporeal life support in pediatric patients with heart failure. Artif Organs 1999; 23:1001–1005.
4. Moler FW, Custer JR, Bartlett RH, Palmisano JM, Akingbola O, Taylor RP, Maxvold N. Extracorporeal life support for severe pediatric respiratory failure: an updated experience 1991–1993. J. Pediatr 1994; 124:875–880.
5. Revenis ME, Glass P, Short BL. Mortality and morbidity rates among lower birth weight infants (2000 to 2500 grams) treated with extracorporeal membrane oxygenation. J Pediatr 1992; 121:452–458.
6. Moler FW, Palmisano JM, Custer JR, Meliones JN, Bartlett RH. Alveolar-arterial oxygen gradients before extracorporeal life support for severe pediatric respiratory failure: Improved outcome for extracorporeal life support-managed patients? Crit Care Med 1994; 22:620–625.
7. Meyer DM, Jessen ME, Results of extracorporeal membrane oxygenation in neonates with sepsis: the extracorporeal life support organization experience. J Thorac Cardiovasc Surg 1995; 109:419–427.
8. UK collaborative ECMO Trial Group. UK collaborative randomised trial of neonatal extracorporeal membrane oxygenation. Lancet 1996; 348:75–82.
9. Lai WW, Lipshultz SE, Easley KA, Starc TJ, Drant SE, Bricker T, Colan SD, Moodie DS, Sopko G, Kaplan S. Prevalence of congenital cardiovascular malformations in children of human immunodeficiency virus-infected women. The prospective P2C2 HIV multicenter study. J Am Coll Cardiol 1998; 32:1749–1955.
10. Kanto WP Jr. A decade of experience with neonatal extracorporeal membrane oxygenation. J Pediatr 1994; 124:335–347.
11. Kulik TJ, Moler FW, Palmisano JM, Custer JR, Mosca RS, Bove EL, Bartlett RH. Outcome-associated factors in pediatric patients treated with extracorporeal membrane oxygenator after cardiac surgery. Circulation 1996; 94:II63–II68.
12. Dalton HJ, Siewers RD, Fuhrman BP, Del Nido PJ, Thompson AE, Shaver MG, Dowhy M. Extracorporeal membrane oxygenation for cardiac rescue in children with severe myocardial dysfunction. Crit Care Med 1993; 21:1020–1028.
13. Duncan BW, Ibrahim AE, Hraska V, Del Nido PJ, Laussen PC, Wessel DL, Mayer JE, Bower LK, Jonas RA. Use of rapid-deployment extracorporeal membrane oxygenation for the resuscitation of pediatric patients with heart disease after cardiac arrest. J Thorac Cardiovasc Surg 1998; 116:305–311.
14. Lee KJ, McCrindle BW, Bohn DJ, Wilson GJ, Taylor GP, Freedom RM, Smallhorn JF, Benson LN. Clinical outcomes of acute myocarditis in childhood. Heart 1999; 82:226–233.
15. Ibrahim AE, Duncan BW, Blume ED, Jonas RA. Long-term follow-up of pediatric cardiac patients requiring mechanical circulatory support. Ann Thorac Surg 2000; 69:186–192.

16. Duncan BW, Hraska V, Jonas RA, Wessel DL, Del Nido PJ, Laussen PC, Lapierre RA, Wilson JM. Mechanical circulatory support in children with cardiac disease. J Thorac Cardiovasc Surg 1999; 117:529–542.
17. Langley SM, Sheppard SV, Tsang VT, Monro JL, Lamb RK. When is extracorporeal life support wothwhile following repair of congenital heart disease in children? Eur J Cardiothorac Surg 1998; 13:520–525.
18. Wernovsky G, Chang AC, Wessel DL. Intensive care. In: Emmanouilides GC, Riemenschneider TA, Allen HD, Gutgesell HP eds. Heart Disease in Infants, Children, and Adolescents—Including the Fetus and Young Adult. Baltimore: Williams and Wilkins, 2000, pp 398–439.
19. Chang AC, Hanley FL, Wernovsky G, Wessel DL. Pediatric Cardiac Intensive Care. Baltimore: Williams & Wilkins, 1998.
20. Wernovsky G, Wypij D, Jonas RA, Mayer JE, Hanley FL, Hickey PR, Walsh AZ, Chang AC, Castaneda AR, Newburger JW, Wessel DL. Postoperative course and hemodynamic profile after the arterial switch operation in neonates and infants: a comparison of low-flow cardiopulmonary bypass versus circulatory arrest. Circulation 1995; 92:2226–2235.
21. Goldman AP, Delius RE, Deanfield JE, De Leval MR, Sigston PE, Macrae DJ: Nitric oxide might reduce the need for extracorporeal support in children with critical postoperative pulmonary hypertension. Ann Thorac Surg 1996; 62:750–755.
22. Wilson JM, Bower LK, Fackler JC, Beals DA, Bergus BO, Kevy SV: Aminocaproic acid decreases the incidence of intracranial hemorrhage and other hemorrhagic complications of ECMO. J Pediatr Surg 1993; 28:536–541.
23. Wessel DL, Adatia I, Giglia TM, Thompson JE, Kulik TJ. Use of inhaled nitric oxide and acetylcholine in the evaluation of pulmonary hypertension and endothelial function after cardiopulmonary bypass. Circulation 1993; 88:2128–2138.
24. Munoz R, Laussen PC, Palacio G, Zienko L, Piercey G, Wessel DL. Changes in whole blood lactate levels during cardiopulmonary bypass for surgery for congenital cardiac disease: an early indicator of moridity and mortality. J Thorac Cardiovasc Surg 2000; 119:155–162.
25. Cheung P-Y, Robertson CMT, Finer NN. Plasma lactate as a predictor of early childhood neurodevelopmental outcome of neonates with severe hypoxaemia requiring extracorporeal membrane oxygenation. Arch Dis Child 1996; 74:F47–F50.
26. Friesen RH, Tornabene MA, Coleman SB. Blood conservation during pediatric cardiac surgery: Ultrafiltration of the extracorporeal circuit volume after cardiopulmonary bypass. Anesth Analg 1993; 77:702–707.
27. Arnold JH, Truog RD, Orav EJ, Scavone JM, Hershenson MB. Tolerance and dependence in neonates sedated with fentanyl during extracorporeal membrane oxygenation. Anesthesia 1990; 73:1136–1140.
28. Arnold JH, Truog RD, Scavone JM, Fenton T. Changes in the pharmacodynamic response to fentanyl in neonates during continuous infusion. J Pediatr 1991; 119: 639–643.
29. Leuschen MP, Willett LD, Hoie EB, Bolam DL, Bussey ME, Goodrich PD, Zach TL, Nelson RM. Plasma fentanyl levels in infants undergoing extracorporeal membrane oxygenation. J Thorac Cardiovasc Surg 1993; 105:885–891.

6

Nursing Management for Children with Cardiac Disease on Mechanical Circulatory Support

Paula J. Moynihan, Dorothy M. Beke, Kim Reiser, and Patricia A. Hickey
Children's Hospital, Boston, Massachusetts

Infants and children with complex congenital heart defects undergoing surgical repair or those with acquired heart disease (i.e., cardiomyopathy) are at risk for developing cardiopulmonary failure that does not respond to maximum conventional therapy (1). Other infants and children at risk for cardiopulmonary failure include those that fail conventional resuscitation techniques during an arrest and those awaiting a heart, lung, or heart-lung transplant. A means to provide gas exchange and biventricular support is essential to achieve optimal, quality outcomes for these patients.

Although mechanical support of the failing circulation may be provided by a variety of devices in the adult population, options for infants and children are limited (2). Adult modalities available include intra-aortic balloon pump counterpulsation, ventricular assist devices, and noninvasive external devices.

The intra-aortic balloon pump augments aortic diastolic flow to increase coronary flow and decrease left ventricular afterload. It is difficult to use in the pediatric population because of problems with femoral artery access, the size of the catheter, synchronous timing with faster pediatric heart rates, and failure to support the right ventricle (1).

Ventricular assist devices provide cardiac support only. The percentage of cardiac output supported by the pump depends on the degree of ventricular dysfunction and is adjusted as needed. These devices have been applied to the adult population and are effective in the adult-sized adolescent, but the variation of cannula size and ability to achieve the desired cardiac output, as well as problems in placing the device, have limited their pediatric use (1).

Noninvasive external devices such as military antishock pants support venous return to the right ventricle by compressing the abdomen. Their advantage is easy application, but disadvantages include respiratory compromise from diaphragmatic compression, mesenteric and renal artery compromise, and blockage of venous access below the device (2).

During the 1980s, extracorporeal membrane oxygenation (ECMO) emerged. This therapy was adapted from intraoperative cardiopulmonary bypass and used in the management of infants and children with respiratory failure. It is now considered standard rescue therapy for this patient population. ECMO provides full respiratory support, and, more importantly for the cardiac patient, it can provide significant hemodynamic support when needed (3).

This chapter discusses ECMO as a viable alternative treatment for infants and children requiring cardiopulmonary support beyond traditional methods. It begins with the preparation and implementation of an ECMO program for cardiac infants and concludes with an in-depth discussion of specialized cardiac patient care issues for those who require this alternative mode of hemodynamic support.

I. EXTRACORPOREAL MEMBRANE OXYGENATION

No specific inclusion or exclusion criteria have been defined for cardiac patients requiring ECMO. Some indications include severe ventricular failure, pulmonary hypertension, and respiratory failure refractory to maximum cardiovascular pharmacological support and mechanical ventilation. Patients fall into three broad groups (4):

1. Failure to wean from cardiopulmonary bypass following surgical repair
2. Severe cardiorespiratory failure in the CICU following surgical repair
3. Myocarditis or cardiomyopathy with severe ventricular failure

Table 1 provides a listing of cardiac patients by diagnosis and age treated with ECMO at Children's Hospital, Boston, during 1998.

There are two options when providing ECMO support: veno-arterial (VA) and veno-venous (VV). VA ECMO (which will be the focus of this chapter) provides cardiac and pulmonary support, while VV ECMO provides pulmonary support (4). (For other comparisons see Table 2). VA ECMO for cardiac support of pediatric patients is increasing as one of the few mechanical devices for smaller patients. However, problems are associated with this device, including variations in the site of cannulation, possible requirements for left ventricular venting, he-

Table 1 Cardiac ECMO Patients, 1998

Patient and Month	Weight (kg)	Diagnosis	Cannula site
Patient #1, 1/98	67	Endocarditis	Chest
Patient #2, 1/98	37	Pretransplant	Chest
Patient #3, 2/98	6.3	VSD/Arrest	Neck
Patient #4, 2/98	14	Stage II/Arrest	Chest
Patient #5, 3/98	3.6	CAVC/Arrest	Neck
Patient #6, 5/98	2.5	HLHS/Arrest	Neck
Patient #7, 5/98	66	Fontan	Chest
Patient #8, 5/98	3.1	DILV	Neck
Patient #9, 6/98	40	TGA, s/p switch	Neck
Patient #10, 6/98	2.5	TOF	Neck
Patient #11, 9/98	2.3	CAVC	Neck
Patient #12, 9/98	2.5	Ebstein's anomaly	Chest
Patient #13, 9/98	15	Cardiomyopathy, s/p transplant	Chest
Patient #14, 9/98	18	AP window, arrest	Neck
Patient #15, 10/98	2.5	Ebstein's anomaly	Chest
Patient #16, 10/98	80	PPA stenosis	Chest
Patient #17, 11/98	15	Dextrocardia, s/p senning	Neck
Patient #18, 12/98	2.3	Ebstein's anomaly	Neck
Patient #19, 12/98	10	Heterotaxy, s/p transplant	Neck
Patient #20, 12/98	6.5	PS, s/p conduit change	Neck

Source: Data obtained from Children's Hospital ECMO Committee.

mostasis and coagulation defects, requirements for ultrafiltration, and difficulties in evaluating cardiac function (2).

The use of this highly technical, mechanical support as a cardiac assist in pediatric cardiac patients requires institutional support and the development of a comprehensive multidisciplinary program. As a resource, ECMO is labor intensive and expensive.

II. PREPARATION AND IMPLEMENTATION

Before an ECMO program can be implemented, many considerations require evaluation and planning. Its initiation in any hospital, or in various critical care units within one hospital, necessitates commitment at all levels of administration and practice (6), specialized equipment and supplies, carefully designed clinical protocols, training of personnel, and a well-defined follow-up program (see Chapter 11).

Table 2 Comparisons of VA and VV ECMO

VA ECMO	
	Provides cardiac and pulmonary support
	Decompresses the pulmonary vascular bed
	Carotid artery is used
	Potential lethality of emboli
	Coronary artery blood flow is derived from the LV ($<\mathrm{Pao}_2$)
VV ECMO	
	Provides only pulmonary support—does not support cardiac function
	Normal pulmonary circulation is maintained
	Can still assess PA pressures—cannot use thermodilution cardiac output
	Provides higher Svo_2 saturations to the PV bed, so it may help decrease PVR and heal the lung
	May require a 20% increase in flow to compensate for ''pump recirculation''
	Requires standard ventricular management
	Selective perfusion is not a problem—myocardial circulation is maintained
	Normal pulsatile pulse contour is maintained
	Carotid artery is spared
	May develop problems with the femoral vein related to chronic venous insufficiency/edema
	Longer cannulation time (two sites)
	Less concern over emboli-returning blood to the venous system

Source: Ref. 31.

Assuming institution support, preparation of the staff and a setting where ECMO is to be performed requires a program-based, multidisciplinary work group (see Table 3). The goals of this work group are to assure:

Smooth implementation
Infection safe environment
Standardization of equipment and protocols
Comprehensive training program for all team members
Process of measuring quality outcomes

Table 3 Membership of the Cardiac ECMO Work Group

Cardiovascular surgeon	CICU medical director
Cardiologist	CV nursing (ICU & OR)
ECMO tech	Anesthesia
Blood bank	Clinical laboratories
Neurologist	Infection control
Biomedical engineering	

Table 4 Dimensions of Care Class Content

I. The ECMO circuit
II. Precannulation management
III. Cannulation/Decannulation: preparation and procedure
IV. Managing patient analgesia and sedation
V. Nursing management of the patient on ECMO
VI. Cycling/Decannulation/Post-ECMO stabilization

A. Orientation Program

Successful implementation of an ECMO program requires a comprehensive education program. In designing this program, all dimensions of care must be included (see Table 4 for class contents). Additionally, the development of a multidisciplinary clinical practice guideline will contribute to a smooth and unified approach.

B. Equipment

A consensus must be reached to standardize all equipment including cannulae and contents of instrument trays and carts. Appendixes A–D contain detailed lists of equipment as organized and utilized at Children's Hospital, Boston. Devoted space for equipment and supplies is a necessity. Orderly storage of the cannulae is best accomplished by using a mobile cart that may be easily wheeled to the bedside (Fig. 1). Maintaining a par level of cannulae may be achieved by assistive staff, trained and familiar with the cart's contents. Additional equipment includes electrocautery, headlight, operating room light, bedside activated clotting time (ACT) machine, and a ''primed'' ECMO circuit (see Chapter 6).

C. Environment

ECMO cannulation is a surgical procedure performed in the intensive care unit (ICU). Ideally, the surgical team should include an operating room nurse. The surgical team controls the sterile environment, which includes the sterile space, instrument tables, suction, and electrocautery. Caps and masks are worn by all personnel within 6 feet of the operative field (5). It may be necessary for an ICU nurse to perform in the role of the surgical nurse. Preparation and training for this role must be part of the education plan. The bed will be raised to facilitate venous drainage once on ECMO. A wooden platform may be needed for staff to care for the patient. A height of 6–9 inches is generally adequate for this platform.

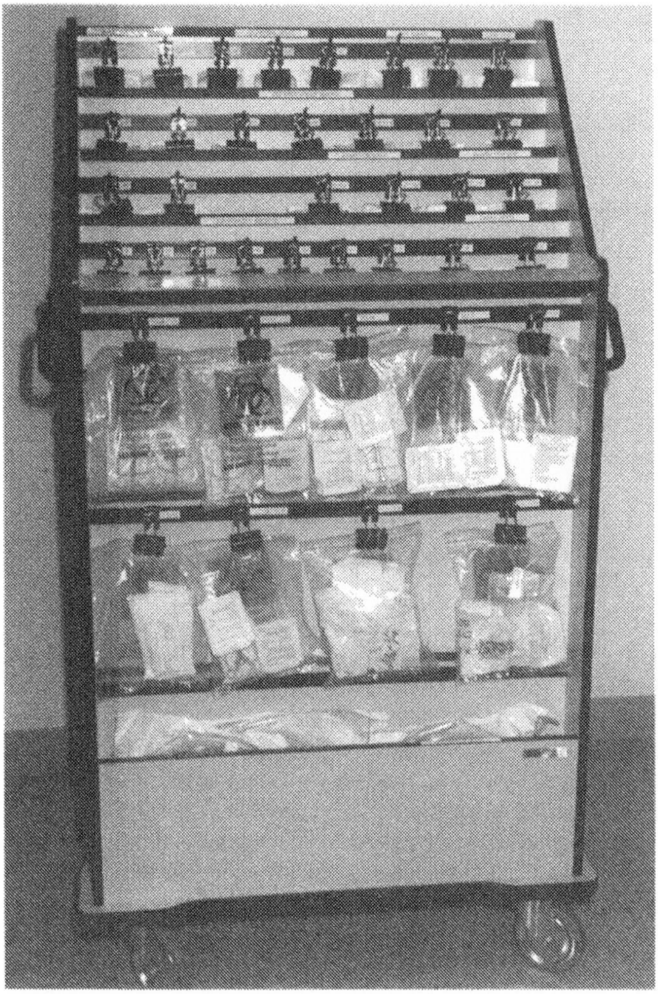

Fig. 1 Datel@ Mobile Cart for cannulae. (Courtesy of the Datel Company, Holland, MI.)

III. PRECANNULATION PREPARATION

Once a decision is made to initiate ECMO therapy, activation of the precannulation protocol begins. Initiation of ECMO may be emergent (the patient must be on ECMO within 30 minutes of the call for ECMO), or it may be routine (the patient is placed on ECMO nonemergently). The cannulation site in cardiac patients who have a closed sternum (closed chest) is through the neck. Infants and children who have undergone cardiac surgery using a sternotomy approach or those in whom the mediastinum has been opened during resuscitation will be cannulated via the right atrium and aorta (open chest) (4).

IV. ACTIVATION OF THE PRECANNULATION PROTOCOL

A. Page System

Once the decision is made, the team is activated by notification through the hospital paging system. The first call is to the ECMO therapist. Other members of the team to be paged include the ICU attending physician, attending cardiac surgeon, cardiac surgical resident, perioperative nurse, the clinical laboratory, and the blood bank. These calls are best made by an administrative associate or another member of the assistive staff. All team members will be notified of the status, emergent or nonemergent.

B. Priming the Circuit

A ''primed'' neonatal circuit is kept ready, at all times, in the CICU (see Chapter 7). All emergent ECMOs are placed on this circuit. If the patient weighs more than 6 kg and is stable on ECMO, he or she will be transferred to the appropriate circuit. If the decision to cannulate is nonemergent, the ECMO specialist prepares and primes the circuit (4). This may be done immediately if the ICU nurse has been trained to perform as the operative nurse.

C. Blood Products

The blood product needs of the patient going on ECMO and while on ECMO are vast. Protocols to standardize the anticipated needs will help the blood bank to meet these demands. The blood bank must be notified immediately if the patient is placed on ''emergent'' ECMO. This will alert them to prepare the following products immediately (if the patient has a current type and cross-match sample): 1 unit type-specific whole blood (WB, <21 days and CMV negative), 2 units pooled platelets (PLT), and 2 units cryoprecipitate; if no type is available, two units of type O-negative packed red blood cells (PRBC, <21 days and CMV negative), 2 units pooled PLT (100 mL), fresh frozen plasma (FFP), and 2 units of cryoprecipitate. These products must be ready for release within 15 minutes. Blood bank orders including a clot for STAT type and cross match for the initial ''prime'' of patients being placed on nonemergent ECMO are as follows: ''Neonatal Pack,'' 500 mL CMV-negative PRBC (less than 7 days), 200 mL FFP, 2 units cryoprecipitate, and 2 units concentrated PLT; ''Pedi Pack,'' 1000 mL

PRBC (less than 7 days), 400 mL FFP, three units cryoprecipitate, and 4 units PLT; and "Adult Pack," 1500 mL PRBC (less than 7 days), 500 mL FFP, 4 units cryoprecipitate, and 6 units PLT (4). Understanding the potential additional needs of the patient on ECMO, the blood bank maintains available typed and cross-matched blood for the patient. While the patient is on ECMO, 5% albumin must always be at the bedside.

D. Precannulation Patient Laboratory Studies

Prior to cannulation the following studies are obtained: complete blood count (CBC), prothrombin time (PT), partial thromboplastin time (PTT), fibrinogen, whole blood potassium (K), ionized calcium (CA), and arterial blood gas (4).

E. Medication Preparation

In addition to routine resuscitation medications, preparation of the following drips is recommended: dopamine, heparin, morphine, apresoline, and aminocaproic acid. Standard preparation of these medications will allow for more timely preparation and delivery.

V. CANNULATION

Following surgical cannulation, the patient is connected to the ECMO circuit. A chest film is obtained to confirm cannula(e) position. Within the first hour of going on ECMO the following blood tests are drawn: hematocrit, platelet count, PT, PTT, fibrinogen level, and postmembrane gas. As VA ECMO flow increases, inotropic support may generally be weaned. Infants generally have a head ultrasound within 24 hours of cannulation.

VI. CARE OF THE PATIENT ON ECMO

The goal of ECMO in patients with low cardiac output is to ensure adequate oxygenation and perfusion of vital organs. VA ECMO unloads the right heart but increases the left ventricular (LV) afterload and wall tension in patients with poor myocardial function (7). As a result, coronary perfusion is potentially compromised. This may be related to inadequate decompression of the LV, aortic valve incompetence, ECMO flow, or the position of the reinfusion aortic cannula. The majority of coronary arterial perfusion occurs via pulmonary venous return in patients with adequate LV ejection (8). Also, oxygen delivery (FiO_2 of at least 40%) with conventional, mechanical ventilation while on ECMO may aid in the coronary oxygenation (8). However, in patients with LV overdistention and poor LV function, the majority of coronary arterial perfusion may actually occur from flow through the aortic reinfusion cannula. ECMO flow rate is ideally adjusted to approximately 80–120 mL/kg/h (5,9), which supports approximately 70–80% of the patient's cardiac output. However, cannula size, circuit resistance, and the patient's volume status may limit the ability to achieve the desired flow rate. Throughout the ECMO course, there is a need to continually assess this critically ill patient and to provide timely interventions to achieve optimal outcomes. Continual nursing assessment of cardiac function includes monitoring of mean arterial blood pressure (MAP), cardiac preload pressures, SvO_2, peripheral perfusion and pulses, and urine output. (For information regarding information on accidental decannulation or mechanical pump failure, see Chapter 6.)

VII. CARDIOVASCULAR ASSESSMENT

A. Heart Rate and Rhythm

Heart rate and rhythm are monitored continuously to assess for abnormalities and changes. Cardiac patients may be prone to arrhythmias that may further inhibit cardiac output. While the need for atrio-ventricular synchrony may not be crucial with otherwise stable hemodynamics, the additional cardiac output and decrease in cardiac preload (filling) pressures achieved with synchrony may provide a critical advantage in weaning patients from ECMO with borderline cardiac function.

Patients with temporary atrial and/or ventricular epicardial pacing wires may benefit from cardiac pacing when indicated. Serum electrolytes are monitored and supplemented as necessary. Antiarrhythmic medications are commonly indicated as well.

In rare circumstances, patients with severe arrhythmias causing marked hemodynamic instability may benefit from the initiation of ECMO to allow for radiofrequency catheter ablation or recovery of the underlying myocardial disease (11).

B. Hemodynamic Pressure Monitoring

Assessment and monitoring of ECMO patients requires arterial and/or central venous intracardiac lines.

1. Decreased MAP

Since the pump flow is nonpulsatile, arterial and intracardiac waveforms dampen and arterial pulse pressure narrows as flow is increased. MAP is continuously assessed while on ECMO. Infants generally require a MAP of 45–65 mmHg (9), and pediatric patients may need a MAP of at least 60 mmHg (5). MAP range is individualized according to the size and age of the patient. Inadequate circulating volume may result in low MAP and cardiac preload pressures with SvO_2 less than 70% and may lead to the inability of ECMO to flow causing ''bladder chatter'' (5). The bladder servo-regulates the pump to stop when there is not enough volume present. Volume expanders are administered to treat hypovolemia (5% albumin, PRBC, or FFP, depending on hematological values). Increased inotropic support improves the MAP by assisting with cardiac ejection if hypovolemia treatment is unsuccessful (11). Other factors contributing to low arterial pressure may include inadequate ECMO flow, sepsis, or oversedation.

2. *Increased MAP*

Large amounts of volume administered during resuscitation, capillary leakage of fluids into the interstitial space, and oliguria or anuria before the initiation of ECMO all contribute to hypervolemia and hypertension (5). The combination of the patient's own cardiac output and the ECMO circuit may also cause hypertension (12). Additionally, nonpulsatile ECMO flow leads to the release of renin. The release of renin stimulates the renin-angiotensin system, which constricts the arteriolar smooth muscles causing retention of sodium and water (13). Elevated MAP may cause bleeding in the anticoagulated patient. Arteriolar dilating medications (apresoline) and short-acting β-adrenergic blocking agents are useful in controlling episodes of hypertension. Other medications may reduce blood pressure including afterload reducing agents, α-adrenergic blocking agents, or phosphodiesterase-inhibiting agents. Patient pain must always be ruled out as a source of hypertension and/or bleeding.

3. *Intracardiac Pressures*

Postoperative cardiac patients may have one or more intracardiac catheters in place. Depending on the cardiac defect and type of procedure performed, there may be a transthoracic right atrial (RA), left atrial (LA), and/or pulmonary artery (PA) catheter in place. These lines may provide information regarding LV overdistention from poor ventricular function and trends in intravascular volume status. Elevations in the RA and LA pressures may be indicative of a problem. Preload pressures are generally low. A rising LA pressure may be demonstrative of deteriorating LV function. Echocardiography is useful in confirming the diagnosis. Treatment options include a balloon atrial septostomy or a left atrial vent via the ECMO circuit (11,14,15). Lowering the LV pressure decreases both mitral regurgitation and elevated LA pressures that may be causing pulmonary hemorrhage or edema. Preexisting atrial or ventricular defects or a patent foramen ovale may serve as LV vents (2). Avoiding LV distention during ECMO therapy may shorten the overall ECMO course (14).

VIII. RESPIRATORY ASSESSMENT

A. Ventilator Settings

Once the patient is on VA ECMO, ventilator settings are adjusted to prevent barotrauma. Settings are reduced and individualized and may include FiO_2 of 21–40%, peak inspiratory pressure of 25 cm H_2O, positive end expiratory pressure of 5 cm H_2O, inspiratory time of 1.0 second, and frequency of 10 breaths per minute (4). Continuous positive airway pressure may be less deleterious than conventional mechanical ventilation for patients with continuous pulmonary airleaks.

B. Chest Radiography

A chest x-ray is done postcannulation, after any unexplained changes in the patient's status, and daily to evaluate the lungs. Generalized opacification of all lung fields within the first 24 hours on ECMO is common. The initial interaction of blood along the surface of the ECMO circuit activates complement, leading to a limited capillary leak syndrome (8). Both the activation of these vasoactive substances and withdrawal of distending airway pressure account for the complete opacification.

C. Pulmonary Toilet

Endotracheal suctioning is individualized for every patient and may include suctioning with manual ventilation every 4 hours as needed with gentle vibrations, if not cannulated transthoracically. Manual ventilation with pulmonary toilet allows for the maintenance of alveolar volume and evaluation of lung compliance (5). Frequency of suctioning may need to be increased depending on amount of secretions or may need to be limited when bleeding is exacerbated by the procedure.

D. Arterial and Venous Blood Gases

Arterial and venous blood gases are monitored. SvO_2 should be greater than 70% to ensure adequate cardiac output and tissue oxygenation by the ECMO circuit. Venous pH should be within normal limits. Arterial saturation of at least 95% with normal arterial pH and $PaCO_2$ of 35–40 are expected. Increasing the ECMO flow rate enables a greater volume of blood to come in contact with the membrane oxygenator, thus elevating PaO_2 levels (5). Increasing the sweep gas decreases $PaCO_2$ levels.

E. Muscle Relaxants

Patients generally benefit from their own respiratory effort. Therefore, muscle relaxants are avoided, but sedatives, analgesics, and paralyzation medications to provide patient comfort, control bleeding, and stabilize hemodynamics are frequently indicated.

IX. ASSESSMENT OF HEMOSTASIS AND COAGULATION

A. Bleeding

Bleeding is one of the most common complications of ECMO (6). In the postoperative patient, fresh incision sites may also be a source of bleeding. All potential sites should be monitored closely—intravenous and arterial catheters, ECMO cannulae insertion sites, chest tubes, incisions, and drains. Sanguinous drainage from all dressings should be weighed when possible and should be considered in calculations of output. Other sites of potential bleeding include the cranium and the abdomen. The abdomen should be assessed for girth changes as well as increasing distention and firmness. Routine head ultrasounds assess for intracranial hemorrhage in infants. Infants are also monitored for increased head circumference and increased tension by palpating the anterior fontanel. Pupil size and reaction should be monitored in all patients. Additional nursing care includes assessment for blood in all body fluids and secretions including stool, urine, gastric drainage, and sputum. Sanguinous drainage from operative sites may be controlled by absorbable gelatin or microfibrillar collagen dressings (5). Control of bleeding from the nasal or oral pharynx may require packing and further evaluation by the otolaryngology team. Heel sticks, venipunctures, rectal probes, injections, and placement of tubes within the patient should be avoided to prevent bleeding once ECMO is initiated. Changing of endotracheal tubes, nasogastric tubes, and urinary catheters must be done cautiously if needed. Discontinuation of arterial and/or venous access may also lead to excessive bleeding.

B. Heparin

The interface of blood with a foreign substance causes proteins to attach to the surface of the ECMO circuit (9). This reaction activates the complement and clotting systems, causing clots to form immediately (9). Therefore, systemic heparinization is required for patients on ECMO. Heparin combines with antithrombin III to inhibit clot formation. Antithrombin III deficiencies may render heparin ineffective and cause increased clot formation (16). The separate infusion of heparin via a circuit bladder port ensures accurate and immediate response to dose changes. Heparin infusion is usually initiated at 10 μ/kg/h.

C. ACT Levels

ACTs are followed hourly and the heparin infusion adjusted to maintain ACT levels of 180–200 seconds. Various factors will influence ACT levels. The ACT may need to be lowered if the patient is experiencing excessive bleeding or increased when weaning from ECMO. Diuresis may lower the ACT because heparin is excreted by the kidneys. Platelets contain heparinase, which destroys heparin and potentially lowers the ACT. If platelet transfusion is indicated, it is not unusual to give one half of the hourly heparin dose as a bolus prior to the transfusion.

D. Tamponade

Pericardial or mediastinal tamponade are potentially life-threatening complications in patients with an open sternotomy incision and transthoracic cannulation sites. Tamponade inhibits venous return to the ECMO circuit and decreases cardiac function (15). The sternotomy site should remain concave in appearance. Signs of tamponade include increased LA and RA pressures with decreased MAP, increased heart rate or decreased electrocardiogram voltage, sudden increase or cessation of chest tube drainage, and a convex or bulging sternotomy patch (2). When tamponade is suspected, immediate exploration of the chest and evacuation of clots by the cardiac surgeon is warranted. If chest tubes from the operative sites are in place, it may be necessary to strip or milk the tubes to avoid clot formation, which may lead to tamponade (2).

E. Aminocaproic Acid

Patients at high risk for intracranial hemorrhage or other bleeding complications may benefit from the administration of aminocaproic acid (17). Patients most at risk are those with profound acidosis (pH <7.1), profound hypoxia, hypotension, previous intracranial hemorrhage, sepsis, or gestational age less than 37 weeks (4,17). Aminocaproic acid prevents fibrinolysis by inhibiting plasminogen activator substance and, to a lesser extent, through the effects of antiplasmin (17). The medication is administered 100 mg/kg over 5 minutes either prior to or immediately postcannulation. It is infused continuously via intravenous route at 30 mg/kg/h (4). Aminocaproic acid is discontinued after 72 hours with cessation of bleeding and when control of coagulation factors is achieved (4). Daily plasminogen activator time is obtained and should be greater than 120 seconds (5).

F. Routine Laboratory Studies

Various hematological factors are assessed routinely and as needed. These include CBC and PLT every 8 hours and PT and fibrinogen levels every 12–24 hours. An infusion of PRBCs (10–20 mL/kg) should be administered for a HCT less than 36%. Albumin 5% should be readily available at the bedside and used as volume replacement when the HCT is greater than 45%. An infusion of FFP, 10–20 mL/kg is administered for PT greater than 16 seconds. Cryoprecipitate replacement of 1–3 units is considered for fibrinogen levels less than 150 mg/dL. The PLT count is generally maintained at 150,000 mm^3 to control bleeding and decrease the risk of intraventricular hemorrhage (4). Platelets are continuously destroyed by ECMO and may need to be replaced more frequently than other blood components (9). Platelets are not optimally infused via the bladder port because they will aggregate in the silicone membrane. If they must be administered via the ECMO circuit, they should be given postmembrane (16). Platelet integrity is best maintained when platelets are not concentrated, thus affording higher levels with transfusion. Often platelets are transfused before invasive procedures to decrease bleeding. After a few days on ECMO, cholestatic jaundice with hepatomegaly may result from platelet aggregation along with other substances within the liver (18). The result of this is obstruction of conjugated bile excretion, however, liver enzymes usually remain within normal limits (18).

X. ASSESSMENT OF FLUIDS, ELECTROLYTES, AND NUTRITION

A. Fluid Management

Renal failure is a common complication for patients on ECMO and occurs with greater incidence among cardiac ECMO patients (7). The kidneys may have been previously compromised in the unstable cardiac patient by a low cardiac output state prior to the initiation of ECMO. Fluid retention from pre-ECMO resuscitation, general anesthesia, or cardiopulmonary bypass contributes to edema. The nonpulsatile flow of the ECMO circuit may also play a role in renal insufficiency. Generally intravenous fluids are restricted to one-half to three-quarters maintenance. When urine output has improved, fluids are increased to full maintenance. Insensible water loss from the patient and from the membrane oxygenator may be included when calculating fluids. Precise calculation of insensible losses cannot be calculated, but an estimated 10% may be added on to account for this (19). Optimal fluid management ensures adequate tissue perfusion, diuresis, calories, and correction of hematological values (13). Minimal hourly urine output in the infant or pediatric patient is 0.5–1.0 mL/kg/h.

B. Diuretic Therapy

Furosemide is usually instituted to promote a negative balance. A continuous infusion (0.2–0.3 mg/kg/h) may be considered rather than bolus doses to avoid sudden shifts in intravascular volume associated with hypotension and decreased cardiac preload (12). The addition of chlorothiazide may add to diuresis. An infusion of renal dose dopamine (2.5–3.0 μg/kg/min) may aid in the perfusion of the kidneys and enhance glomerular filtration. While on diuretics, serum potassium and electrolytes are followed closely and supplemented as needed.

C. Ultrafiltration

Ultrafiltration, via the ECMO circuit, may be needed if the diuretic regime proves inadequate. Ultrafiltration has minimal effects on serum electrolytes, but coupled with diuretics the blood urea nitrogen (BUN) and creatinine may become elevated. Dialysis may also be initiated via the ECMO circuit for rising creatinine levels accompanied by hyperkalemia and anuria (12).

D. Nutrition

Adequate calories (80–100 kcal/kg/d) and nutrition may be achieved using parenteral nutrition. Parenteral nutrition can be infused via the ECMO bladder port. Intralipid infusion is not recommended through the bladder port. In determining nutritional status, additional studies include a total protein and albumin. The administration of ranitidine to inhibit gastric secretions and antacids to regulate gastric pH may be therapeutic.

XI. NEUROLOGICAL ASSESSMENT

Acidosis, hypoxia, low cardiac output, cardiac arrest prior to ECMO, or systemic anticoagulation on ECMO all pose threats to neurological integrity. Alterations in the neurological status may be subtle and may include hemodynamic instability, seizures, and/or unequal size and reaction of the pupils. Infants may also exhibit a bulging anterior fontanel.

A. Head Ultrasound

A head ultrasound should be obtained in infants within 24 hours of cannulation and every 48 hours thereafter unless patient status warrants greater frequency. Large intracranial bleeds may preclude continuation of ECMO.

B. Hypothermic Cooling

Mild hypothermia may be helpful in preventing further central nervous system insult (20), especially in patients who have required resuscitation before the initiation of ECMO. Cooling core body temperature to 34°C for the first 24 hours and maintaining normothermia during the first several days may be therapeutic in preserving neurological integrity (14).

XII. INFECTION

Signs of infection may be difficult to determine. Usual indicators of infection are unreliable on ECMO. Thrombocytopenia results from platelet destruction by the circuit, and the core body temperature is affected by the circuit heat exchanger (12). Patients on ECMO receive prophylactic antibiotic coverage predisposing them to fungal infections. Mycostatin administration may be useful in avoiding the overgrowth of fungus, and postoperative cardiac patients may be at greater risk for infection secondary to ''open'' sternotomy incisions, intracardiac lines, prolonged mechanical ventilation, and possible immunosuppression resulting from cardiopulmonary bypass. White blood cell count and differential should be obtained and assessed daily, and routine blood, endotracheal aspirates, and urine cultures should be obtained every other day and as indicated (21).

XIII. COMFORT

A. Medications

Sedation while on ECMO is essential to promote comfort, decrease agitation, and avoid accidental decannulation by the patient. Signs of discomfort in patients may include increases in the heart rate, increased MAP, changes in pupillary size, diaphoresis, and tears from the eyes (22). In addition, patients who are not pharmacologically paralyzed may have increases in respiratory rate, changes in respiratory pattern, facial grimacing, and withdrawal from painful stimuli (22). Continuous infusions or bolus doses of both narcotics and benzodiazapines should decrease levels of pain and stress. If sublimaze is used, increases in the daily dosage may be necessary to maintain analgesia because sublimaze binds quickly to the oxygenation membrane (23). Tolerance to the medication necessitates as much as a 10% increase in the drug on a daily basis (24). Benzodiazapines provide sedation and amnesia. Sedation, analgesia, and paralyzing medications make the neurological examination a challenge (25). Therefore, medication dosages are provided to achieve optimal levels of comfort but may need to be readjusted to adequately examine the patient's neurological status.

B. Comfort Measures

Care is clustered to allow for periods of decreased patient stimulation. Environmental factors such as excess noise and bright lights are minimized (26). Pediatric patients are usually placed on a low-airflow bed to help maintain skin integrity. Gel pillows are often used under the occiput to prevent skin breakdown. Pressure points are assessed routinely, and the patient is moved slightly to change position if possible. Passive range of motion and changes in position help to maintain skin integrity and prevent muscle contractures. Maintenance of intact skin and mucosa is achieved by providing routine skin care and gentle oral hygiene with mouth rinse.

XIV. FAMILY CARE

One of the most stressful experiences for any parent is to have a critically ill child in an intensive care unit connected to an array of invasive equipment. They often face overwhelming feelings of anxiety, fear, helplessness, and hopelessness (27). Fears of death and brain injury provoke extreme anxiety for family members (27). All these emotions are reinforced when a child is on ECMO. Children are often placed on ECMO after cardiac arrest, and the family has no time to prepare. The unfamiliar setting, equipment, and faces all contribute to heightened stress. Before the family visits for the first time following cannulation, the nurse should meet them away from the bedside and explain to them what they are about to see (12). Honest and open communication between the nurse and family is central to developing a trusting relationship. Parents need hope within reason. Concrete explanations of the equipment, alarms, and the staff caring for their child may help to alleviate some of the anxiety (12). Parents should be encouraged to visit, touch, and talk to their child, as well as assist with simple care needs such as skin care. Ongoing information is provided by the nurse, and a time is set aside daily for updates by other members of the multidisciplinary team. The social worker and chaplain are often very important members of this team.

XV. TRIAL ON DECREASED FLOW RATES

After recovery on ECMO, patients are trialed on lower flows with assessment of cardiac function by echocardiography (21,28), observation of systemic pulsatile, blood pressure, SvO_2, heart rate, rhythm, and conduction. Generally, the patient will need inotropic support and some volume during the trial to maintain adequate systemic blood pressure and atrial pressures. If the patient tolerates the lower flow, with signs of recovered function and increased systemic flow, he or she may be decannulated.

XVI. WEANING THE PATIENT FROM ECMO

There are several ways to wean a patient from ECMO. The most common mode for cardiac patients is to gradually reduce the flow rate over a period of time. This is accomplished by decreasing flow rates by 10–20 mL/min increments every 1–2 hours or, during a faster wean, reducing the flows by 60–70 mL/min. During flow reduction, the patient is continually assessed, ventilator settings are readjusted, inotropic support generally increased, and sedation and a muscle relaxant administered (5). During cycling, if the patient shows signs of decompensation or is hemodynamically unstable, the previous flows are resumed and ventilator and inotropic support readjusted. Once the patient is cycled to a flow of 30–50 mL/min (idle flow rates), the bridge of the circuit will be clamped and an echocardiogram will be performed to assess cardiac function (21). Vital signs, oxygen saturation, and SvO_2 are measured at this time. If the patient has been supported at the idle flow rates for 2–4 hours and remains hemodynamically stable, subsequent deterioration is unusual (6). Evaluation by cardiac catheterization may be necessary for patients who are refractory to weaning (4).

The primary nursing responsibility during the cycling process is to evaluate the patient's response and tolerance to weaning. It is critical to document vital signs, RA and LA pressures, arterial and venous blood gases, ventilator settings, and changes in inotropic support (4). If the patient's recovery is obvious during the bridge clamping, he or she will remain on the low flow rates and plans will be discussed with the team and family to decannulate the patient.

XVII. PREPARATION FOR DECANNULATION

Patients with pulmonary failure exhibit positive outcomes by improvement in blood gases, chest x-ray, and ventilator settings. Attempting to evaluate cardiac function in patients dependent on maximum VA ECMO flow may be challenging (4). The indication for weaning from ECMO is evidence of potential hemodynamic independence. Determining the patient's readiness for decannulation is dependent upon the patient's intrinsic ventricular function, RA and LA pressures, and ventricular afterload.

Decannulation is a planned procedure involving a great deal of preparation. The patient is medicated with sublimaze and pharmacologically paralyzed. The ventilator settings are adjusted to support respiratory function in the low-flow state and the endotracheal tube is properly positioned for access under the drapes. All intravenous infusions, except heparin, that have been infusing via the circuit must be transferred to other central or peripheral access sites. Anticipating the increasing need for inotropes requires that adequate volumes of these medications must be readily available, placed inline, and accessible before draping. If the patient is being paced or pacing may be necessary, the pacing wires must be attached to the pacemaker and readily available. Access to a large-bore angiocath or central line to deliver emergency medications, blood and/or volume, or analgesia is essential, as well as access to the arterial line for serial blood gas analysis during the procedure. Having a unit of RBCs at the bedside in anticipation of bleeding or for volume resuscitation is recommended.

XVIII. DECANNULATION

Decannulation is a surgical procedure performed in the ICU. The same strict principles of antisepsis followed in the operating room apply. Nursing responsibilities include monitoring and managing the patient's clinical status, documentation of vital signs, administration of medications or colloids, and titrating inotropes. Two units of PLT are given after the cannulae are removed (13). If the patient was cannulated through the neck, attempts may be made to reconstruct the vessels rather than ligate them (29). If the patient was cannulated transthoracically through the sternotomy incision, the surgeon may opt to wait 24–48 hours postcannulation to close the sternum, especially if the patient has not diuresed adequately. Decannulation should not be a long procedure (<2 hours), and every effort should be made to allow the parents to visit as soon as possible.

XIX. PATIENT STABILIZATION POSTCANNULATION

Initially, low cardiac output is a common problem following decannulation. Improving cardiac output is dependent on maintaining adequate atrial pressures, titrating inotropes, and adding vasodilators for afterload reduction. Crystalloid, colloids, and blood products may be administered. Signs of good end-organ perfusion include brisk capillary refill time, adequate pulses, urine output of 1 mL/kg/h and stable arterial blood gases. SvO_2 should be maintained at 60–75% (30). A falling SvO_2 warrants investigation to determine what factors are contributing to decreased oxygen delivery (shunting, hypoxia, anemia) or to increased oxygen demands (sepsis, pain, inadequate sedation). A chest x-ray is done in the immediate postcannulation period to evaluate lung fields. Laboratory studies performed include CBC, PLT, PT, PTT, fibrinogen, serum electrolytes, and arterial blood gases. Blood studies are followed every 4–6 hours until values have stabilized. Initially the patient may continue sedation and chemical paralysis. When the patient demonstrates satisfactory pulmonary function, adequate gas exchange, and hemodynamic stability, a weaning plan from the ventilator may be initiated. Maintenance fluids should be adjusted to meet the patient's requirements, and a nutrition plan should commence soon after decannulation. Enteral feeds may be poorly absorbed in the immediate recovery period but should be considered because they offer less risk of infection than parenteral feeds. Many opportunities for infection exist: the ''open'' sternum, invasive lines, and indwelling tubes and catheters. Daily CBC with differential should be obtained and blood cultures drawn if the patient is exhibiting signs of sepsis. Prophylactic antibiotics are continued until the sternum is closed and the chest tubes removed.

XX. SUMMARY

The pediatric cardiac patient requiring ECMO therapy has many complex needs. The entire critical care team is responsible for the patient's continuous evaluation and identification of any complications that could hinder the patient's survival. Care begins with a well-planned program that is designed to utilize ECMO as a temporary measure that can be initiated in the critical care setting as emergently as necessary. Although costly, ECMO has proven to be a valuable medical intervention for infants and children who otherwise have high predicted mortality. Parents coping with the grief and pain of a dying child with few treatment options should be offered this therapy. Knowledgeable and aggressive care by a collaborative team can make the difference. The authors have shared their experience in the hope that staff in other centers will benefit from this discussion.

APPENDIX A: ECMO CART INVENTORY/SUGGESTED PAR LEVELS

Top Drawer
Scrub brushes (4)
Betadine ointment (2)
Bacitracin ointment (2)
Betadine solution (1)
Alcohol (1)
Esmark dressings
Benzoin (2)

Drawer Two
Bovie pads; adult/baby
Hand-held bovies
Asepto syringes (2)
Pump kit (1)
Straight connector $1/4 \times 3/8$ (2)
Y connector $1/4 \times 1/4 \times 3/8$ (3)

Drawer Three
Baby tourniquets (2 pkgs.)
Weitlander retractors (1 sm. & 1 med.)
Baby chest retractor (1)
Haight chest retractor (1)
Fine C clamp (1)
Pump tubing clamps (1 adult, 1 infant)
Castro needle holders (2 sets)
Arterial and venous line clamps, $1/4 \times 3/32$ and $3/8 \times 3/32$ (2 sets)

Drawer Four
Medium clips (1 box)
Large clips (1 box)
#11 blades (1 box)
#15 blades (1 box)
Bone wax (1 box)
Thrombin/gelfoam (4 each)
Ioban drapes
Extra pump tubing (arterial and venous)

Drawer Five
Sutures—one box each
- 5-0 prolene RB-2 multipack
- 6-0 prolene BV-1 multipack
- 5-0 prolene RB-1
- 4-0 prolene RB-1
- 4-0 ethibond RB-1
- 3-0 ethibond RB-1
- 3-0 ethibond BB
- 2-0 ethibond V-7
- 2-0 ethibond ties
- #2 silk
- 3-0 vicryl SH
- 3-0 ethilon PS-2
- 4-0 ethilon PS-2

Wire Cart (use as back table)

Basic Setup (on wire cart)
ECMO Custom pack
Pediatric drape
ECMO instrument set
Blue towel pack
Prep set
Bovie pad to size
Sutures appropriate to size (see below)

Baby Sutures and Extras (in plastic bag)
Esmark dressing
Asepto syringe
Medium clip
Large clip
#2 silk ties
2-0 ethibond ties
4-0 ethibond RB-1
3-0 ethibond BB
2-0 ethibond V-7
4-0 prolene RB-1
5-0 prolene RB-2 multipack
6-0 prolene BV-1 multipack
4-0 ethilon PS-2 (2)

Adult Sutures and Extras (in plastic bag)
Asepto syringe
Medium clip
Large clip
#2 silk ties
2-0 ethibond ties
3-0 ethibond ties
3-0 ethibond BB
2-0 ethibond V-7
4-0 prolene RB-1
5-0 prolene RB-2 multipack
6-0 prolene BV-1 multipack
Bone wax
3-0 ethilon PS-2 (2)

PLEASE REMEMBER to send arterial and venous line clamps to CPD after patient comes off ECMO.

APPENDIX B: MEDIASTINAL CART INVENTORY

Drawer One
6 cm × 7 cm tegaderms
10 cm × 12 cm tegaderms
4 in. × 5 in. bioclusive dressing
4 in. × 10 in. bioclusive dressing
Bacitracin ointment
Betadine ointment
Raytex sponges
6 in. × 6 in. Esmark bandages
6 in. × 4 yd. Esmark bandages
Culture tubes
Small red vessel loops
Cotton umbilical tape
Bone wax

Drawer Two
21 × ¾ butterfly
4-way stopcocks
Medtronic pressure catheter set
Argyle umbilical vessel catheters
19 gauge intracath
Suture boots
Size 100 gelfoam
Box of 12 Surgicel
Thrombin
20 gauge Arrow catheters
22 gauge Arrow catheters

Drawer Three
0 vicryl CT-1
2-0 vicryl CT-1
3-0 vicryl SH
3-0 vicryl PS-1
4-0 vicryl PS-2
3-0 ethilon PS-2
4-0 ethilon PS-2
4-0 prolene BB
5-0 prolene BB
6-0 prolene BV-1
7-0 prolene BV-1
5-0 prolene RB-2 multipack
6-0 prolene BV-1 multipack
2-0 ethibond V-7
2-0 ethibond ties
#2 silk ties
3-0 tevdek T-2
4-0 tevdek T-3
5-0 tevdek T-3
2-0 temporary pacing wires BB
2-0 temporary pacing wires SH

Drawer Four
ValleyLab handheld bovie pencil (4)
Suction tubing (2)
Yankauer suction tip (4)
Instruments—Jakes (2)
C-clamp (2)
Weitlander retractor (2)
Episiotomy scissors (1)
Metzenbaum scissors (1)
Asepto syringes (5)
Hemaclips—Small (10)
Medium (10)
Large (10)

Drawer Five
#1 sternal wires (1 bx)
#3 sternal wires (1 bx)
#5 sternal wires (1 bx)
35 cm × 35 cm Ioban drape (5)
60 cm × 45 cm Ioban drape (5)
ValleyLab REM bovie pads—Infant (4), Adult (4)

APPENDIX B: Continued

Biogel gloves—$6\frac{1}{2}$ (10)
7 (10)
$7\frac{1}{2}$ (10)
8 (10)
Alcohol (2)
Betadine solution (2)
Benzoin (2)
Haight retractor (1)
Large Finachetto retractor (1)
Chest retractor (1)

APPENDIX C: CARDIAC ECMO INSTRUMENT TRAY

ITEM	QTY	ITEM	QTY
Sm. towel clips	4	#7 knife with mounted #11 blade	1
Jones towel clip	2	4 × 4 Raytec sponge	10
7″ tenotomy scissors	1	$7\frac{3}{4}$″ castro needle holder	2
Wire cutter scissors	1	Sm. neonatal clamp	1
6″ med. Ryder needle holder	1	Fine C clamp 35-4458	1
6″ fine Ryder needle holder	2	Sm. hvy. C clamp 35-4815	1
Sternal needle holder	1	Hvy. Lge. C clamp 35-8417	1
6″ Hegar needle holder	1	Neonatal vascular clamp	4
Cvd. Mosquito clamp	4	Str. med. length vascular clip	2
Str. snaps	6	Angl. med. length vascular clip	2
Rankin clamp	2	Andrews suction tip	1
Schnidt	1	Fine Andrews suction tip	1
Short right angle	1	Small pump line clamp	2
$7\frac{3}{4}$″ right angle	1	Large pump line clamp	2
Paddle forcep (fcp)	2	Line clamp $\frac{3}{8} \times \frac{1}{16}$	2
$7\frac{3}{4}$″ fine Debakey fcp	2	Line clamp $\frac{3}{8} \times \frac{3}{32}$	1
$7\frac{3}{4}$″ med. Debakey fcp	2	Medium clip applier	1
Adson tooth forcep	1	Large clip applier	1
Edna clamp	2	10 mm tourniquet	2
Baby Finochietto retr	1	14 mm tourniquet	3
Right angle retractor	2	Monel basin	1
Sharp Senn retractor	1	Custard cup	1
Small Weitlander retr	1	Straight Mayo scissors	1
Sponge stick with 4 × 4 Raytec sponge in jaws	1	Line clamp $\frac{1}{4} \times \frac{1}{16}$	2
Line clamp $\frac{3}{8} \times \frac{1}{2}$	1	Color-coded orange/brown/yellow	
#3 knife handle with mounted #15 blade	1	$7\frac{1}{4}$″ Metzenbaum scissors	1

Revised 10/98

APPENDIX D: MEDIASTINAL INSTRUMENT TRAY

ITEM	QTY	ITEM	QTY
Small towel clips	4	#7 knife with mounted #11 blade	1
Jones towel clips	2		
Straight Mayo scissors	1	12″ × 16″ tray lined with blue towel	1
7″ Metzenbaum scissors	1		
7″ tenotomy scissors	1	4 × 4 Raytec sponge	10
6″ med. Rydel needle holder	1	Castro needle holder	2
6″ fine Ryder needle holder	2	CVD. Jake	1
Sternal needle holder	1		
6″ Hegar needle holder	1		
Cvd. Mosquito clamp	4		
Wire cutter scissors	1		
Rankin clamp	2		
Schnidt	1		
Short right angle	1		
7¾″ right angle	1		
Paddle forcep (fcp)	2		
7¾″ fine Debakey fcp	2	Put sponge stick & towel clips in L.P. pan	
7¾″ med. Debakey fcp	2		
Adson tooth forcep	1		
Baby Finochietto retr	1	Color-coded orange/yellow	
Right angle retractor	2		
Sharp Senn retractor	1	DUST COVER	
Small Weitlander retr	1	L.P. pan with monel basin and custard cup; towel to cover bottom of pan	
Sponge stick with 4 × 4 Raytec sponge in jaws	1		
#3 knife handle with mounted #15 blade	1	*Do not wick monel basin & custard cup*	
Andrews suction tip	1		

Revised 3/98

REFERENCES

1. Dalton HJ, Siewers RD, Fuhrman BP, et al. Extracorporeal membrane oxygenation for cardiac rescue in children with severe myocardial dysfunction. Crit Care Med 1993; 21:1020–1028.
2. Suddaby EC, O'Brien AM. ECMO for cardiac support in children. Heart Lung 1993; 5:401–407.
3. Hilt T, Graves DF, Chernin JM, et al. Successful use of extracorporeal membrane

oxygenation to treat severe respiratory failure in a pediatric patient with a scald burn. Crit Care Nurse 1998; 18:63–72.
4. Multidisciplinary Intensive Care Unit. ECMO Clinical Practice Guideline. Boston: Children's Hospital, 1996.
5. Curley MAQ, Thompson, JE, Molengrafy J, et al. Oxygenation/Ventilation. In: Curley MAQ, Smith JB, Maloney-Harmon PA, eds. Critical Care Nursing of Infants and Children. Philadelphia: WB Saunders Co., 1996:249–319.
6. Klein MD, Whittlesey GE. ECMO in the hospital setting. In: Zwischenberger JP, Bartlett RH, eds. Extracorporeal Cardiopulmonary Support in Critical Care. Ann Arbor: ELSO, 1995:191–203.
7. Fasules JW. Extracorporeal life support for infants and children with cardiac disease. In: Zwischenberger JB, Bartlett RH, eds. Extracorporeal Cardiopulmonary Support in Critical Care. Ann Arbor: ELSO, 1995:445–497.
8. Fauza D, Hines M, Wilson J. Hemodynamics, perfusing, and blood volume. In: Zwischenberger JB, Bartlett RH, eds. Extracorporeal Cardiopulmonary Support in Critical Care. Ann Arbor: ELSO, 1995:73–86.
9. Bower L, Wilson J. Extracorporeal life support. In: Barnhart S, Czervinski M, eds. Perinatal and Pediatric Respiratory Care. Philadelphia: WB Saunders Co., 1995: 376–398.
10. Walsh E. Personal communication.
11. DelNido P. Extracorporeal membrane oxygenation for cardiac support in children. Ann Thorac Surg 1996; 61:336–339.
12. Caron E, Berlandi J. Extracorporeal membrane oxygenation. Nurs Clin North Am 1997; 32:125–140.
13. McDermott B, Curley MAQ. Extracorporeal membrane oxygenation: current use and future direction. AACN Clin Issues 1990; 1:348–364.
14. Duncan B, Ibraham A, Hraska V, et al. Use of rapid-deployment extracorporeal membrane oxygenation for the resuscitation of pediatric patients with heart disease after cardiac surgery. J Thorac Cardiovasc Surg 1998; 116:305–311.
15. Klein M, Whittlesley G. Extracorporeal membrane oxygen therapy for cardiac disease. In: Arensman R, Cornish J, eds. Extracorporeal Life Support. Boston: Blackwell Scientific Publications, 1993:302–315.
16. Short B. Clinical management of the neonatal ECMO patient. In: Arensman R, Cornish J, eds. Extracorporeal Life Support. Boston: Blackwell Scientific Publications, 1993:195–206.
17. Wilson J, Bower L, Fackler J, et al. Aminocaproic acid decreases the incidence of intracranial hemorrhage and other hemorrhagic complications of ECMO. J Ped Surg 1993; 28:536–541.
18. Bartlett R, Lilley R. Physiology of extracorporeal life support. In: Arensman R, Cornish J, eds. Extracorporeal Life Support. Boston: Blackwell Scientific Publications, 1993:89–104.
19. Heulitt M, Packard C. ECLS and fluid, electrolyte, and renal function. In: Zwischenberger JB, Bartlett RH, eds. Extracorporeal Cardiopulmonary Support in Critical Care. Ann Arbor: ELSO,, 1995:123–136.
20. Lanier W. Cerebral metabolic rate and hypothermia. J Neurosurg Anesth 1995; 7: 216–221.

21. Ziomek S, Harrell J, Fasules J, et al. Extracorporeal membrane oxygenation for cardiac failure after congenital heart operation. Ann Thorac Surg 1992; 54:861–868.
22. Laussen P, Hickey P. Principles of sedation and analgesia. In: Chang A, Hanley F, Wernovsky G, Wessel D, eds. Pediatric Cardiac Intensive Care. Baltimore: Williams and Wilkins, 1998:85–93.
23. Caron E, Maquire D. Current management of pain, sedation, and narcotic physical dependency of the infant on ECMO. J Perinat Neonat Nurs 1990; 4:63–74.
24. Arnold J, Truog R, Scavone J, Fenton T. Changes in the pharmacologic response to fentanyl in neonates during continuous infusion. J Pediatr 1991; 119:639–643.
25. DuPlessis A. Neurologic disorders. In: Chang A, Hanley F, Wernovsky G, Wessel D, eds. Pediatric Cardiac Intensive Care. Baltimore: Williams and Wilkins, 1998: 369–386.
26. Estrada E. ECMO for neonatal and pediatric patients: state-of-the-art and future trends. Pediatr Nurs 1992; 18:67–73.
27. Hickey P, Atz T. Perspective in the cardiac intensive care unit. In: Chang A, Hanley F, Wernovsky G, Wessel D, eds. Pediatric Cardiac Intensive Care. Baltimore: Williams and Wilkins, 1998:519–523.
28. Martin GR, Short BL. Doppler echocardiographic evaluation of cardiac performance in infants on prolonged extracorporeal membrane oxygenation. Am J Cardiol 1998; 62:929–934.
29. Aldolph V, Bonis S, Faltman K, et al. Carotid repair after pediatric extracorporeal membrane oxygenation. J Pediatr Surg 1990; 25:867–869.
30. Hazinski MF. Cardiovascular disorders. In: Hazinski MF, ed. Nursing Care of the Critically Ill Child. St. Louis: Mosby-Year Book Inc., 1992:117–394.
31. Curley MAQ, Smith JB, Maloney-Harmon PA, eds. Critical Care Nursing of Infants and Children. Philadelphia: WB Saunders Co., 1996.

7

Management of the Extracorporeal Membrane Oxygenator Circuit for Children with Cardiac Disease

Lynne K. Bower
Children's Hospital
Boston, Massachusetts

I. THE ECMO CIRCUIT

The extracorporeal membrane oxygenator (ECMO) circuit is composed of several disposable and nondisposable components. The disposable components consist of the tubing, bladder, membrane, heat exchanger, and cannulas. Most institutions have preassembled sterile tubing pacs manufactured to their specifications. The ideal system should promote laminar flow, require minimum blood volume, be constructed for longevity, and be mobile for intrahospital transport.

Blood flow through a typical veno-arterial (VA) circuit is as follows; blood is drained by gravity from the venous cannula to the bladder. From there it is pumped through the membrane and heat exchanger before it is reinfused via the arterial cannula. The veno-venous circuit follows the exact same pattern except that the reinfusion cannula is inserted into a vein.

Choosing the appropriate circuit size is dependent on the weight of the child. The larger the membrane surface area, the greater the potential gas exchange. However, the larger the surface area of the membrane, the higher the platelet consumption and the greater the priming volume, which will hemodilute the patient. In general, the flow requirements are approximately 120 mL/kg/min for neonates, 75 mL/kg/min for children, and 50 mL/kg/min for adults.

A. Cannulas

The ECMO circuit begins and ends with the cannulas. The cannulas chosen dictate the maximum flow rates that the system can achieve. Older children have a larger assortment of cannulas available. Different cannula manufacturers have different flow capabilities, side hole locations, wire reinforcement, tip configuration, and radiopaque markings. Cannulas with identical external diameters may have markedly different flow capabilities. Optimal flow characteristics of the cannulas can be compared by their M number (1). The M number is a standardized method for comparing the flow-pressure relationships in vascular devices. A device with a low M number indicates lower resistance and higher potential flows.

The ideal cannula should be thin-walled, stiff enough for insertion, kink resistant, marked to determine length, and radiopaque. The lower portion of the venous cannula has multiple side holes for optimal drainage, while the arterial cannula is shorter in order to reduce resistance. In larger children, most venous and arterial cannulas can be interchanged depending upon the situation.

The traditional access for VA ECMO is through the right internal jugular vein into the lower portion of the right atrium. The arterial cannula is inserted into the right common carotid artery and should lie at the junction of the innominate artery and aorta. The head is maintained in a midline position to decrease cerebral venous congestion caused by angulation of the left internal jugular vein. In postoperative cardiac patients, the transthoracic approach is commonly chosen.

The largest drainage cannula that can be safely inserted into the vein is selected. Drainage is also dependent on venous cannula position, right atrial filling pressure, and the height of the patient above the bladder. Subtle manipulations of these variables may be necessary to optimize flow. The most common causes of a decrease in venous return are malposition of the venous cannula, kinking of the cannula, shift of the mediastinum, or a hypovolemic state.

The reinfusion cannula dictates the maximum flow rate that can be safely infused (2). Because hemolysis can occur at system pressures exceeding 350 mmHg, it is important to select a reinfusion cannula large enough to manage the anticipated flow rate but no larger (3). If the cannula placed through the right common carotid artery is too large, flow to the right subclavian artery may be obstructed, resulting in less perfusion to the right arm (4). Since some preferential flow does occur irrespective of cannula size, blood pressure and blood gas monitoring in the right arm should be avoided. A reinfusion cannula larger than necessary may result in minimum back pressure to the membrane oxygenator, potentially allowing microbubbles to cross from a higher pressure gas phase into the blood phase. These bubbles can accumulate over time and may embolize.

In transthoracic cannulation, the cannulas are inserted directly into the ascending aorta and the right atrium. When interpreting cannula position on chest x-ray, it should be realized that different cannula manufacturers place the radiopaque markings used to identify cannula placement in different positions relative to the tip. High flows towards the aortic valve can cause aortic regurgitation and damage the valve. An echocardiogram may confirm cannula placement and flow direction (5,6). In small children, transthoracic cannulation allows for only a limited portion of the venous cannula to occupy the right atrium. Consequently, a cannula with side holes may not be appropriate in these situations. In larger children and when left ventricular vents are required, additional cannulas can be spliced into the circuit. However, the extra connectors are a prime site for clot formation. These additional cannulas usually contribute to lower flow rates and should always be inspected to assure that they have not clotted.

VA ECMO support can also be accomplished by percutaneous cannulation of the femoral vein and artery. This technique avoids ligating the vessels, thereby maintaining drainage and perfusion to the leg. It also has the advantage of minimizing bleeding from the cannulation site because it avoids a surgical cutdown. However, in a poorly perfused state, identifying the vessels can be difficult, and this technique should be avoided when a strong pulse cannot be identified (7).

Prevention of lower limb ischemia is a concern when femoral vessels are used for VA support. This may be accomplished by inserting a small cannula distal to the arterial infusion cannula to perfuse the lower limb (8).

Both the femoral and transthoracic routes of cannulation eliminate the issues of carotid artery ligation. Interrupting cerebral blood flow in pediatric ECMO has not been well studied, and massive ischemic infarcts have resulted from carotid ligation in older patients.

B. Bridge

The bridge connects the venous and arterial lines to one another and is located near the cannulas (3). During trials off ECMO, it allows the circuit to be isolated from the patient while maintaining blood flow to prevent stagnation and circuit thrombosis. The bypass bridge is clamped while the patient is on ECMO. It requires brief periods of unclamping to prevent blood in the bridge from stagnating. Opening and closing the bridge has been shown to cause changes in cerebral blood flow (9).

C. Tubing and Connectors

The tubing commonly used in ECMO circuits is composed of polyvinyl chloride (PVC) (3). Depending upon the patient's flow requirements, the internal diameter can be $^1/_4$, $^3/_8$, or $^1/_2$ in. with a wall thickness of either $^1/_{16}$ or $^3/_{32}$ in.

There are various types of polycarbonate connectors in the circuit. Connectors may be straight, y'ed, graduated, or contain luer-lock fittings. Any connection in the circuit provides an area for turbulent flow. Limiting the amount of connectors will limit potential sites for clot formation.

D. Bladder

The bladder is a seamless small reservoir composed of thin pliable silicone (3). It allows the roller pump to pull from this small reservoir instead of the right atrium. If there is an acute decrease in venous drainage, the bladder will collapse upon itself, preventing excessive negative pressure from being transmitted to the heart. The bladder also prevents negative pressure from pulling the vessel wall into the cannula. In addition, the bladder serves as a collecting port for small amounts of air. Two ports are built into the top for purging air and for continuous IV infusions. The bladder is the most dependent component of the circuit and is prone to thrombus formation. A larger reservoir is unacceptable during ECMO because blood becomes stagnant and clots. Newer bladders have become more streamlined to minimize clots. Currently the blaldder has a maximum inlet and outlet port of $^3/_8$ in. When high flow rates (>3 L/min) are anticipated, $^1/_2$-in.-diameter tubing on the venous drainage limb is used to improve flow capabilities. This decrease in diameter from the $^1/_2$ in. venous limb to the $^3/_8$ in. bladder inlet impedes flow. To circumvent this, a bridge is placed around the bladder, which reduces the resistance and increases potential flow. Some of the blood flow is shunted around the bladder, while the remainder continues through the bladder for servo-regulation. This bridge also allows a clotted or damaged bladder to be replaced without stopping the circuit.

E. Pumps

There are two types of pumps available for use with ECMO: the roller pump and the centrifugal pump.

1. Roller Pump

The roller pump is a positive displacement pump. It functions on the principle of compression and displacement (3). Flow is produced by compressing a segment of tubing between two roller heads spaced 180 degrees apart and a back plate. Volume is displaced as the rollers travel the length of the raceway (the segment of tubing contained within the pump head). A second roller begins compressing the tubing as the first roller is reaching the end.

The output of the roller is dependent upon the size of the tubing, rotations per minute, and proper occlusion. Occlusion is the amount of pressure the roller heads exert on the tubing to prevent fluid from slipping backwards. Most roller pumps require manual adjustment of the occlusion prior to use. Over time the occlusion can loosen, resulting in a lower delivered flow rate. This can be identified by both lower membrane pressures and lower systemic blood pressure.

The section of tubing housed between the pump heads and the back plate is referred to as the raceway. It is under continuous strain from the roller heads. To prevent breakdown, the tubing needs to be advanced to a new section at a predetermined time interval. This is referred to as "walking the raceway." A consensus has not been reached between centers regarding when to walk the raceway (10). At our institution the raceway is walked at 120 hours if flow rate is <1 L/min, 72 hours if flow rate is <2 L/min, and 48 hours if flow rate is >2 L/min. Another approach to maximize the longevity of the raceway tubing is to use a larger-diameter tubing in the raceway. The larger volume in this tubing decreases the RPMs needed to achieve a given flow rate. Tubing composed of a stronger polymer, known as Super Tygon S65HL, is ideal for high flow rates (11). It is a chemically altered PVC material that is resistant to wear. Due to its high cost, it is commonly used only for the raceway.

The major advantage of the roller pump is its constant flow output. Another advantage is reduced hemolysis at low flow rates. A disadvantage is that a roller pump is not pressure dependent. If excessive pressure builds up within the system, the pump will continue to operate until the problem is recognized or rupture occurs.

For safe operation, a roller pump requires the incorporation of a venous servo-regulation system—either a bladder box or pressure-monitoring system.

a. Bladder Box

The bladder box is the safety mechanism for a roller pump circuit. The purpose of the bladder box assembly is to prevent the pump's flow rate from exceeding the venous drainage (3). It is composed of brackets to support the silicone bladder and a microswitch, which rests on the bladder surface. When the bladder collapses, the microswitch is released and interrupts the electrical signal stopping the pump. When the problem is corrected (i.e., more volume or a lower set flow rate), the bladder reexpands and depresses the microswitch, thus restoring the pump's electrical current.

b. Pressure System

An alternative to the bladder box is a servo-regulated pressure-monitoring system (12,13). A pressure transducer is connected between the patient and the bladder. When flow diminishes, the pressure in the venous line decreases until a predetermined level is reached. At this point, the pressure monitoring system either reduces the pump's speed if there is partial obstruction or stops the pump if there is a complete obstruction.

2. *Centrifugal Pump*

The centrifugal pump is a kinetic pump, which transfers energy to the blood by a rapidly rotating cone. Blood passes through a vortex created by the spinning motion of the cone and is forced through the outlet. It automatically responds to the resistance against which it pumps. As line pressure increases, flow will decrease. This pressure-limited feature prevents pumping against a high-pressure head and eliminates potential system rupture. Flow is ultimately dependent upon the pump's preload, afterload, size of the rotating cone, and the pump speed (14).

The centrifugal pump cannot generate excessive positive pressure in the system. Another advantage of this system is the elimination of the venous servoregulating system and the raceway. This pump exerts a negative pressure on incoming blood and is not dependent upon the passive filling of the venous side of the pump. Therefore, gravity drainage is not a concern. However, this characteristic can also be a disadvantage (15). When venous drainage is inadequate, significant negative pressure as high as −200 to −700 mmHg can be transmitted to the right atrium and the blood, leading to hemolysis. Hemolysis is reported to be higher at low blood flow rates (300 mL/min) with centrifugal pumps compared to roller pumps.

3. *M Pump*

Another type of nonocclusive roller pump, used by Chevalier et al., is a pediatric tidal flow ECMO system (16). Recently modifications of Chevalier's pump have been made, and it is now manufactured and marketed in the United States as the M pump (17).

The M pump has a three-prong rotor with a stretched distensible silicone rubber chamber around it. The pumping chamber passively fills with venous blood distending the chamber while the rotors push the blood forward. A plexiglass box surrounds the rotor and pumping chamber. Suction can be applied to the box, which eliminates the need for gravity dependence. If venous return is inadequate, the pumping chamber collapses, eliminating any negative pressure.

If a distal occlusion occurs, the rubber chamber becomes round. The distended shaped chamber prevents the turning rotor from generating any forward flow, and maximum pressure cannot exceed 300 mmHg. This prevents rupture from occurring. With more clinical experience, this pump may become the ideal pump for long-term use.

F. Oxygenators

1. Membrane Oxygenators

Most ECMO experience has been with the silicone rubber membrane originally designed by Kolobow (18). It has a flat silicone rubber envelope, wound in a spiral coil around a polycarbonate spool. Two compartments are separated by a semipermeable membrane, one for blood and one for gas. The gas compartment also contains a spacer screen for mixing the gas and increasing gas transfer. Blood flows on the other side of the membrane, while O_2 diffuses across the membrane into the blood.

Similarly, CO_2 in the blood diffuses through the membrane into the gas compartment, where it is flushed out by the continuous flow of the ventilating gas (3). This ventilating gas is referred to as the ''sweep gas'' and is regulated by a flowmeter from an oxygen blender and occasionally by an additional flowmeter from a carbogen (5% CO_2/95% O_2) source.

a. Gas Exchange

Gas transfer across the membrane is dependent upon the type of gas, thickness of the membrane, surface area, and the partial pressure differences (driving pressure) of the gases across the membrane. Gas exchange can be further characterized by either the transfer rate or the blood film thickness (3).

b. Transfer Rate

The transfer rate is the driving pressure of the gas times the permeability of the membrane to that gas. The driving pressure causes the gases to diffuse from a high pressure to a low pressure. The greater this differential, the greater the rate of exchange. Similarly, the more permeable the membrane is for a particular gas, the greater the gas exchange of that gas (19).

If the sweep gas on the membrane is 100% oxygen, the oxygen pressure difference between the gas side and blood side is high. This pressure difference drives oxygen into the blood. The carbon dioxide driving pressure is significantly smaller. To compensate for this small driving pressure, the membrane is composed of silicone rubber, which is six times more permeable to CO_2 than to O_2 (Fig. 1).

c. Blood Film Thickness

The transfer rate of oxygen is limited by the blood film thickness between the membrane's layers. Red cells closest to the membrane become saturated with oxygen first. Over time, oxygen diffuses deeper into the blood, finally reaching the red cells in the outermost layer. Blood must remain in contact with the mem-

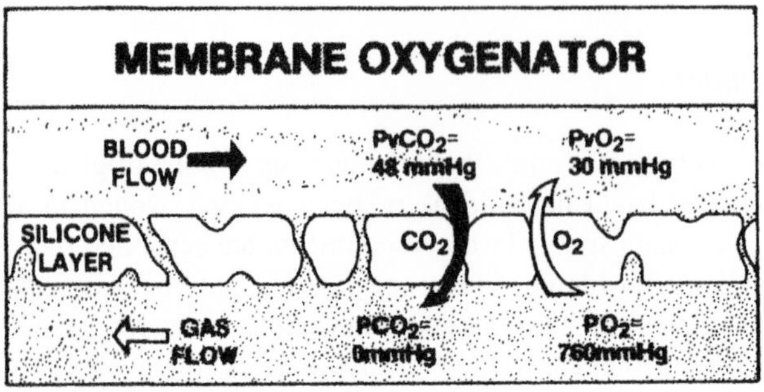

Fig. 1 Gas exchange at the blood-membrane interface. Note that the driving pressure for oxygen is much higher than the driving pressure for carbon dioxide.

brane long enough for complete saturation to occur. This limitation is referred to as the ''rated flow'' (20). Every oxygenator has a rated flow, which should never be exceeded. If higher blood flow rates are required, a larger membrane is needed.

d. CO_2 Transfer

Carbon dioxide transfer is not dependent upon the blood film thickness or the blood flow rate. It is dependent upon the sweep gas flow rate, the surface area of the membrane, and the driving pressure (18).

The rate at which the equilibrated gas can be exchanged for fresh gas with a lower CO_2 concentration has a direct effect on CO_2 elimination. Consequently, the higher the sweep gas flow rate, the lower will be the arterial PCO_2 (19).

CO_2 clearance can be decreased by water accumulation in the gas compartment of the membrane, which occurs due to the temperature difference between the blood and gas phases. The warm blood and cooler gas encourages condensation. For this reason, a minimum sweep gas flow rate is required to continuously flush the condensation out the gas exhaust port. If the minimum sweep gas rate results in too much CO_2 removal, addition of carbogen (5% CO_2/95% O_2) to the sweep gas will help maintain normocarbia.

Water accumulation affects CO_2 because CO_2 builds up in the water barrier, thereby decreasing the driving pressure for CO_2 transfer. This accumulation can be treated by transiently occluding and releasing the outflow gas port of the membrane, known as ''coughing'' the membrane (19). Temporarily increasing the sweep gas rate will also expel more water droplets, however, there is a flow limit to the sweep gas. Excessive gas flow will place the gas compartment under a higher pressure than the blood compartment, resulting in gas embolism. Gas embolism can also occur if the gas exhaust port becomes occluded. The gas compartment pressure should never exceed the blood compartment pressure. A pop-off safety release valve calibrated between 50 and 100 mmHg can be placed on the sweep gas inflow line to assure this.

Monitoring the difference between premembrane PCO_2 and postmembrane PCO_2 is important because a decreasing CO_2 transfer rate can be an early indicator of membrane malfunction (increased thrombus formation, excessive water accumulation) (19). Water expulsion from the membrane contributes to insensible water loss from the patient. This has been estimated to be 5–10 mL/m^2 of membrane per hour at 37°C.

e. Pressure Drop

Each oxygenator also has a rated pressure drop across the membrane, which, if exceeded, may result in membrane rupture. Pressure drop results from the resistance to blood flow produced by the membrane. It is obtained by subtracting the outlet pressure (postmembrane pressure) from the inlet pressure (premembrane pressure). This pressure difference can increase with internal clotting, higher blood flow rates, and an increase in blood viscosity. Continuous monitoring of the pre- and postmembrane pressures allows for assessment of the membrane's internal resistance (19). An increase in clot formation within the membrane will result in a higher premembrane pressure and no change in the postmembrane pressure. Conversely, a change in cannula resistance (kink or position change) will be reflected in both pre- and postmembrane pressures.

f. Surface Area

Oxygen and carbon dioxide are also affected by the surface area of the membrane. The larger the patient, the more surface area is required for adequate oxygenation and ventilation. Membrane oxygenators are available up to a surface area of 4.5 m^2. Patients weighing more than 60 kg may need two membranes parallel to one another in the circuit for optimal gas exchange. Both membranes should have pre- and postmembrane pressures monitored. If membrane pressures increase, each membrane should be briefly isolated to assess which one is responsible for the higher resistance. In this duel configuration, a failing membrane may be isolated and replaced without interrupting patient support.

2. Hollow Fiber Membrane Oxygenator

Another type of oxygenator used less frequently for ECMO is the hollow fiber membrane. This membrane has woven capillary tubes composed of microporous polypropylene. The microporous openings are 3–5 μm in diameter, which allows for a transient direct interface between the blood and the gas. Gas can pass through the capillaries while blood flows around them. Some manufacturers design these membranes with the blood flowing inside the capillaries and gas outside them. However, the high blood flow resistance of this configuration makes it less suitable for extended use.

In addition, after the initiation of ECMO, proteins build up in these small pores, eliminating the direct blood/gas contact. Over time the pores lengthen due to the pressure exerted on them, which results in serum leakage and a further decrease in gas exchange (21). These two problems make hollow fiber membranes unsuitable for extended ECMO runs.

However, because the microporous material has excellent gas exchange capabilities, low resistance, and is easy to prime, it is ideal as part of an emergency circuit. It also has the ability to be bonded with heparin, which is ideal in postoperative patients (22). Some centers use the heparin-bonded hollow fiber membrane in patients with bleeding complications despite the fact that it must be replaced every 8–48 hours, depending upon its function.

Heparin-bonded circuits are occasionally used for ECMO support to decrease the use of heparin administration and clot formation. It has been shown that clotting activation is delayed during the first 6 hours of use but then returns to the same level as a non–heparin-bonded circuit (23).

a. Heat Exchanger

Heat is lost through the oxygenator due to the cooling effects of the sweep gas, water evaporation, and from the exposed surface area of the tubing. A disposable heat exchanger warms the blood and maintains the body temperature at 37°C (3). A water pump circulates and regulates water temperature through the heat exchanger. The circulating water has no direct contact with the blood and is pumped countercurrent to the blood flow to achieve maximum heat transfer. The water bath temperature should never exceed 42°C to avoid protein denaturation and thermal trauma to the blood elements. Typically the water bath temperature is set at least 1°C warmer than the desired body temperature due to the surface cooling through the tubing. The heat exchanger is also used to cool the patient in order to decrease oxygen consumption.

Heat exchangers are available in different sizes. They can be incorporated into larger membranes or can be free-standing. Some centers bypass the heat exchanger when they are integrated with the membrane. This is because free-standing heat exchangers are easier to prime and are manufactured using longer-lasting stainless steel components rather than aluminum. Furthermore, the free-standing heat exchanger may be positioned postmembrane, which allows it to serve as a trap for air coming from the membrane.

II. PRIMING

Prior to placing a patient on ECMO, the circuit has to be prepared by a process referred to as priming. Priming is divided into four stages: carbon dioxide flush, vacuum, crystalloid infusion, and blood prime (3).

Carbon dioxide is flushed through the circuit for a minimum of 2 minutes. This step flushes the air out of the circuit and replaces it with CO_2, which is highly soluble in blood, thereby decreasing the risk of microbubbles.

Line vacuum is applied to the gas ports of the membrane for a minimum of 5 minutes (19). The tubing and reservoirs will gradually collapse, pulling the CO_2 from the blood compartment to the gas compartment of the membrane. This step exposes more of the membrane's surface area to full contact with the blood, optimizing gas exchange. The negative pressure also facilitates the filling of the circuit with fluid.

Next, an electrolyte solution is added and the circuit is filled in a step-by-step fashion, expelling air as each section of the circuit is fluid primed (19). Once completely filled, the vacuum is disconnected and the pump is turned on to circulate the fluid prime. All air must now be removed from the circuit. Special attention should be directed towards the membrane and heat exchanger to assure that they are bubble free. Albumin is then added to the circuit and circulated. Albumin coats the internal surface of the circuit and transiently prevents platelet adhesion and activation (24). Next the water bath is attached to the heat exchanger, warming the blood to 37°C.

The prime is then slowly drained and replaced with packed red blood cells and fresh frozen plasma (25). Most institutions have their own blood product recipe and treatment protocol for the prime. Finally, the blood is treated with heparin for anticoagulation, THAM to normalize pH, and calcium gluconate to reverse the citrate effect of stored blood. Once circulating, oxygen flow is briefly added to the membrane and a blood gas, activated clotting time (ACT), ionized calcium and potassium are obtained from the circuit. Abnormal values are adjusted until they are in the acceptable range (26).

In emergency situations, initiating ECMO support with a crystalloid prime may be necessary to save time. When this occurs, the ECMO circuit still needs to be treated with albumin and heparin. Prior to connecting a patient to ECMO, their coagulation factors are usually deficient (25). Further hemodilution will cause a greater deficiency with a non–blood-primed circuit. Blood products should be expeditiously administered when available to decrease the potential for bleeding. An ultrafiltration device can be connected to the circuit to adjust the patient's volume status and reverse hemodilution and coagulopathy (27,28). There is not a standard insertion site for the ultrafiltration device. A common configuration is to connect the drainage line prior to the membrane and reinfuse into the bladder.

Some centers have resorted to prepriming the ECMO circuit with a saline solution for up to 30 days. This prolonged exposure has been reported to lead to circuit degradation (29).

III. CIRCUIT MANAGEMENT

Following the initiation of ECMO support, platelets and cryoprecipatate are administered to the patient (25). ACTs are drawn every 15 minutes until stabilization occurs. Once the ACT is below 250 seconds, a continuous heparin infusion is connected to the circuit and started at 20 units/kg/h (30). Blood gases from the patient and the circuit are obtained and evaluated for oxygen delivery. Adjustments in the ECMO blood flow rate and sweep gas are made to achieve a $PaCO_2$ of 40–45 mmHg and a PaO_2 of >60 mmHg. Adequate oxygen delivery is verified by a PvO_2 of >34 mmHg (or saturation >70%) without metabolic acidosis. If an intracardiac communication or left ventricular drainage cannula exists, the MvO_2 from the circuit will be inaccurate, and an alternative site in the patient should be used to assess oxygen delivery. Once stable, arterial and venous blood gases are analyzed at least once a shift and after changes in ECMO flow rate or sweep gas. At our institution, a postmembrane blood gas is initially drawn to assess the membrane's function and then repeated in situations when a decrease in the membrane's efficiency is suspected.

After ECMO flow is established, a chest x-ray is obtained to identify cannula position, and the integrity of all connections is assured. All blood products and medications that are given via the circuit are administered prior to the bladder. Continuous infusions can be given via the ports on top of the bladder. Blood sampling usually occurs at a postbladder connection. Nothing should be administered beyond the heat exchanger to eliminate accidental injections of air (30).

Platelets adhere to the silicone of the membrane oxygenator. Therefore, they are administered either directly to the patient or after the membrane. Most centers infuse fat emulsion solutions through a separate line. The patient's central access line is the prefered site. Cracked stopcocks are the most frequently reported problem with direct circuit infusion of lipids (31).

IV. SAFETY CHECK

At the beginning of each shift, the cannulation site is inspected for oozing and cannula security (30). If neck vessels have been cannulated, the head is maintained midline to optimize cerebral flow. The occipital area is inspected for breakdown and a gel pad is placed under the head (32).

Table 1 Accessory Monitoring Devices used on Cardiac ECMO Patients

Devices	Manufacturer most reported	None used
Air bubble detector	Shiley caps 24%	44%
Oxygenator pressure monitor	Stockett-Shiley 64%	0%
SVO2/ABG Monitoring	CDI 52% Oximetrix 22%	0%
Ventilation gas analyzers	Mini Ox 21%	33%
Gas pop-off valves	27%	—

Every 4 hours a safety check of the ECMO circuit is performed. This entails a detailed inspection of the circuit for clot formation and both visual and audible alarm verification (30).

Prime areas for clot formation are the venous cannula, all connection sites, the bridge, venous limb, raceway section, bottom and top of the membrane, and bottom and top of the heat exchanger (33,34). If an ultrafiltration filter is in line, proper drainage is assured and any clot formation is documented. The bridge is also unclamped every 15 minutes to flush it and inspected for thrombus (30).

Alarm verification includes the pump and the pressure-monitoring system (i.e., membrane pressures). Pressure transducers are calibrated at the beginning of every shift. The correct raceway tubing diameter is verified on the pump.

Accessory monitoring devices, such as indwelling oxygen saturation and blood gas monitors, flow probes, gas pop-off valves, and air detectors, are available for the circuit. Each institution has its own philosophy concerning monitoring devices. Some believe the more the better, while others believe that using more devices leads to additional potential complications. The Extracorporeal Life Support Organization (ELSO) Committee of Devices and Techniques offers the results of a national survey for the use of equipment but does not imply a standard of care (Table 1).

V. TECHNICAL CONSIDERATIONS IN WEANING AND DECANNULATION

Prior to a trial off ECMO, all vasopressors infusing into the circuit are switched to a patient access site (30). The ventilator support is increased, cardiac drugs are optimized, while the ECMO support is slowly decreased. When the patient is clamped off, the bridge is unclamped and the sweep gas is disconnected from the membrane. Vital signs and oximetry are closely monitored. Arterial blood gases are obtained and oxygen delivery is assessed. If the patient is to remain off the circuit for an extended period of time (>15 min) the cannulas are flushed periodically by briefly returning the patient to bypass for a few seconds. During long trials off, both the patient and the circuit ACT should be monitored.

Once it is determined that the patient can be decannulated, the procedure is performed at the bedside. All IV infusions except heparin are changed over to the patient's access. When the surgeon is ready, the patient is disconnected from the circuit. Depending on the patient's size, 2–6 units of platelets may be given to the patient to promote adequate hemostasis.

Some centers do not remove the cannulae after discontinuation from the circuit. These patients are at high risk for developing thrombi, which can lead to severe embolic events (35). Therefore, retaining the cannulas should be discouraged and reserved only for patients at high risk for requiring a second ECMO course.

After decannulation, the patient is referred to a follow-up program within the hospital for further evaluations. Depending upon the integrity of the carotid artery, reconstruction of the vessel can be attempted (36).

VI. MECHANICAL COMPLICATIONS

ELSO is the professional group for health care professionals and scientists studying prolonged extracorporeal circulation for cardiac and pulmonary failure. One of ELSO's major responsibilities is to maintain a large central database of reported ECMO cases known as the ELSO Registry (37).

The incidence of oxygenator failure is reported by the ELSO registry to range between 4 and 20% depending on the age category (neonatal, pediatric, adult). Some centers use membrane pressure and blood gas monitoring to diagnose failure. Other centers use platelet count, plasma free hemoglobin, and fibrin split products to demonstrate consumptive coagulopathy that may be caused by an oxygenator with increased clot formation. Significant clot formation in the circuit or membrane may promote a coagulopathy by the activation of complement, white blood cells, platelets, or red blood cells that adhere and lyse on the fibrin strands (38). High circuit pressures (too high a blood flow rate for the reinfusion cannula or increased membrane resistance due to thrombus) will shear red blood cells, causing hemolysis and lead to an elevated plasma free hemoglobin.

Plasma free hemoglobin should be obtained daily, especially when the centrifugal pump is used. Significant elevation in free hemoglobin has prompted some centers to change either the whole circuit (increasing thrombus formation) or the pump's cone if using the centrifugal pump. If a roller pump's occlusion is significantly tight or loose, hemolysis can also occur leading to an elevated free hemoglobin (30).

In cardiac failure the mechanical complications reported to the ELSO Registry are listed in Table 2.

One of the first responsibilities of the bedside ECMO clinician is to be aware of the patient's ability to support themselves if a mechanical complication occurs. This knowledge can dictate how a situation is handled. One also needs to determine if the complication requires immediate removal of the patient from the circuit or if temporary actions can be performed until everyone is prepared. Air seen in the reinfusion line, cannula dislodgement, and an occluded venous line require immediate removal from ECMO. Other complications (e.g., failing membrane, air prior to heat exchanger, clot, pump failure) can be treated with different interventions before removal is necessary (39).

The proper method of removing a patient from ECMO is to clamp the venous line, open the bridge, and clamp the arterial line. Sweep gas is disconnected from the membrane and the pump is turned off. The patient's respiratory support is increased while all blood pressure–dependent drugs are administered to the patient instead of the circuit. Volume boluses should be available for hypotensive episodes. Once the problem with the circuit has been corrected, the blood flow through the circuit is reestablished and the circuit assessed again prior to initiating ECMO.

If air is seen in the reinfusion line, a clamp is immediately placed near the cannula and the pump is shut off. The bridge is opened and the venous

Table 2 Mechanical Complications During Cardiac ECMO

Complications	# Reported	% Reported
Oxygenator Failure	235	7.7%
Raceway Rupture	3	0.1%
Other Tubing Rupture	50	1.6%
Pump Malfunction	48	1.6%
Heat Exchanger Malfunction	21	0.7%
Clots: Oxygenator	31	1.0%
Bridge	23	0.8%
Bladder	30	1.0%
Hemofilter	19	0.6%
Other	47	1.5%
Air in Circuit	13	0.4%

Source: ELSO Registry Report July 1999.

line is then clamped. Again the patient's respiratory and cardiac support is increased and continuously monitored while the problem is being corrected. If it is suspected that air has entered the reinfusion cannula, placing the patient in the Trendelenburg position may divert any infused air away from the cerebral circulation. Attempts should also be made to aspirate air from the reinfusion cannula prior to reestablishing ECMO. Decreasing the circuit temperature to 35°C and treating the patient for increased cerebral pressure should be considered.

The following suggestions are our institution's policy for when to change an entire ECMO circuit versus when to change the membrane only. The exact procedures for responding to mechanical complications should be dictated by the type of equipment each center employs and the experience of the bedside ECMO specialist.

The entire ECMO circuit is changed if any of the following occur:

1. Premembrane pressures > 350 mmHg with no changes in the postmembrane pressure along with the presence of clots identified in other areas of the circuit
2. Inability to remove CO_2 despite maximum sweep gas flow rate along with the presence of clots in other areas of the circuit
3. Unexplained coagulopathy/platelet consumption or high plasma-free hemoglobin
4. Gas to blood leak from the membrane
5. More than 120 hours of continuous amicar use (institutional policy due to circuit complications that occur with extended use) (40)

Only the membrane should be changed if any of the following occur:

1. Premembrane pressure > 350 mmHg with no changes in postmembrane pressures (circuit without clot formation)
2. Inability to remove CO_2 despite maximum sweep gas flow rate (circuit without clot formation)
3. Blood to gas leak that does not seal over (i.e., frank blood vs. pink condensation) without clot formation in the circuit

REFERENCES

1. Montoya JP, Merz SI, Bartlett RH: A standardized system for describing flow/pressure relationships in vascular access devices. Trans Am Soc Artif Internal Organ 1991; 34:4–8.
2. Van Meurs KP, Mikesell GT, Seale WR, Short BL, Rivera O. Maximum blood flow

rates for arterial cannulae used in neonatal ECMO. Trans Am Soc Artif Internal Organ 1990; 36:679–681.
3. Bartlett RH: Extracorporeal life support for cardiopulmonary failure. Curr Probl Surg 1990; 27(10):261–750.
4. Alexander AA, Mitchell DG, Merton DA, et al. Cannula-induced vertebral steal in neonates during extracorporeal membrane oxygenation: detection with color Doppler US. Radiology 1992; 182(2):527–530.
5. Nagaraj HS, Mitchell KA, Fallat ME, Groff DB, Cook LN. Surgical complications and procedures in neonates on extracorporeal membrane oxygenation. J Pediatr Surg 1992; 27:1106–1109; discussion 1109–1110.
6. Rais-Brahrami K, Martin GR, Schnitzer JJ, Short BL. Malposition of extracorporeal membrane oxygenation cannulas in patients with congenital diaphragmatic hernia. J Pediatr 1993; 122 (5 Pt 1):794–797.
7. Mair P, Hoermann C, Moertl M, et al. Percutaneous venoarterial extracorporeal membrane oxygenation for emergency mechanical circulatory support. Resuscitation 1996; 33(1):29–34.
8. Yoshimura N, Ataka K, Nakagiri K, et al. A simple technique for the prevention of lower limb ischemia during femoral veno-arterial cardiopulmonary support. J Cardiovasc Surg 1996; 37(6):557–559.
9. Liem KD, Kollee LA, Klaessens JH, Geven WB, Festen C, DeHaan AF. Disturbance of cerebral oxygenation and hemodynamics related to the opening of the bypass bridge during veno-arterial extracorporeal membrane oxygenation. Pediatr Res 1995; 38(1):124–129.
10. Faulkner S. ELSO techniques survey. Presented at the Extracorporeal Life Support Organization Meeting, Ann Arbor, MI, 1995.
11. Toomasion JM, Kerby KA, Chapman RA, et al. Performance of a rupture-resistant polyvinylchloride tubing. Proc Am Acad Cardiovasc Perfusion 1987; 8:56–59.
12. Atkinson JB, Emerson P, Wheaton R, Bowman CM. A simplified method for autoregulation of blood flow in the extracorporeal membrane oxygenation circuit. J Pediatr Surg 1989; 24(3):251–252.
13. Setz K, Kesser K, Kopotic RJ, Cornish JD. Comparison of a new venous control device with a bladder box system for use in ECMO. ASAIO J 1992; 38(4):835–840.
14. Green TP, Kriesmer P, Steinhorn RH, et al. Comparison of pressure-volume-flow relationships in centrifugal and roller pump extracorporeal membrane oxygenation systems for neonates. ASAIO Trans 1991; 37(4):572–576.
15. Steinhorn RH, Isham-Schopf B, Smith C, Green TP. Hemolysis during long-term extracorporeal membrane oxygenation. J Pediatr 1989; 115(4):625–630.
16. Chevalier JY. Extracorporeal respiratory assistance for pediatric acute respiratory failure. Crit Care Med 1993; 21(9 suppl):S382–383.
17. Montoya JP, Merz SI, Bartlett RH. Laboratory experience for the novel, non-occlusive, pressure regulated parastoltic blood pump. ASAIO J 1992; 38:M411.
18. Kolobow T, Bowman RL: Construction and elimination of an alveolar membrane artificial heart-lung. Trans Am Soc Artif Internal Organ 1963; 9:238.
19. Bartlett RH. Extracorporeal Membrane Oxygenation Technical Specialist Manual. 9th ed. Ann Arbor, MI: University of Michigan, 1988.

20. Galletti PM, Richardson PD, Snider MT. A standardized method for defining the overall gas transfer performance of artificial lungs. ASAIO Trans 1972; 18:359.
21. Visser C, de Jong DS. Leakage across hollow-fiber membrane in oxygenators: a pilot study. Perfusion 1996; 11(5):389–393.
22. Toomasian JM, Hsu LC, Hirschl RB, et al. Evaluation of Duraflo II heparin coating in prolonged extracorporeal membrane oxygenation. Trans Am Soc Artif Internal Organ 1988; 34:410–414.
23. Urlesberger B, Zobel G, Rodl S, et al. Activation of the clotting system: heparin-coated versus non-coated systems for extracorporeal circulation. Int J Artif Organs 1997; 20(12):708–712.
24. Adrian K, Mellgren K, Skogby M, et al. The effect of albumin priming solution on platelet activation during experimental long-term perfusion. Perfusion 1998; 13(3): 187–191.
25. McManus ML, Kevy SV, Bower LK, Hickey PR. Coagulation factor deficiencies during initiation of extracorporeal membrane oxygenation. J Pediatrics 1995; 126(6): 900–904.
26. Cheung PY. Normalization of priming solution ionized calcium concentration improves hemodynamic stability of neonates receiving venovenous ECMO. ASAIO J 1996; 42(6):1033–1034.
27. Sell LL, Cullen ML, Whittlesey GC, Lerner GR, Klein MD. Experience with renal failure during extracorporeal membrane oxygenation: treatment with continuous hemofiltration. J Pediatr Surg 1987; 22(7):600–602.
28. Heiss KF, Pettit B, Hirschl RB, et al. Renal insufficiency and volume overload in neonatal ECMO managed by continuous ultrafiltration. Trans Am Soc Artif Internal Organ 1987; 33:557–560.
29. Riley BJ, Sapatnekar S, Cornell DJ, Anderson J, Walsh-Sukys MC. Impact of prolonged saline solution prime exposure on integrity of extracorporeal membrane oxygenation circuits. J Perinatol 1997; 17(6):444–449.
30. Multidisciplanary Intensive Care Unit. ECMO Clinical Practice Guideline, Children's Hospital, Boston, 1996.
31. Buck ML, Ksenich RA, Wooldridge P. Effects of infusing fat emulsion into extracorporeal membrane oxygenation circuits. Pharmacotherapy 1997; 17(6):1292–1295.
32. Curley MAQ, Thompson JE, Molengraf J, et al. Oxygenation/ventilation. In: Curley MAQ, Smith JB, Maloney-Harmon PA, eds. Critical Care Nursing of Infants and Children. Philadelphia: W.B. Saunders Co., 1996:249–319.
33. Zwischenberger JB, Nguyen TT, Upp JR, Jr., et al. Complications of neonatal extracorporeal membrane oxygenation. Collective experience from the Extracorporeal Life Support Organization. J Thorac Cardiovasc Surg 1994; 107(3):838–848; discussion 848–849.
34. Upp JR Jr, Bush PE, Zwischenberger JB. Complications of neonatal extracorporeal membrane oxygenation. Perfusion 1994; 9(4):241–256.
35. McKay VJ, Stewart DL, Massey MT, et al. Retaining extracorporeal membrane oxygenation cannulae after extracorporeal support in the neonate: is it safe? J Pediatr Surg 1997; 32(5):703–707.
36. Moulton SL, Lynch FP, Cornish JD, et al. Carotid artery reconstruction following neonatal extracorporeal membrane oxygenation. J Pediatr Surg 1991; 26(7):794–799.

37. ECMO Registry Report of the Extracorporeal Life Support Organization. Ann Arbor, MI: 1998.
38. Stammers AH, Fristoe LW, Christensen K, et al. Coagulopathic-induced membrane dysfunction during extracorporeal membrane oxygenation: a case report. Perfusion 1997; 12(2):143–149.
39. Faulkner SC, Chipman CW, Baker LL. Troubleshooting the extracorporeal membrane oxygenator circuit and patient. J Extracorp Technol 1993; 24(4):120–129.
40. Wilson JM, Bower LK, Fackler JC, et al. Amicar decreases the incidence of intracranial and other hemorrhagic complications of ECMO. J Pediatr Surg 1993; 28: 536–541.

8
Management of the Ventricular Assist Device Circuit for Pediatric Cardiac Patients

David M. Farrell, Robert A. LaPierre, Robert J. Howe, and Gregory S. Matte
Children's Hospital, Boston, Massachusetts

I. INTRODUCTION

The pediatric experience with ventricular assist has lagged behind that of the adult industry. Adaptation of adult circuits for use with pediatric patients resulted in lower flow velocity and increased risk of thromboembolism. With the development of a pediatric centrifugal pump head by Medtronic Bio-Medicus, Inc. (Eden Prairie, MN) in the late 1980s, it became possible to provide a safe, effective means of ventricular support for infants and children.

We began our experience with ventricular assist in 1991. The initial goal in developing a protocol was to design a circuit that would be simple in design and hence able to be set up quickly and easily. We identified the factors of durability, reliability, and prime volume as key factors in deciding which type of pump to employ for our system. We have used the Bio-Medicus constrained vortex centrifugal pump system for this application from the inception of the program. This simplicity in design allowed for a reduction in hemodilution, heparinization, radiant heat loss, and damage to the formed elements of blood. This system provides nonpulsatile flow and is sensitive to changes in both preload and afterload.

Subsequently, other nonpulsatile flow impeller devices such as the Hemopump and the intraventricular axial flow pump have been employed for pediatric use. Recently manufacturers have begun miniaturizing pulsatile ventricular devices for pediatric use. We have had minimal contact with these devices, as they are currently not FDA approved. Therefore we will limit our discussion to the management of our current system.

II. CIRCUIT DESIGN

There are many different circuit designs that are used clinically. There are the nonpulsatile pumps such as roller pumps, which are used primarily in extracorporeal membrane oxygenation (ECMO), along with Bio-Medicus (centrifugal pump), and the Hemopump (impeller device). Some of the pulsatile systems that have been used successfully in adults are now being miniaturized for use in the pediatric population. These include the Berlin Heart ventricular assist device (VAD) (Mediport Kardiotechnik, Berlin, Germany), Medos-HIA (Stolberg, Germany) ventricular support system, and the Abiomed BVS5000 (Danvers, MA).

At The Children's Hospital, Boston, we use the Medtronic Bio-Medicus system to perform ventricular support. Depending on the size of the patient and the flow that we want to achieve, we use either the BP50 or the BP80 cone. The BP50, which has $^1/_4$ in. connections, is used at a maximum flow of 1500 cc/min. The BP 80, which has $^3/_8$ in. connections, is used for patients requiring blood flow greater than 1500 cc/min.

III. CIRCUIT CONSTITUENTS

The actual circuit design is very simple. Along with the Bio-Medicus cone are the following items:

Bio-Medicus electromagnetic flow probe (DP-38 for $^3/_8$ in. tubing, and DP-38P for $^1/_4$ in. tubing)
Two 8-foot pieces of appropriate size tubing for the bio head, with a wall thickness of $^3/_{32}$ in.
Cannulae (one for inflow, one for outflow)

All of the above items are Carmeda coated (Medtronic, Inc., Cardiopulmonary Division, Anaheim, CA).

The above-described items are the main components of the VAD circuit. Other miscellaneous items are used during circuit setup and priming, including:

Custom Bently BCR2500 cardiotomy reservoir (Baxter Health Care Corp, Irvine, CA) with 12 in. length of $^3/_8 \times ^3/_{32}$ in. tubing on the outlet port

Table 1 Boston Children's Hospital Basic Left Ventricular Assist Device (LVAD) Circuit Components

1/4 inch VAD setup	3/8 inch VAD setup
3/8 × 1/4 inch connector (cardiotomy to 1/4 inch inflow line)	3/8 × 3/8 inch connector (cardiotomy to 3/8 inch inflow line)
1/4 × 1/4 luer lock connector for flushing	1/4 × 3/8 inch luer lock connector for flushing
1/4 inch tube holding forcep for securing the tubing to the table	3/8 inch tube holding forcep for securing the tubing to the table

and a prime line attached to a SQ40S filter (Pall Biomedical, Inc., Fajardo, PR)
Filtered gas line for CO_2 flushing the circuit prior to priming
1 L Plasmalyte®A pH 7.4 (Baxter Health Care Corp. Deerfield, IL) with 25 mg heparin
CO_2 tank for flushing the circuit
2 ft 1/4 × 1/16 in. tubing
Small prep table for the circuit.
Sterile linen bundle (including several towels, gloves, gown, and fan draw)

Table 1 lists the items that differ between the 1/4 and the 3/8 in. VAD setups.

IV. PRIMING THE VAD CIRCUIT

When the perfusionist is directed to set up and prime a VAD circuit, the equipment listed above is collected and opened in a sterile fashion. Usually two people are involved in this process. The sterile linen bundle is opened on the prep table, and everything except the cardiotomy, Plasmalyte, cannulae, and the CO_2 tank is placed on the prep table. The cardiotomy is opened and placed in its holder (attached to the Bio-Medicus® Bio-Console cart). The Plasmalyte is heparinized and spiked with the SQ40S filter. A clamp is placed below the outlet of the cardiotomy, and the 1 L bag of Plasmalyte is added.

One person scrubs and gowns for the sterile portion of the circuit priming. The first 8-foot length of tubing is attached to the inlet of the cone, while a second 8-foot length of tubing is attached to the outlet. Approximately 15 inches past the outflow of the head, the tubing is cut and the electromagnetic flow probe is inserted. This distance ensures laminar flow through the probe while minimizing interference from the rotary magnet of the console. A size-appropriate luer lock connector is connected to the end of the outflow line, and the 2-foot length of ¼ in. tubing is attached, clamped, and handed off to the other perfusionist, who connects it to a suction port on the cardiotomy. The gas line is attached to the luer lock connector, handed off, and the circuit is CO_2 flushed for approximately 1–2 minutes. Once the circuit has been gassed, the gas line is disconnected, the luer lock is recapped, the appropriate connector is attached to the inflow line, and that is passed off the table and connected to the ⅜ in, outflow line of the cardiotomy.

An effort is made to maximize the length of sterile tubing remaining on the sterile field. At the time of cannulation, the surgeon determines the length that is actually needed. Quite often the inflow and outflow lines are reduced to 4–5 feet in length. We find that this provides safe, adequate length for transportation, patient positioning, and intensive care unit (ICU) management. The lines are attached to the table using clamps designed by Cardiovascular Instrument Corporation (Wakefield, MA). These are very effective in keeping the tubing immobilized during ICU management and transport.

At the time priming is initiated, a clamp is placed between the centrifugal head and the flow probe. This will be used to control the speed of priming the circuit. The outlet line from the cardiotomy is raised above the fluid level in the reservoir, and the clamp is released. The appropriate connector is debubbled, and the fluid is slowly allowed to follow the path to the head. The sterile perfusionist determines the speed. The head is raised or lowered to allow for the fluid to advance or retreat down the lines. Once the Plasmalyte has started entering the head, the head is slowly turned so that the outlet of the head is in the highest position to allow the air to escape. Once the fluid has filled the entire head and continued past the flow probe, the line is clamped and the head is given a couple of hard shakes to dislodge any air that may be trapped. If air is seen, it is walked up the line, the clamp is opened, and the air is allowed to pass the clamp. The line is then reclamped, and this procedure is repeated until the head appears to be free of air.

At this point, the clamp is opened and the Plasmalyte is allowed to continue the rest of the way to the cardiotomy. The centrifugal head is then handed off and attached to the console, trying to keep as much of the line as possible on the table. Flow is established and the lines are debubbled starting at the outlet of the cardiotomy. Once the lines have been debubbled up to the head, a clamp is placed on the outflow line of the centrifugal pump, the pump flow is turned off, and the head is quickly removed, shaken, and inspected for air. If air is seen, it is walked up the head to the outlet, the head is then put back in the console, flow is turned on, and the clamp is removed so that the air is sent back to the cardiotomy. This procedure is repeated until all air has been removed. This can be accomplished very quickly depending on how fast the unit was allowed to prime.

Once the circuit has been successfully primed and debubbled, the sterile circuit is isolated. The cardiotomy is removed from the Bio-Medicus console and discarded. Sterile labels are applied to the inflow and outflow lines that are passed from the centrifugal head to the field for added safety during cannulation. The flow probe transducer is applied, clamped out, and calibrated. At this point, the circuit is delivered to the table. The lines are handed to the surgeons and the console is placed as close to the table as possible.

V. CANNULATION

The cannulae used for ventricular assist are surgeon dependent in many institutions. Regardless of this subjectivity, there are certain cannulae characteristics that are universally ideal for VADs. These characteristics are listed in Table 2. With these characteristics in mind, we use Bio-Medicus arterial and venous cannulae the majority of the time. Bard (C. R. Bard, Inc., Haverhill, MA) arterial and Medtronic DLP (Medtronic DLP, Inc., Grand Rapids, MI) venous cannulae are occasionally used as well. Additionally, one must also consider utilizing the cannulae currently in use for the postcardiotomy cardiogenic shock patient being converted to ventricular assistance from cardiopulmonary bypass (CPB).

The cannulation sites for ventricular assist in infant and pediatric patients do not vary greatly. Typically for left ventricular assist, the left atrial appendage or the superior pulmonary vein is cannulated to provide centrifugal pump inflow. The ascending aorta then serves as the pump outflow (Fig. 1) Generally for right ventricular assist, the right atrial appendage is cannulated to provide centrifugal pump inflow while the main pulmonary artery is cannulated to serve as pump outflow. For the CPB patient being converted to ventricular assist in the operating room, the CPB cannulation sites and/or cannulae may be used depending on their location and whether or not the chest will be closed for transport to the intensive care unit.

Table 2 Ideal Characteristics of Cannulae for VADs

Maximal inside to outside diameter ratio
Nonthrombogenic
Flexible without kinking
Clear color for visual inspection
Venous: multiple side holes

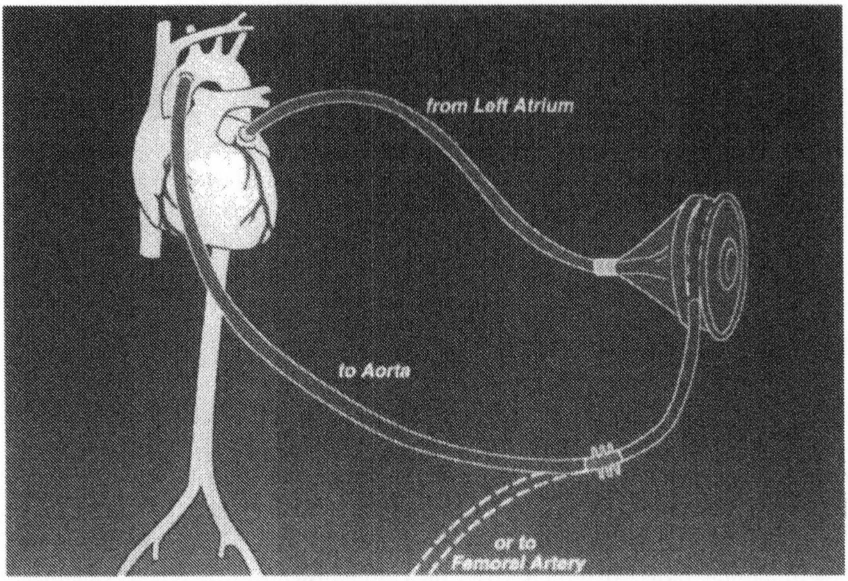

Fig. 1 Boston Children's Hospital basic Left Ventriclar Assist Device (LVAD) circuit.

VI. INITIATION OF SUPPORT

Following cannulation, an air-free connection is made between the pump circuit and the cannulae. Once the proper circuit set-up is verified, ventricular assist can be initiated. The revolutions per minute (rpm) of the centrifugal head are increased prior to removing the outflow clamp. This is done to prevent back flow upon initiation of support. Flow is established while observing the circuit and pertinent patient parameters. For left ventricular assist, the left atrial pressure (LAP) and arterial blood pressure (ABP) are primarily followed. Within the limits of the centrifugal pump, circuit, and patient preload, an increase in pump rpm and thus flow will decrease the LAP and increase the ABP. For right ventricular assistance, the central venous pressure (CVP) and pulmonary arterial pressure (PAP) are primarily followed. Once again within limits, an increase in pump flow will decrease the CVP and increase the PAP. Generally speaking, a balance is sought for maintaining the LAP and/or CVP below a defined limit while maintaining the ABP and/or PAP above a defined limit.

The balance obtained between ventricular preload and afterload is unique to each patient. Upon initiating support, it is important to integrate the volume and pharmacological management of the patient with the ventricular support. While it is beyond the scope of this chapter to describe this integration in depth, it is important to note that for optimal VAD support, pump preload must be adequately maintained.

Once this acceptable balance is found, we define the pump flow–to–rpm ratio. This relationship can be a helpful diagnostic tool for the duration of support. For example, the need for increased rpm to maintain the same pump flow without a change in arterial blood pressure may indicate an outflow tubing or cannula problem. Overall, this parameter is followed with respect to preload and systemic vascular resistance to monitor the patient-pump circuit.

VII. CIRCUIT MONITORING

Typically, we distinguish between two types of patients for VAD support. These are (a) postcardiotomy, failure-to-wean patients and (b) medical ICU patients who are refractory to medical management.

VIII. HEPARIN

A. Postcardiotomy Patients

After termination of bypass and the initiation of the VAD, the patient remains fully heparinized until the hemodynamics are satisfactory. At the surgeon's direction, the anesthesiologist will administer protamine. The patient's activated clotting time (ACT) is reduced to high normal values. These values will be maintained until hemostasis is under control, which may take several hours. After hemostasis is achieved, low-dose heparin is administered through an infusion line to maintain mildly elevated ACT values between 220 and 240 seconds, when using a Hemochron 401 (International Technidyne, Edison, NJ) and P214/P215 glass activated tubes. Boluses of heparin can be given on an as-needed basis if the ACT drops too low. Prior to weaning off the VAD, heparinization is increased to achieve higher ACTs due to the reduction in flow through VAD and the potential of thrombosis due to stagnation.

B. Nonpostcardiotomy Patients

These patients receive 50 units/kg of heparin, one quarter of the prebypass heparinization dose, given as a bolus prior to cannulation. During cannulation, a blood sample is obtained to ensure adequate ACT elevation. After the initiation of VAD support, the ACT measurements are maintained at mildly elevated values as stated above.

IX. ALARMS

In trying to maintain simplicity in design and function of the VAD circuit, we have limited the use of mechanical alarms to the high- and low-flow alarms that are integrated into the Bio-Medicus console. Setting the high- and low-flow alarms 20% higher and lower, respectively, has yielded safe margins of management, since the flow can frequently change in response to alterations in blood flow, pressure, and/or resistance. The simplicity in design and function that we use requires substantial and consistent visual, auditory, and tactile monitoring. Visual checks of the circuit include detection of chattering lines and fibrin strands at connector sites as well as at the centrifugal head itself. Color changes at connector sites may be an indication of fibrin clot formation. Auditory checks include listening to the centrifugal head for vibration noises as well as any other sounds that may indicate changes or problems with the circuit. Tactile checks include feeling the line coming from the patient to the head to determine if the line is chattering. This may be a situation where the preload is inadequate or the cannula is obstructed. Another check is to place one's hands on the centrifugal head itself to feel for vibrations or heat changes from the spinning magnet.

After termination of VAD support, we typically drain the circuit through gauze sponges. Visual examination of the sponges and the circuit around connector sites and cone is performed to identify the presence of clots. This information is used for ongoing evaluation of the VAD management protocol.

X. PATIENT MONITORING

A. Atrial Pressure

Well-placed, functioning pressure lines are of paramount importance to successfully monitor and manage the physiological parameters of a patient on a VAD. Left and right atrial lines must be positioned and functioning prior to the initiation of flow from the VAD. In the setting of an LVAD, the left atrial pressure reveals the off-loading of volume from the left ventricle. The amount of ventricular off-loading required is determined by the physician and is based on the amount of recovery time needed for the myocardium and the amount of work they would like the heart to perform. The atrial filling pressure should not be allowed to drop below zero in order to prevent cavitation and subsequent air entrainment in the VAD circuit. The right atrial pressure is monitored to assess whether the right ventricle is functioning properly or progressing into failure.

B. Arterial Pressure

After initiation of the VAD, the ventricle becomes off-loaded, and flow is increased until the arterial waveform is diminished. The waveform is diminished due to the continuous laminar flow from the VAD. The physician determines the range of mean arterial pressures for each patient based on the patient's specific anatomy and physiology. Once the hemodynamics on the VAD are acceptable, inotropic support can be weaned to allow the myocardium sufficient time to recover. Leaving the patient on inotropic support increases the work the heart must perform and therefore increases the oxygen demand and consumption. Weaning the inotropes reduces the oxygen demand and allows the myocardium to replenish its stores of high-energy phosphates.

Inotropic support can be restarted if the right ventricle begins to fail or when myocardium has recovered and it is deemed that the patient can be weaned from the VAD. Prior to the initiation of weaning, inotropic support may commence, enabling the heart to take over progressively more work.

C. Electrocardiogram

The EKG should be monitored to ensure adequate delivery of oxygen to the compromised myocardium. If the heart fibrillates, there will be a loss of flow to the atrial cannula, with the potential of cavitation and the concomitant reduction in VAD output. Filling pressures and the EKG are also good assessments for the development of right-sided failure.

XI. WEANING

If the injury to the myocardium is reversible, there are usually signs of recovery within 48–120 hours. Once it is felt that the patient is ready to be weaned from support, conditions are optimized to support the rested myocardium. Inotropic therapy is reinstituted or increased. Afterload reduction therapy and antiarrhythmic therapy may be employed. The weaning process results in decreased flow velocity in the circuit. This decrease in flow velocity and the need to leave the cannulae in place transiently after weaning necessitates increased anticoagulation.

Once pharmacology is optimized and the intensivist and surgeon are present, the support flow is reduced incrementally. Echocardiography may be employed to assess myocardial function during the weaning process. If myocardial recovery is sufficient and hemodynamics are stable, the patient is decannulated.

XII. SUMMARY

Ventricular support utilizing a simple centrifugal support system has been shown to be effective in pediatric patients. However, further developments in technology may provide greater benefits. These emerging technologies may provide pulsatile flow, greatly reduced prime volumes, and more automation resulting in less intensive management.

REFERENCES

1. Duncan BW, Hraska V, Jonas RA, Blume ED, del Nido PJ, Wessel DL, Laussen PC, LaPierre RA, Wilson JM. Mechanical circulatory support for pediatric cardiac patients. J Thorac Cardiovasc Surg 1999; 117:529–542.
2. del Nido PJ, Duncan BW, Mayer JE, Jr., Wessel DL, Lapierre RL, Jonas RA. Left ventricular assist device improves survival in children with left ventricular dysfunction after repair of anomalous origin of the left coronary artery from the pulmonary artery. Ann Thorac Surg 1999; 67:169–172.
3. Meliones JN, Custer JR, Snedecor S, Moler FW, O'Rourke P, Delius RE. Extracorporeal life support for cardiac assist in pediatric patients. Circulation 1991; 84(suppl III):III-168–III-172.
4. Karl TR, Sano S, Horton S, Mee RBB. Centrifugal pump left heart assist in pediatric cardiac operations. J Thorac Cardiovasc Surg 1991; 102:624–630.
5. Marcus B, Atkinson JB, Wong PC, Chang AC, Wells WJ, Lindesmith GG, Starnes VA. Successful use of transesophageal echocardiography during extracorporeal membrane oxygenation support as a bridge to pediatric heart transplantation. Circulation 1994; 90(part 2):II-66–II-69.

9

Use of Rapid Deployment Extracorporeal Membrane Oxygenation for the Resuscitation of Children with Cardiac Disease after Cardiac Arrest

Brian W. Duncan
Children's Hospital and Regional Medical Center and University of Washington School of Medicine, Seattle, Washington

I. INTRODUCTION

Cardiac arrest may complicate the course of any child with cardiac disease, particularly in the postoperative period after congenital heart surgery. These children represent the most critically ill subset of an already challenging patient population. Conventional cardiopulmonary resuscitation (CPR) in adults and children has often yielded dismal results (1,2). Mechanical circulatory support has been utilized in adult patients with cardiac arrest in a number of settings but without significant improvement in outcome (3–5). The use of extracorporeal membrane oxygenation (ECMO) to resuscitate children suffering cardiac arrest after cardiac surgery has demonstrated better results than in many other pediatric patient groups (6,7). In this chapter, the use of ECMO to resuscitate children with cardiac disease who suffer cardiopulmonary arrest will be reviewed by analyzing our results with the development of a "rapid resuscitation" ECMO circuit followed by a review of the literature that pertains to this area. Although critically ill, the available data suggest that pediatric patients with cardiac disease who suffer cardiac arrest represent a salvageable group, which might do best with an aggressive approach.

II. COMPONENTS OF A RAPID RESUSCITATION ECMO PROGRAM

Based on these considerations we developed a modified ECMO circuit, made personnel immediately available, and streamlined the priming process to expeditiously institute support in pediatric cardiac patients who suffered cardiac arrest refractory to conventional CPR (8).

A. Components of the Rapid Resuscitation ECMO Circuit

The rapid resuscitation circuit is modified from the standard ECMO circuit to allow the institution of support within 15 minutes of notification of its need. Maintained in the intensive care unit on a cart with a battery power supply, the circuit is completely mobile and can be wheeled to any location in the hospital. The circuit is maintained by a vacuum and CO_2-primed with a 0.8 m^2 membrane oxygenator (Avecor Cardiovascular, Inc., Plymouth, MN) in line. This oxygenator is capable of supporting flows of 1.2 L/min suitable for children up to 10 kg. For larger children up to 25 kg, a 1.5 m^2 membrane is spliced into the circuit (1.8 L/min maximum flow rate).

When needed for resuscitation of patients that suffer cardiac arrest postoperatively, direct aortic and atrial cannulation via the chest usually provides the most expeditious means of instituting support while allowing the performance of effective, open CPR. In patients that have arrested in settings other than the postoperative period, femoral or neck cannulation is performed at the discretion of the surgeon. The rapid resuscitation circuit is Normosol (Abbott Laboratories, Abbott Park, IL) primed with the addition of 50 cc of 5% albumin and debubbled at the bedside. Normosol has been substituted for the standard saline prime in the rapid resuscitation circuit to minimize electrolyte disturbances with the institution of support. The circuit is connected to the cannulas and ECMO support is initiated.

B. Addition of Blood Components

When deployment of the rapid resuscitation ECMO circuit is requested, the blood bank is also notified to procure blood products for addition to the circuit. If blood products are not available when cannulation is complete, support is initiated with the crystalloid primed circuit and then 200 cc packed red blood cells, 100 cc fresh frozen plasma, and 2 units of cryoprecipitate are added to the circuit when available. For those patients who have support instituted with a crystalloid primed circuit, blood is usually available for addition to the circuit within 15–60 minutes of the institution of support. Blood is then added to the circuit and crystalloid volume is removed using a one-for-one syringe exchange transfusion. We use the Amicon (W. R. Grace and Co., Beverly, MA) ultrafiltration system to further remove crystalloid volume as blood products are added, once hemodynamics on support have stabilized.

C. Rapid Resuscitation ECMO Team

A key component of the rapid resuscitation program is the maintenance of personnel in the hospital at all times for the institution of urgent ECMO support. If a pediatric cardiac patient suffers cardiac arrest and there is no response to standard resuscitative measures after 10 minutes, a cardiologist or cardiac surgeon initiates a call for rapid resuscitation ECMO. On-call members of cardiac surgery, cardiology, and cardiac nursing are notified that emergency ECMO is required. The circuit is then transported to the patient's bedside and priming is initiated while cannulation is proceeding.

III. ANALYSIS OF RESULTS FOR RAPID RESUSCITATION ECMO

We reviewed the course of 11 patients that were treated with rapid resuscitation ECMO during 1996 (8). All children were in full cardiopulmonary arrest, receiving CPR at the time of ECMO cannulation. We compared these patients to 7 historical controls who were resuscitated with the standard ECMO circuit prior to development of the rapid resuscitation approach.

A. Demographics and Setting of Support

Demographic data for the patients treated with rapid resuscitation ECMO are listed in Table 1. Seven of the 11 patients were less than one year of age, while 3 of the 11 were less than 30 days of age. Nine of the 11 patients had support instituted in the postoperative period (Table 2). Patient 2, with pulmonary atresia, intact septum, experienced sudden ventricular fibrillation during an otherwise stable preoperative course. After stabilization and diagnostic cardiac catheterization on ECMO, the patient was transported to the operating room, where conver-

Table 1 Patient Characteristics

Sex	3 female, 8 male
Age	109 days (2 days–4.6 years)[a]
Weight	4.9 kg (2.5–15.6 kg)
Time after surgery (N = 9)	10 hours (2–192 hours)
Hours on ECMO	65 hours (2–210 hours)
Days chest open	6.5 days (0–27 days)
Days intubated	13.5 days (4–78 days)
Total hospital days	29.5 days (10–65 days)

[a] Median values are listed with ranges in parentheses.
Source: Ref. 8.

Table 2 Diagnoses, Procedures, and Outcomes

Patient	Setting	Age (days)	Weight (kg)	Diagnosis	Procedure	Outcome
1	Postop	207	4.9	DORV-VSD	Baffle of VSD to aorta	Survived
2	Preop	5	2.9	PA-IVS	TAP, RMBTS	Survived
3	Postop	2	4.5	HLHS	Norwood procedure	Died
4	Postop	12	2.9	Heterotaxy, PA	LMBTS	Survived
5	Postop	567	10.5	Mitral regurgitation	Mitral valve repair	Died
6	Cath lab	1667	15.6	TOF-PA	Coiling of aortopulmonary collaterals	Survived
7	Postop	109	4.9	Transitional AV canal	Patch closure of ASD, VSD; mitral valve repair	Survived
8	Postop	631	10.5	Corrected TGA, PA	IVC-TV baffle; VSD-aorta baffle; RV-PA conduit	Survived
9	Postop	1120	12.0	Rejection	Status post cardiac transplant	Late death
10	Postop	58	2.5	TOF	TOF repair (VSD closure; TAP)	Died
11	Postop	39	3.3	Truncus arteriosus	Truncus arteriosus repair (VSD closure, RV-PA conduit)	Died

DORV = Double outlet right ventricle; VSD = ventricular septal defect; PA = pulmonary atresia; IVS = intact ventricular septum; TAP = transannular patch; MBTS = modified Blalock-Taussing shunt; HLHS = hypoplastic left heart syndrome; TOF = tetralogy of Fallot; ASD = atrial septal defect; TGA = transposition of the great arteries; IVC = inferior vena cava; TV = tricuspid valve; RV-PA = right ventricle-pulmonary artery.
Source: Ref. 8.

sion to standard cardiopulmonary bypass for surgical repair was performed. Due to hypoxia postoperatively ECMO was continued via chest cannulation. The patient was subsequently weaned and survived. Patient 6 with tetralogy of Fallot and pulmonary atresia had support instituted in the cardiac catheterization laboratory following cardiac arrest due to hypoxia while aortopulmonary collaterals were being coiled. This patient was resuscitated with ECMO and eventually discharged with definitive repair being performed during a subsequent hospitalization. The diagnoses of the 7 historical control patients included ventricular septal defect with aortic coarctation, tricuspid atresia, transposition of the great arteries, transposition of the great arteries with ventricular septal defect, severe mitral regurgitation after repair of a transitional atrioventricular canal, total anomalous pulmonary venous return, and complete atrioventricular canal.

B. Nonsurvivors

Patient 3 was a patient with hypoplastic left heart syndrome that suffered ventricular failure and cardiac arrest after a Norwood procedure (Table 2). This patient was successfully resuscitated with ECMO and was eventually weaned from support. This patient subsequently expired due to multisystem organ failure after cardiac transplantation. Patient 5 suffered cardiac arrest due to progressive left ventricular failure after mitral valve repair. After resuscitation with ECMO the patient was unable to be weaned from support and underwent cardiac transplantation. This patient subsequently developed a mycotic aneurysm of the aortic anastomosis of the cardiac allograft, which resulted in the patient's demise. Patient 10 was an infant with multiple congenital anomalies who suffered sudden cardiac arrest the night after repair of tetralogy of Fallot, presumably due to arrhythmia. During cannulation there were significant time periods when open cardiac compressions were discontinued. This resulted in severe hypoxic damage to all organ systems, and ECMO was electively discontinued the following day. This was the only patient in this series in whom ECMO was not successfully weaned. Patient 11 was a child with sudden cardiac arrest after truncus arteriosus repair, possibly due to a pulmonary hypertensive crisis. ECMO was instituted and eventually weaned successfully, however, within 24 hours of discontinuing ECMO the patient developed supersystemic pulmonary artery pressures that failed to respond to conventional measures. ECMO was again instituted via neck cannulation for an additional 6 days, at which point the patient developed overwhelming mediastinal sepsis resulting in his demise. Patient 9 represents the only late death in this series. This patient was born with hypoplastic left heart syndrome and underwent cardiac transplantation for progressive ventricular dysfunction at 3 years of age after a Norwood procedure and a subsequent bidirectional Glenn shunt. This patient suffered cardiac arrest during an episode of severe rejection and was successfully weaned from ECMO after treatment of the rejection episode. The patient was discharged from the hospital with mild hypoxic encephalopathy but eventually developed disseminated lymphoma, resulting in death.

C. Sites of Cannulation

Seven patients were cannulated in the immediate postoperative period through the chest. Patient 8 suffered cardiac arrest the night following surgery after a complex reconstruction for corrected transposition of the great arteries with pulmonary atresia and was cannulated through the chest. This patient was subsequently converted to a left ventricular assist device after a successful resuscitation and a brief period (2 hours) of ECMO support. Patient 11 was cannulated in the immediate postoperative period through the chest and was successfully weaned from ECMO but was recannulated via the neck on postoperative day 8 as discussed above. Patients 4 and 9 suffered cardiac arrest 10 and 8 days after cardiac surgery, respectively, and were cannulated through the neck. Patient 2 was cannulated preoperatively through the neck and was recannulated through the chest for postoperative support as detailed above. Patient 6 had ECMO initiated in the cardiac catheterization laboratory via sheathes in the femoral vessels while neck cannulation was being performed and was subsequently converted to neck cannulation.

D. Complications

Cardiovascular complications (Table 3) included two patients that required cardiac transplantation due to lack of return of native cardiac function on ECMO and

Table 3 Complications

Complication	Number of patients
Cardiovascular	4
Pulmonary	3
Gastrointestinal	3
Renal failure	2
Neurological	4
Hemorrhage	2
Any infection	5
Positive blood cultures	3
Mediastinitis	3
Pneumonia	2
Mechanical	1

Source: Ref. 8.

two cases with significant ventricular ectopy. The three pulmonary complications included single cases of pulmonary infarction, pulmonary hemorrhage, and a pneumothorax. The gastrointestinal complications included upper gastrointestinal hemorrhage due to gastritis, nutritional failure requiring gastrostomy tube placement, and one patient with unexplained chronic elevation of liver function tests. There were two cases of renal failure requiring dialysis. One of these patients had recovery of renal function by the time of hospital discharge, while one of these patients did not recover renal function prior to death. Neurological complications occurred in four patients and included two cases of mild hypoxic encephalopathy, one patient with choreoathetosis, and one patient with seizures. The single mechanical complication was due to aortic cannula dislodgment 30 minutes after support was initiated. The patient was quickly recannulated successfully.

E. Outcome

Figure 1 compares the median duration of CPR in patients receiving rapid resuscitation ECMO with seven historical control patients resuscitated with a stan-

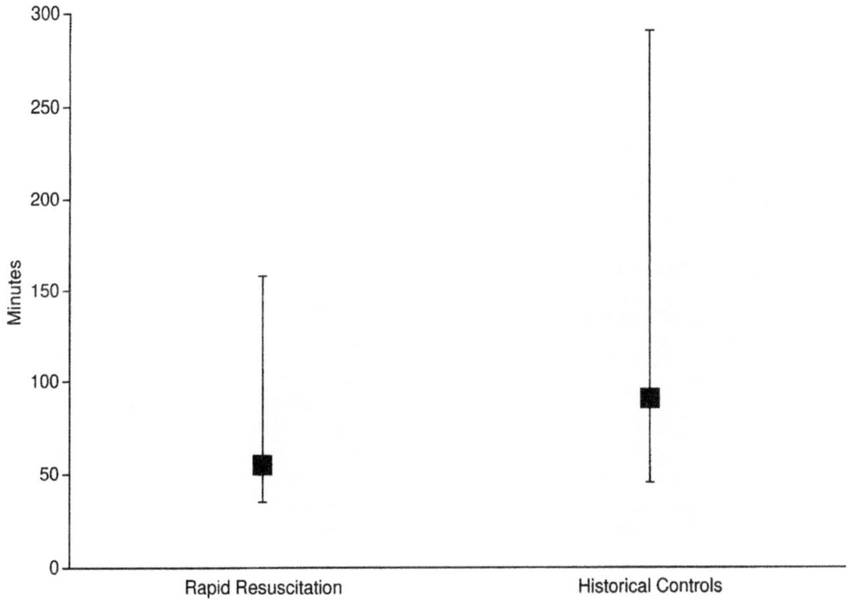

Fig. 1 Duration of CPR for patients resuscitated with rapid resuscitation ECMO circuit since February 1996 (N = 11) compared with historical controls resuscitated with standard ECMO circuit prior to 1996 (N = 7); $p = 0.085$. (From Ref. 8.)

dard ECMO circuit prior to 1996. The median duration of CPR for the rapid resuscitation group was 55 minutes (range 20–103 min) and was 90 minutes (range 45–200 min) for the historical controls. The duration of CPR was more than 30 minutes less with the rapid resuscitation circuit ($p = 0.085$). The duration of CPR for survivors [58 min (range 25–103 min)] and nonsurvivors [51 min (range 20–83 min)] in the rapid resuscitation patients was not significantly different ($p = 0.63$). Figure 2 compares the outcomes between the rapid resuscitation patients and the historical controls. A single patient in the rapid resuscitation group failed to wean from ECMO. The hospital survival in the rapid resuscitation group [7/11 survivors; 64% (CL 45–81%)] represents a substantial improvement over the historical control group [2/7 survivors; 29% (CL 10–55%)] ($p = 0.15$). Figure 3 demonstrates the NYHA functional status in the six long-term survivors after rapid resuscitation ECMO. All but one survivor is in NYHA class 1, with one patient in class II. One of the six long-term survivors demonstrates mild neurological impairment, while one child is moderately impaired (Fig. 4).

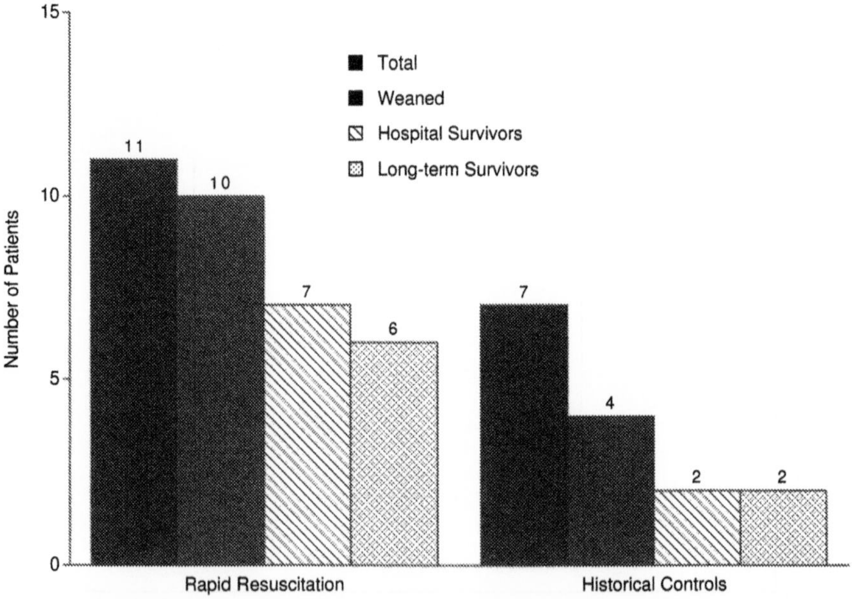

Fig. 2 Outcomes for rapid resuscitation ECMO patients and historical controls. Total patients undergoing ECMO resuscitation, patients successfully weaned from ECMO, in-hospital survivors, and long-term survivors are demonstrated for both groups. (From Ref. 8.)

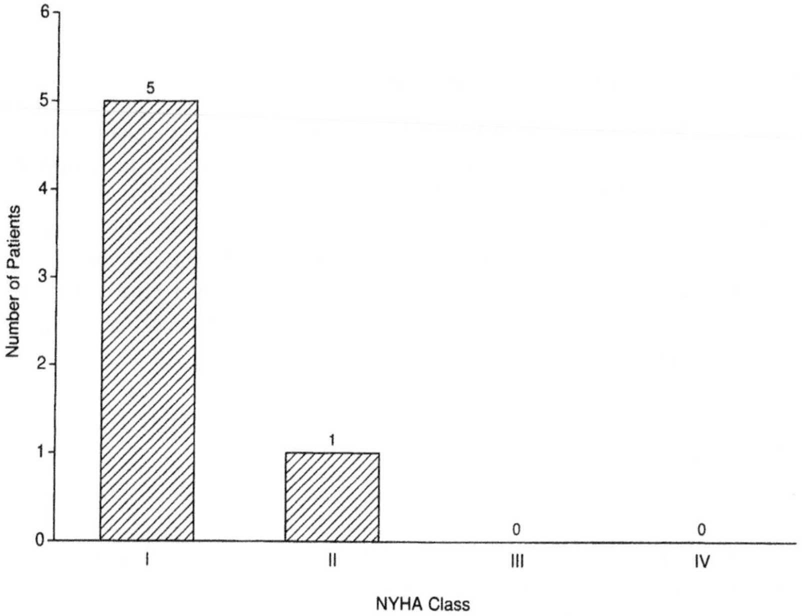

Fig. 3 New York Heart Association (NYHA) classification of six long-term survivors after ECMO rapid resuscitation. (From Ref. 8.)

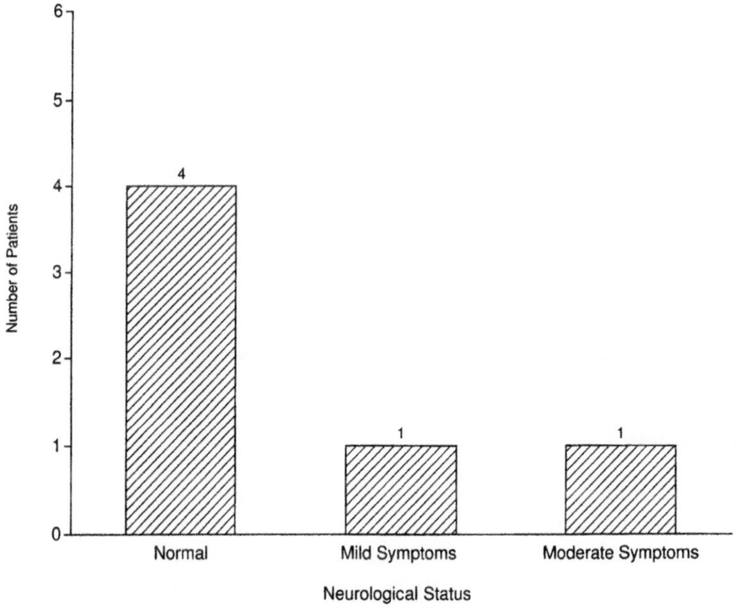

Fig. 4 Neurological status of six long-term survivors after ECMO rapid resuscitation. (From Ref. 8.)

F. Prime Composition and Outcome

Data regarding the composition of the ECMO prime at the time of institution of support is available for 8 of the 11 patients. Six of these 8 patients had support instituted with crystalloid, while 2 had support instituted with a blood primed circuit. Of the 6 patients that received ECMO support with a circuit initially primed with crystalloid, 5 (83%) were successfully weaned from support and 4 (67%) survived to hospital discharge. Both patients supported with a blood-primed ECMO circuit were successfully weaned from support, and one of these patients (50%) survived to hospital discharge.

IV. DISCUSSION

A. General

Mechanical circulatory support for the resuscitation of patients suffering cardiac arrest has gained increasingly widespread use in a number of settings (3–5,9,10). The application of mechanical circulatory support for this indication has arisen due to the dismal outcome of conventional resuscitative measures in these patients (11,12). Despite initial enthusiasm for ECMO in the setting of cardiac arrest in adults, substantial mortality persists in most reports (4). However, previous reports using ECMO to support pediatric cardiac patients suffering cardiac arrest suggest that their outcomes may be better, justifying an aggressive approach in their resuscitation (6,7). The reasons for better outcomes in pediatric cardiac patients may relate to witnessed arrests in an intensive care unit setting, the use of effective, open CPR in postoperative patients, and a greater degree of core cooling during cardiac arrest in children compared to adults. In addition, the etiology of cardiac arrest in these children is often due to a transient arrhythmia or other reversible causes, such as pulmonary hypertensive crisis. The impact of core cooling and effective CPR is supported by the data in the present study, where 10 of 11 patients were successfully weaned from ECMO with excellent end-organ function. Only a single patient had evidence of significant hypoperfusion during resuscitation requiring termination of support due to advanced end-organ failure.

B. Other Reports

Our experience is similar to results reported by del Nido where 11 children suffered cardiac arrest after cardiac surgery and were resuscitated with ECMO (7). In this experience, cardiac arrest accounted for 33% of all indications for ECMO support. ECMO support was expeditiously instituted with a circuit that was maintained assembled but unprimed after a mean CPR duration of 65 minutes (range

20–110 min). Six patients (55%) survived to hospital discharge with no long-term sequelae in any of the survivors. The authors stated that the outcome for patients with cardiac arrest was better than patients supported for severe postoperative cardiac dysfunction without cardiac arrest (55% vs. 33% survival, respectively). These results support the concept that these patients are salvageable and deserve an aggressive approach during resuscitation with prompt institution of ECMO if conventional resuscitative measures fail.

Interestingly, a recent review of the ELSO Registry for neonates with respiratory failure who required CPR prior to ECMO support found a substantial percentage of these patients survived (61%), with nearly two thirds of these patients demonstrating grossly normal neurological outcomes (13). These results led the authors to conclude that cardiac arrest should not be a contraindication to ECMO in neonates with respiratory failure. The overall good results obtained for ECMO resuscitation of children with cardiac and noncardiac disease are quite different from the dismal results reported for conventional CPR in children that suffer cardiac arrest in the intensive care unit (14,15). Prompt normalization of cardiac output provided by ECMO may be responsible for improved survival rates in ECMO resuscitated children compared with pediatric medical patients treated with conventional CPR.

In fact, we believe that the most important factor in the successful resuscitation of these patients is the prompt establishment of an adequate cardiac output. This rapid resuscitation approach begins with a prompt decision to institute ECMO support in patients who have not responded to routine resuscitative measures after cardiac arrest. We currently initiate a call for rapid resuscitation ECMO for our patients who suffer cardiac arrest if CPR is unsuccessful after 10 minutes. Other important components of this approach include using a modified ECMO circuit to facilitate rapidly instituting support and creating an organized team to minimize response times. Although having 24-hour in-house coverage by personnel who can perform priming is a distinct advantage to the success of these programs, hospitals can still increase the speed and efficiency of the institution of ECMO in emergency situations without costly additional personnel. Most centers can improve response times for ECMO resuscitation by relatively simple means. These include providing a clear line of communication for notification of the ECMO team in the event of a cardiac arrest, establishing efficient protocols for mobilizing operating room resources to the patient's bedside for cannulation, and establishing logical and simple storage for circuit components and related equipment. We have found that the most important ingredient for decreasing response times is facilitating communication by standardized protocols to ensure that the diverse personnel (surgery, operating room staff, nursing, blood bank, perfusion or other priming personnel) required to provide ECMO in an emergency setting can be quickly and efficiently mobilized.

C. Crystalloid Versus Blood Priming of the Circuit

In our prior experience we found that routine priming of the ECMO circuit led to delays in the institution of support. A source of significant delay was consistently incurred while waiting for blood products and the subsequent blood-priming step. We currently institute support with a crystalloid primed circuit if blood is not available to establish adequate hemodynamics as quickly as possible. The majority of the patients in this series had support instituted with a crystalloid primed circuit without apparent detriment to end-organ function. Blood is added to the circuit when it becomes available, which is usually within 30 minutes of the institution of ECMO. We have not used O-negative or type-specific blood, however, if excessive delays in receiving cross-matched blood occur, the use of non–cross-matched blood products could be considered. Ultrafiltration can be performed as blood is added to remove crystalloid volume from the circuit when hemodynamics have stabilized.

D. Further Management

Once support is instituted this patient population requires meticulous management. Temporary ventricular dysfunction is often profound. We aggressively monitor for left ventricular distention by transesophageal echocardiography and measurement of left-sided filling pressures. We incorporate a left atrial vent into the circuit or perform balloon atrial septostomy if left ventricular distention occurs. Balloon atrial septostomy may be performed in the cardiac catheterization laboratory or at the bedside under echocardiographic guidance (16). If left ventricular distension is avoided, many of these patients can be expected to require relatively brief periods of ECMO support, providing further evidence of the reversible nature of the etiology of cardiac arrest in the majority of these cases.

E. Complications

The complications and deaths in our series are an indication of the gravity of the clinical condition of these patients. Bleeding complications are common in patients undergoing postoperative mechanical circulatory support, and in our previous analysis excessive blood loss was a risk factor for in-hospital death (17). Mediastinal sepsis was also a common source of morbidity and mortality in this patient population. Two of the four deaths in our series were due to mediastinal infections that were undoubtedly due to the fact that the majority of these children were cannulated through the chest (8). The development of percutaneous systems for femoral cannulation for children may eliminate lengthy periods where the chest is open leading to a decrease in the incidence of mediastinitis in these patients.

Neurological complications were less common in the 11 rapid resuscitation patients than might be predicted, attesting to the importance of effective CPR and prompt ECMO institution. We further attempt to lessen the impact of central nervous system ischemia suffered during resuscitation by aggressive, controlled hypothermia (18). This begins at the time of cardiac arrest by placing ice around the patient's head during cannulation while CPR is performed. We then maintain patient temperature at 34°C or less during the first 24 hours of support and avoid temperature elevations above 37°C at any time during the first few days of support. Long-term neurological follow-up will be necessary to determine the ultimate functional status of these children.

V. SUMMARY

Pediatric cardiac patients who suffer cardiac arrest appear to represent a subset of patients with a potentially favorable outcome. Apparently reversible etiologies of cardiac arrest in these patients may be quickly diagnosed and treated during brief periods of ECMO support. The most important factor leading to a successful outcome in these children is the prompt institution of ECMO to provide a normal cardiac output. We have developed a portable ECMO circuit that can be ready for the institution of support within 15 minutes of cardiac arrest. Using this system for resuscitation has resulted in survival of 7 of 11 (64%) of pediatric cardiac patients suffering cardiac arrest. This "rapid resuscitation" ECMO circuit is maintained vacuum and CO_2-primed in the intensive care unit at all times and is portable with a battery power supply allowing it to be quickly utilized in any location throughout the hospital. The rapid resuscitation team is made up of on-call members of cardiology, cardiac surgery, and cardiac nursing. If standard CPR is unsuccessful within 10 minutes of cardiac arrest, the circuit is moved to the patient's bedside and crystalloid priming is initiated while cannulation is proceeding. If cannulation is completed prior to the availability of blood products, ECMO flow is initiated with a crystalloid-primed circuit and blood products are added when available. The excess crystalloid volume is removed as blood is added to the circuit with exchange transfusions by hand and use of ultrafiltration after the hemodynamics have stabilized. We believe that establishing a normal cardiac output provided by ECMO is the most important factor in successful resuscitation of these children, even if the hematocrit is low at the institution of support with a crystalloid-primed circuit.

REFERENCES

1. Fiser DH, Wrape V. Outcome of cardiopulmonary resuscitation in children. Pediatr Emerg Care 1987; 3:235–238.

2. Von Seggern K, Egar M, Fuhrman BP. Cardiopulmonary resuscitation in a pediatric ICU. Crit Care Med 1986; 14:275–277.
3. Grambow DW, Deeb GM, Pavlides GS, Margulis A, O'Neill WW, Bates ER. Emergent percutaneous cardiopulmonary bypass in patients having cardiovascular collapse in the cardiac catheterization laboratory. Am J Cardiol 1994; 73:872–875.
4. Dembitsky WP, Moreno-Cabral RJ, Adamson RM, Daily PO. Emergency resuscitation using portable extracorporeal membrane oxygenation. Ann Thorac Surg 1993; 55:304–309.
5. Phillips SJ, Zeff FH, Kongtahworn C, et al. Percutaneous cardiopulmonary bypass: application and indication for use. Ann Thorac Surg 1989; 47:121–123.
6. Dalton HJ, Siewers RD, Fuhrman BP, et al. Extracorporeal membrane oxygenation for cardiac rescue in children with severe myocardial dysfunction. Crit Care Med 1993; 21:1020–1028.
7. del Nido PJ, Dalton HJ, Thompson AE, Siewers RD. Extracorporeal membrane oxygenator rescue in children during cardiac arrest after cardiac surgery. Circulation 1992; 86(suppl II):II-300–II-304.
8. Duncan BW, Ibrahim AE, Hraska V, et al. Use of rapid-deployment extracorporeal membrane oxygenation for the resuscitation of pediatric patients with heart disease after cardiac arrest. J Thorac Cardiovasc Surg 1998; 116:305–311.
9. Goldman AP, Kerr SJ, Butt W, et al. Extracorporeal support for intractable cardiorespiratory failure due to meningococcal disease. Lancet 1997; 349:466–469.
10. Laub GW, Banaszak D, Kupferschmid J, Macgovern GJ, Young JC. Percutaneous cardiopulmonary bypass for the treatment of hypothermic circulatory collapse. Ann Thorac Surg 1989; 47:608–611.
11. Ballew KA, Philbrick JT, Caven DE, Schorling JB. Predictors of survival following in-hospital cardiopulmonary resuscitation. Arch Intern Med 1994; 154:2426–2432.
12. Zaritsky A. Outcome of pediatric cardiopulmonary resuscitation. Crit Care Med 1993; 21(suppl):S325–S327.
13. Doski JJ, Butler TJ, Louder DS, Dickey LA, Cheu HW. Outcome of infants requiring cardiopulmonary resuscitation before extracorporeal membrane oxygenation. J Pediatr Surg 1997; 32:1318–1321.
14. Torres A, Pickert CB, Firestone J, Walker WM, Fiser DH. Long-term functional outcome of inpatient pediatric cardiopulmonary resuscitation. Pediatr Emerg Care 1997; 13:369–373.
15. Zaritsky A, Nadkami V, Getson P, Kuehl K. CPR in children. Ann Emerg Med 1987; 16:1107–1111.
16. O'Connor TA, Downing GJ, Ewing LL, Gowdamarajan R. Echocardiographically guided balloon atrial septostomy during extracorporeal membrane oxygenation (ECMO). Pediatr Cardiol 1993; 14:167–168.
17. Duncan BW, Hraska V, Jonas RA, et al. Mechanical circulatory support in children with cardiac disease. J Thorac Cardiovasc Surg 1999; 117:529–542.
18. Lanier WL. Cerebral metabolic rate and hypothermia: their relationship with ischemic neurologic injury. J Neurosurg Anesthesiol 1995; 7:216–221.

10

The Use of Mechanical Circulatory Support in the Treatment of Myocarditis and Cardiomyopathy

Desmond Bohn
The Hospital for Sick Children, Toronto, Ontario, Canada

I. INTRODUCTION

The relationship between infection and cardiac function was first recognized in the early 1800s when diphtheria was linked with chronic heart failure. Since this original description, the causal relationship between inflammation and heart failure has been clearly identified in many other disease processes and labeled as either myocarditis or cardiomyopathy. This in turn has led to some lack of clarity in the medical literature as to diagnosis, treatment, and outcome in patients presenting in acute or chronic heart failure without a precisely defined etiology. Common practice has been to apply the term "cardiomyopathy" to heart disease where an ischemic, congenital, rheumatic, or hypertensive etiology has been excluded. This remains unsatisfactory, however, since the term "cardiomyopathy" is frequently applied to patients with acute myocarditis. With the advent of endomyocardial biopsy and the increasing use of echocardiography, further attempts have been made to achieve a consensus on classification according to morphometry. Based on echo/angiography appearance, cardiomyopathies can be classified into dilated cardiomyopathies, where both left and right ventricles are dilated with poor function; hypertrophic cardiomyopathy, characterized by hypertrophy of the ventricles with pronounced thickening of the interventricular septum; and restrictive cardiomyopathy, which is characterized by reduced diastolic volume with preserved systolic function. In many ways, a more satisfactory classification is to view cardiomyopathies according to their biopsy or postmortem findings (Table 1).

Table 1 Classification of Cardiomyopathies

Inflammatory/Immune cardiomyopathy
Acute viral myocarditis
coxsackie
adenovirus
influenza A
cytomegalovirus
mumps
Cardiac allograft rejection
Hypersensitivity myocarditis
HIV
Chagas' disease
Infiltrative cardiomyopathies
Glycogen storage diseases
Hemochromatosis
Thalassemia
Miscellaneous specific cardiomyopathies
Carnitine deficiency
Endomyocardial fibroelastosis
Arrhythmic
Chemotherapy induced
Peripartum
Nonspecific cardiomyopathies
Idiopathic dilated cardiomyopathy
Familial (metabolic) cardiomyopathy

II. ETIOLOGY AND NATURAL HISTORY

Acute viral myocarditis is a form of inflammatory or autoimmune cardiomyopathy, the most commonly associated pathogen being the enteroviruses, typically the coxsackie B3 strain. The identification of this virus as the causative microorganism is based on either viral culture from blood, nasopharyngeal secretions, cerebrospinal fluid (CSF), urine, or stool, or viral serology titers throughout the course of the disease (1–7). However, identification of an enterovirus either by serology or by culture does not necessarily prove a causal relationship between the microorganism and myocarditis, as a majority of the population will have been exposed to these viruses. In addition, even in children dying in florid heart failure secondary to myocarditis, identification of either virus or viral particles in the myocardium at autopsy is a rare event. More recently, the introduction of more sophisticated viral tests on myocardial tissue such as in situ hybridization and polymerase chain reaction (PCR) have led to a much higher diagnostic yield.

Martin et al. (4) showed that with the use of PCR, the diagnostic yield from endomyocardial biopsy specimens can be as high as 68%, with a much higher incidence of myocarditis secondary to adenovirus compared with previous reports. The same group identified the mumps virus as a causative organism in patients with autopsy-proven fibroelastosis (5). The classical natural history of the disease begins with the typical symptoms of a flu-like illness (fever, rhinorrhea, gastrointestinal disturbance). Following the subsidence of the systemic infection, patients frequently present with symptoms of congestive heart failure, sometimes accompanied by cardiac rhythm disturbance (8). In the most severe forms, particularly in children, the presentation may be of acute circulatory collapse and sudden death (9–12). The prognosis seems to bear some relationship to age. In the multicenter immunosuppressive trial of adult patients with a clinical diagnosis of myocarditis, mortality was 20% at one year and 56% at 4.3 years (13). It is estimated that approximately one third of long-term adult survivors will require transplantation. The natural history of acute myocarditis in children is somewhat different in that the majority of the patients who survive the acute phase seem to have restoration of normal cardiac function and remain asymptomatic (14–16). In young children presenting with dilated cardiomyopathy without a preceding history of myocarditis, the most common etiology is familial, the most frequent inheritance being autosomal dominant (17,18). These patients may be asymptomatic until a hypermetabolic state such as an infection precipitates an episode of acute heart failure, frequently in the first 6 months of life. Most deaths in this diagnostic group seem to occur in the first 2 months, while those that survive may demonstrate improved function within a 2-year period after presentation (19). In older children the cardiomyopathy may be secondary to a previously undiagnosed viral myocarditis with a better long-term survival (20).

III. PATHOGENIC MECHANISMS

Much of our knowledge of the pathogenic mechanisms of viral myocarditis comes from the murine model infected with the coxsackie B or encephalomyocardial virus (3). Viral invasion of the myocardium leads to a complex series of immunological reactions, which result in myocyte damage and the release of inflammatory cytokines into the circulation causing worsening myocardial function. In the initial phase virus enters via the gastrointestinal tract, localizes in the lymph nodes, and then travels to the host's spleen. From there it is spread via the blood stream to the myocardium, where it is localized in the perivascular regions of the myocardium (3). This results in an intense immune response typified by lymphocytic infiltration and myocyte necrosis, features that form the basis of the Dallas criteria for the diagnosis of acute viral myocarditis (21). The persistence of virus in the myocardium is not essential for the acute immune reaction, but virus has been demonstrated in murine models with the subsequent development of dilated cardiomyopathy (22–24). Also, with the introduction of more sophisticated viral detection techniques, a higher rate of viral identification in the myocardium has been achieved (25,26). In a study of 120 human subjects who underwent myocardial biopsy for the investigation of a possible infective cardiomyopathy, one third of the patients had enteroviruses identified by in situ hybridization (27). The mortality in those who were virus positive was 25% versus 4% for those who were virus negative.

The host's immune system plays a large role in the pathogenesis of acute viral myocarditis, in both a positive and a negative way. In the murine model inoculated with coxsackie virus, T cells and natural killer cells can be identified early in the disease followed by macrophages later (28). In the human subject, on the other hand, the myocardium is infiltrated with T lymphocytes and macrophages while the B lymphocytes and natural killer cells are absent (29). Important insights into these competing mechanisms have been gained from the use of specific antibody techniques in the murine model and more recently by the use of the "knock-out" mouse model. This has shown that the T cells (CD4 and CD8) play an important role in the immune response to viral infection of the myocardium and that in the absence of T cells the immunological damage is attenuated (30).

Viral invasion of the myocardium is also associated with increased release of cytokines into the circulation and worsening myocardial function. The myocardial dysfunction seen early in this disease is more likely due to this process rather than direct destruction of myocytes. The important cytokines are TNF-α, which is produced in large quantities by both the immune cells and the myocardium, interleukin-1α, and interleukin-1β, all of which have been shown to be present in either human subjects or the murine model of myocarditis (31–33). Of these, probably the most important is TNF-α, as it is the most commonly identified with myocarditis, in both the human subject and the experimental model, and has been the most extensively studied in this and other diseases. Matsumori et al. (31) reported elevated levels of TNF-α in 46% of patients with acute myocarditis who had undergone endomyocardial biopsy. The influence of this particular cytokine on myocardial function in myocarditis and eventual outcome has been demonstrated in the murine model, where TNF-α was infused in mice who were infected with encephalomyocarditis virus. Animals infused with TNF-α prior to infection had a higher viral content in the myocardium compared with controls (32). The infusion also increased the severity of the lesions as estimated by histology. The infusion of anti-TNF antibody improved the survival in the animals if given prior to the infection. TNF-α has been shown to inhibit myocyte beta-adrenergic responsiveness (34). It is now known that in sepsis most of the negative inotropic effects of TNF-α on the myocardium are mediated through the induction of inducible nitric oxide synthase (iNOS). This has been demonstrated both in septicemia and in cardiomyopathy (35–37), potentiating the immune response and inducing apoptosis in cells. Habib et al. (33) showed increased levels of both iNOS and TNF-α in biopsy specimens of patients with cardiomyopathy and in explanted hearts of patients undergoing cardiac transplantation for end-stage cardiomyopathy. Excessive NO production can lead to microvascular dysfunction and blockade of NO synthesis, while the use of calcium channel blockers in the murine model has been shown to decrease the extent of myocardial lesions (38). The inhibition of superoxide dismutase has also been shown to decrease the myocardial injury in acute viral myocarditis (39). Activation of the sympathetic nervous system leads to depletion of intracardiac catecholamines with a worsening of myocardial dysfunction. The beneficial effects of sympathetic blockade and inhibition of angiotensin-converting enzyme have also been demonstrated in the murine model of myocarditis (40–45). Finally, one of the most interesting developments in the murine model of viral myocarditis has been the use of a serine elastase inhibitor, which results in almost complete inhibition of myocardial injury (46).

IV. CLINICAL PRESENTATION AND DIAGNOSIS

The clinical presentation of myocarditis or cardiomyopathy may vary from acute cardiovascular collapse in a child thought to be previously healthy or only mildly ill to the more gradual onset of symptoms of congestive heart failure. Acute viral myocarditis is one of the leading causes of sudden and unexplained death in children outside the first year of life (9) and in infants is sometimes mistakenly diagnosed as sudden infant death syndrome (47). There may be few symptoms referable to the cardiovascular system, although there is frequently a prodromal history of a flu-like illness, which precedes the onset of heart failure by periods of between a few days to 4–6 weeks. In children the symptomatology is frequently gastrointestinal upset with nausea and vomiting. This is frequently mistakenly diagnosed as gastroenteritis, but a history of diarrhea is frequently lacking. The presumptive diagnosis of gastroenteritis can lead to an attempt at rehydration with intravenous fluids, which only compounds the heart failure. Although it is generally assumed that the gastrointestinal symptoms are a manifestation of viral disease of the gastrointestinal tract, it may be that the nausea and vomiting are due to gut ischemia associated with poor perfusion. Acute viral myocarditis can also present with severe cardiac rhythm disturbances (8,16,48–50), which include ventricular tachycardia, ectopic atrial tachycardia, atrial flutter, and third degree heart block with syncope (51). Abnormal clinical findings, in the absence of an arrhythmia, may be relatively few. Patients with a dilated cardiomyopathy are frequently tachycardic with a third heart sound. The chest x-ray may show pulmonary venous congestion or edema in children presenting with severe heart failure, but in acute viral myocarditis the heart size is frequently normal and an increase in the cardiac silhouette may indicate the presence of a pericardial effusion or a diagnosis of dilated cardiomyopathy. The most common ECG changes are ST flattening and T-wave inversion with low QRS voltages (<5 mm) seen in 80% of cases of myocarditis (14,16). In the most severe cases the typical echocardiography findings are an ejection fraction of <20%, a shortening fraction of <10%, increased left ventricular (LV) end-diastolic dimension, and increased thickness of both the posterior wall of the LV and the interventricular septum (14,16,52). Mitral regurgitation secondary to dilatation of the valve annulus is sometimes seen. The measurement of cardiac enzyme levels is not helpful in making the diagnosis of myocarditis because the CK-MB levels are rarely elevated. An elevation of cardiac troponin I (cTnI), a marker of myocyte necrosis, has been reported in one third of patients with biopsy-proven myocarditis compared with an elevation of CK-MB in only 6% (53). A definitive diagnosis of viral myocarditis in life can only be confirmed by endomyocardial biopsy.

V. ENDOMYOCARDIAL BIOPSY AND HISTOLOGY

The original pathological description of cardiomyopathy was based on necropsy findings of myocyte injury together with inflammatory cells within the interstitial spaces of the myocardium (myocarditis) or fibrosis and myocyte hypertrophy (dilated cardiomyopathy). Virus was rarely identified within the myocardium, and in many of the autopsies the diagnosis was incidental to other systemic diseases. The introduction of endomyocardial biopsy has increased our ability to observe the natural history of the cardiomyopathies and led to the introduction of innovative therapies such as immunosuppression and transplantation. However, even when tissue was made available for diagnosis, there has been considerable disagreement between cardiac pathologists about the histological criteria for the diagnosis of viral myocarditis (54). In order to achieve uniformity in the pathological diagnosis for the purpose of a large trial of immunosuppressive therapy, a group of cardiac pathologists agreed on the so-called Dallas criteria, which defined acute myocarditis as lymphocytic infiltration with myocyte necrosis (*definitive*) and lymphocytic infiltration with interstitial edema (*borderline*) (21). This has now become the generally accepted standard. Patients presenting with new onset cardiomyopathy frequently undergo cardiac catheterization and endomyocardial biopsy with five to six tissue samples usually taken from the right ventricle.

The role of endomyocardial biopsy in the diagnostic evaluation of patients with cardiomyopathy is not without risk and remains a subject of some controversy. Factors pro biopsy are summarized as follows.

1. *Treatment*: to differentiate between viral myocarditis, where immunosuppressive therapy may be used and cardiomyopathy where it is not indicated.
2. *Prognosis*: the outcome with viral myocarditis is better than dilated cardiomyopathy, especially in children (14–16).
3. *Decision algorithm for transplant and/or mechanical circulatory support*: mechanical circulatory support in patients with acute myocarditis should be considered as a definitive therapy in the first instance because of the high rate of recovery of myocardial function. Mechanical support in patients with dilated cardiomyopathy is used as a bridge to transplantation.

Factors contra biopsy are as follows:

1. *High incidence of false-negative results*: the disease may be focal or involve primarily the epicardial heart surface and therefore may be missed by a biopsy even with multiple sections. In a postmortem study that compared autopsy-proven myocarditis with samples taken from the heart by endomyocardial biopsy, a false-negative rate of up to 50% was found (55). In addition, in only 10% of patients with a clinical diagnosis of myocarditis in the adult multicenter immunosuppression trial was this diagnosis confirmed at biopsy (13).
2. *Potential risk*: these patients frequently have very poor myocardial function. Complications include myocardial perforation (small infants at higher risk) and arrhythmias.
3. *Lack of evidence of efficacy for immunosuppressive therapy*: a large multicenter adult trial of immunosuppressive therapy in adults with myocarditis failed to show improved survival (13). Therefore the need for a tissue diagnosis is less imperative.

With the advent of mechanical circulatory support and the increasing use of transplant for end-stage cardiac disease, the issue of whether or not to biopsy has become more than an academic discussion point. Generally speaking, the more acute the presentation, the more likely the biopsy will be positive for lymphocytic infiltration (56). Although the diagnosis of myocarditis can never be excluded by biopsy, the diagnostic yield seems to be higher in children than adults. In a study by Webber et al. (50) of children undergoing endomyocardial biopsy for dilated cradiomyopathy, a positive tissue diagnosis of myocarditis was made 100% of the time in children where the history was less than 6 weeks duration. It has also been suggested that the diagnostic yield can be increased if the biopsy is done within the first 72 hours of presentation (57). Although the procedure is not without risk, it can be done even in patients on extracorporeal support. Indeed, in this group the information is particularly important in terms of early listing for transplantation (cardiomyopathy) versus prolonged mechanical support in the first instance (myocarditis).

VI. THERAPY

A. Inotropes and Afterload Reduction (Pharmacological)

Patients presenting with acute heart failure or cardiogenic shock due to myocarditis are at risk from sudden death. Acute circulatory collapse frequently occurs within the first 24 hours of admission if pharmacological therapy is not introduced to improve cardiac function.

The hemodynamics are characterized by poor contractility and high systemic vascular resistance. Milder forms of cardiomyopathy with ejection fractions of >30% may be managed with oral angiotensin-converting enzyme (ACE) inhibitors, with digoxin reserved for specific rhythm disturbances. In more severe cases systemically administered antifailure therapy is required. The ideal inotrope would enhance contractility without increasing heart rate (myocardial oxygen consumption), would be nonarrhythmogenic, and could be infused peripherally. The ideal vasodilator would be administered systemically with minimal effect on blood pressure.

Although there are few human studies comparing different inotropes and dilators in the setting of cardiomyopathy (58,59), important insights into their effects can be gained from the trials in the murine model of myocarditis, which demonstrate that both calcium channel blockers and angiotensin inhibitors can decrease the amount of injury resulting from viral invasion of the myocardium (38–43,60). The application of these findings to humans with myocarditis is limited by the fact that most patients present after the acute infective phase of the disease has passed. Human studies of captopril in myocarditis and idiopathic dilated cardiomyopathy (IDC) are mostly uncontrolled case series (61–64). Lewis and Chabot (61) reported improved one-year survival in children treated with captopril compared with those who did not in a nonrandomized study. In adults with dilated cardiomyopathy captopril treatment has been associated with a reduction in mitral regurgitation (62) as well as increased heart rate variability and decreased urinary aldosterone excretion (63,64). The ACE inhibitor enalapril has also been used in several randomized controlled trials of heart failure, which have included patients with IDC, and have demonstrated reduced mortality and hospitalizations (65,66).

Calcium channel blockers have also been shown to ameliorate the myocardial injury in the murine model of myocarditis (67). Human studies also suggest some benefit in patients with IDC. The randomized trial by Packer et al. (68) demonstrated a decreased risk of death by 46% compared to placebo, while a second randomized trial showed that when amlodipine was used in addition to captopril and digoxin there was a decreased incidence of pump failure and sudden death (69).

With the exception of digoxin, inotropic agents increase contractility either by promoting synthesis of intracellular cyclic AMP (sympathomimetic agents) or by retarding its degradation (phosphodiesterase inhibitors). Of the widely available sympathomimetic agents, both dopamine and dobutamine will cause increased heart rate and dopamine is known to increase pulmonary capillary wedge pressure in the setting of ischemic heart disease. The beta sympathomimetic agents also produce tachycardia. There are a number of trials of the intravenous phosphodiesterase inhibitor milrinone (58,59,70,71), which show a hemodynamic benefit despite the fact that long-term treatment with the oral preparation was associated with adverse effects in large randomized controlled trials of IDC (72).

Activation of the sympathetic nervous system is a fundamental pathogenic process in viral myocarditis. Beta blockade has been shown to decrease the extent of myocardial injury and improve survival in the murine model of coxsackie myocarditis, presumably by relief of vasospasm (45). Patients with dilated cardiomyopathy and chronic heart failure have been shown to have reduced sensitivity to beta-adrenergic stimulation because of downregulation of beta receptors due to either chronic adrenergic overstimulation (73,74) or the development of anti-β-receptor antibodies (75). Metoprolol has been shown to have a more favorable effect on hemodynamics than captopril in a nonrandomized study of patients with IDC (76). Trials of beta blocker therapy in IDC have shown improved cardiac function and quality of life without increasing survival (77,78).

B. Afterload Reduction (Increased Intrathoracic Pressure)

One of the most interesting developments in the management of heart failure in the past few years has been the recognition of the beneficial effect that raised intrathoracic pressure has on LV afterload (for review see Ref. 79). This has led in turn to the use of nasal or mask CPAP in adults with congestive heart failure. Studies by Bradley et al. (80) and Naughton et al. (81) have shown symptomatic improvement associated with the unloading of the respiratory muscles. Unlike pharmacological afterload reduction, it does not cause hypotension unless the patients are hypovolemic. It is now increasingly used in children with acute myocarditis or dilated cardiomyopathy. These patients frequently present with very reduced ejection fractions and are at their maximum of reserve compensatory mechanisms, and sedating them for endotracheal intubation and conventional ventilation can precipitate an acute decompensation and cardiac arrest.

C. Immunosuppressive Therapy

In the acute murine model infected with virus, the use of steroids limits the extent of the intense immune response to viral invasion of the myocardium but may increase mortality when given in the acute viremic phase of the illness (3,82). It is difficult to translate this to the human because at the time of presentation the virus is frequently no longer active. There are several uncontrolled series that suggest a benefit from immunosuppressive therapy in adults (48,83,84) and one that suggests harm (85). Despite this, the debate about the efficacy of immunosuppressive therapy in the adult with viral myocarditis remains unresolved. There have been two prospective randomized studies in adults. The study by Parrillo et al. (86) used prednisone in adult patients with dilated cardiomyopathy and demonstrated only marginal benefit in terms of improved ejection fractions in the steroid group. A second large multicenter trial, for which the Dallas criteria were developed, randomized 111 patients to receive either conventional therapy or prednisone with either azothiaprine or cyclosporine (13). The primary endpoint was an improvement in LV ejection. There was no difference between treatment and control groups. Furthermore the mortality in the entire group was 20% at one year and 56% at 5 years, much higher than reported in pediatric series. There is also a single case series of 10 patients with dilated cardiomyopathy given gamma globulin (IVIG) (83). Although only one patient had myocarditis on biopsy, nine showed improvements in ejection fraction with only one death.

The evidence for efficacy in pediatric acute myocarditis is somewhat more persuasive but far from conclusive. Several uncontrolled series suggest benefit (14–16,49,57,87). Survival rates with restoration of normal cardiac function are reported without transplantation in up to 80–100% of patients in retrospective series of biopsy-proven myocarditis treated with immunosuppression (16,57,87). A retrospective case-control series in which IVIG was used reported a higher probability of normal cardiac function at one year but no improvement in survival compared with historical controls (88). The single prospective study in children with myocarditis was a matched-cohort study where patients received either conventional (supportive) treatment or one of three immunosuppressive regimes (prednisone, prednisone + azothiaprine, or prednisone + cyclosporine) for a mean of 8 months (52). The investigators reported better outcomes in patients who received the combination immunosuppressive therapy. Significant methodological flaws in this study were highlighted in a recent meta-analysis of all the published studies of immunosuppression trials in viral myocarditis (89). The authors of this overview concluded that efficacy for immunosuppression was lacking. However, the responses to therapy in children, where the disease seems to present in a more acute and fulminant fashion, seems to differ from adults, in whom the onset is more insidious and progresses more frequently to a chronic dilated cardiomyopathy. One could conclude that there is some evidence for efficacy of immunosuppression in children with acute viral myocarditis, but this remains to be tested in a properly designed prospective trial.

VII. MECHANICAL SUPPORT

The use of mechanical circulatory support with extracorporeal membrane oxygenation (ECMO) or ventricular assist devices (VADs) can be life saving in patients with myocarditis or cardiomyopathy presenting in cardiogenic shock. Although the technique is highly invasive with the potential for significant technical and patient complications, there are now well-documented cases of the successful use of mechanical support in patients following prolonged cardiac arrest both after repair of congenital heart disease (90) and in acute myocarditis with intact neurological survival and restoration of normal cardiac function without the need for transplantation (91). A successful approach to these patients requires careful consideration at several key points in a decision algorithm regarding the institution of mechanical circulatory support, management while on support, and consideration for weaning from support versus the need for cardiac transplantation.

A. Choice of Device

There are two options for mechanical support in acute myocardial failure: to use a pumping device with an oxygenator or to use a ventricular assist device to support either the left ventricle (LVAD), right ventricle (RVAD), or both ventricles (BIVAD) without an oxygenator. There is a wealth of experience with the use of ECMO to support children with cardio-respiratory failure. The Extracorporeal Life Support Organization (ELSO) Registry database now contains over 17,000 patients, most of whom have been neonates managed with ECMO for acute respiratory failure. The potential advantages to using this mode of support are familiarity with the technique in pediatric centers, the opportunity to avoid trans-sternal cannulation, the provision of biventricular support with two peripheral cannulation sites as opposed to the four required for BIVAD, and the presence of an oxygenator when hypoxemia complicates the clinical picture. The potential disadvantages are increased destruction of platelets and greater heparin requirements leading to bleeding, which may be particularly problematic if there has been a recent sternotomy. There also may be inadequate unloading of the left heart, which may necessitate a balloon or blade atrial septostomy or opening the sternum to place a left atrial vent. Although most ECMO centers use a roller pump system, others prefer to use a centrifugal pump, which allows for the flexibility to use either the ECMO or VAD option. Using a LVAD or BIVAD has the advantages of automatically unloading the left heart by draining the left side, and since there is no oxygenator in the circuit, less anticoagulation requirements, decreased destruction of platelets, and fewer circuit-related complications. The principal disadvantage is that cannulae have to be placed within the chest, which can result in significant bleeding and the risk of infection. The devices that have been used clinically to support patients with cardiomyopathy/myocarditis are listed in Table 2.

B. Cannulation: Sites and Technique (ECMO and LVAD)

ECMO provides greater flexibility in allowing rapid institution of support from a number of sites, utilizing vessels in the neck, groin, or chest, while the use of VAD necessitates transthoracic cannulation. The institution of ECMO via transthoracic cannulation provides excellent venous drainage and allows the direct insertion of a left atrial drainage cannula (vent). Due to the possible need for transplantation in many of these patients, neck or groin cannulation, while maintaining an intact chest cavity, is preferable to decrease the risk of infectious complications. For the institution of ECMO, most neonates and small children (<10 kg) are cannulated via the carotid artery and internal jugular vein because the femoral vessels are too small to accept adequate size cannulae. In older children, adolescents, and adults the femoral vessels are frequently used due to concerns of cerebral ischemia that may result from cannulation of the carotid artery. The placement of cannulae in the neck vessels for ECMO is via an oblique incision in the right side of the neck with the venous cannula advanced so that the tip is in the mid-right atrium and the tip of the arterial cannula at the junction of the innominate artery and the aorta arch. Both vessels are tied off proximally. For femoral cannulation the venous cannula is advanced so that the tip is at the IVC right atrial junction and the arterial cannula is advanced so that the tip is at the aortic arch. When the trans-sternal approach is used for ECMO, the venous cannula is placed directly into the right atrium with a left atrial vent and the arterial cannula is placed in the ascending aorta. When LVAD is used the venous drainage cannula is placed through the left atrium or superior pulmonary vein. The pneumatic VAD systems use a trans-sternal atrial-to-aortic connection.

C. Patient Management on Mechanical Support

The major objective in mechanical support is "heart rest." Therefore, for ECMO-supported patients the development of left-sided cardiac distension must be assiduously avoided by monitoring left-sided filling pressures and imaging the heart with echocardiography. If left ventricular distension is documented, decompression with balloon atrial septostomy or direct venting of the left ventricle by placement of a drainage line via the left atrial appendage or right superior pulmonary vein must be instituted. Balloon atrial septostomy can be performed in the cardiac catheterization laboratory or at the bedside under echocardiographic guidance

Table 2 Mechanical Circulatory Assist Devices—Pediatric Applications

Assist device	Type of assist	Pump type	Comments
Sarns (Ref. 104)	ECMO	Roller	Extensive experience with ECMO for adults and children
Medtronic (Ref. 91)	ECMO, LVAD, BIVAD	Centrifugal	Adult and pediatric experience for ECMO and VAD
Berlin Heart (Ref. 102,105)	BIVAD	Pneumatic	Adult and pediatric applications
Abiomed (Ref. 106)	BIVAD	Pneumatic	Adult and pediatric applications
BVS 5000 (Ref. 106)			
Thoratec (Ref. 106)	VAD	Pneumatic	Adult and pediatric applications
Medos H.I.A. (Ref. 107)	VAD	Pneumatic	Adult and pediatric applications
Hemopump		Implantable with electronic external drive	Adult application only
Pierce-Donachy (Ref. 108)		Pneumatic	Adult application only; pediatric application in development

(92,93). Adequate coronary artery oxygenation on ECMO support should be provided by continuing to provide ventilatory support when significant ventricular ejection occurs, which ensures that pulmonary venous and hence coronary arterial blood will be fully saturated. Avoiding left ventricular distension and providing fully saturated coronary blood flow gives ECMO-supported patients an excellent chance for recovery of native ventricular function. Many institutions prefer to use ECMO in patients who require support for severe acute myocarditis due to its ability to be instituted via peripheral cannulation and the presence of an oxygenator for use in those patients with significant arterial hypoxemia. Flow rates for ECMO and VAD depend on patient size and may be limited by unfavorable venous cannula position, small cannula size, thrombus within the cannula, and hypovolemia. With the centrifugal pump systems negative pressures of >20 cmH_2O in the venous line, frequently accompanied by "chattering" in the lines, indicates inadequate venous return to the pump and will result in hemolysis. A mixed venous (SvO_2) saturation of 65–70% and a normal blood lactate are indications of adequate pump flow. In-line SvO_2 measurements with an oximetric catheter in the venous line is useful for this purpose but can only be interpreted when the left atrial vent is clamped. During mechanical assistance inotropes may be discontinued but vasodilator therapy should be continued. Anticoagulation is maintained with a continuous heparin infusion with the objective of an ACT in the range of 180–220 seconds, which usually results in a heparin level of 3–5 units/mL. The platelet count should be kept at >100,000.

D. Mechanical Support: Definitive Therapy Versus Bridge to Transplantation

Despite profound ventricular dysfunction at presentation, many patients with myocarditis have sufficient return of ventricular function to allow device weaning and demonstrate normal ventricular function in nontransplanted survivors. In addition, reports have suggested that prolonged mechanical circulatory support may result in the recovery of ventricular function in dilated cardiomyopathy due to favorable influences on the neurohormonal cardiovascular milieu and unloading of the left ventricle resulting in normalization of ventricular geometry—a process termed "reversible remodeling" (94,95). It is probable that the institution of mechanical circulatory support in patients with severe, acute myocarditis can favorably impact these same factors, resulting in ventricular recovery after relatively brief periods of support. However, a competing interest is the need to successfully procure a donor heart for those patients that fail to demonstrate substantial return of ventricular function. Due to the scarcity of donor organs in the pediatric age group, timely listing for transplantation provides for the best chance for successful organ procurement. The period of support that optimally balances these competing interests should be highly individualized in each patient. An attempt should be made to identify patients who have return of native ventricular function sufficient for discontinuation of support by repeated attempts at weaning. The return of a pulsatile arterial waveform is an important sign marking the beginnings of return of function. At the time that weaning is attempted, all available diagnostic modalities should be brought to bear on the decision-making process. Visualization of myocardial contractility with surface or transesophageal echocardiography should be performed with each weaning attempt while monitoring the response of hemodynamic parameters (heart rate, blood pressure, atrial filling pressures). It should be noted that echo estimation of cardiac function is load dependent and requires adequate atrial filling. In addition, ventricular contractility on echocardiography remains markedly abnormal in many of these patients despite their ability to be weaned. In each case the synthesis of all of the clinical parameters listed above will determine the suitability for weaning. In borderline cases, patients may be maintained with the cannulas clamped in place for several hours with intermittent flushing while maintaining full systemic heparinization in order to safely assess stability after weaning from mechanical support.

Identifying those patients that will require the use of ECMO or VAD as a bridge for transplantation is a clinical determination based on failure after repeated attempts at weaning as described above. Extended periods of support have been used successfully for both acute myocarditis and idiopathic dilated cardiomyopathy. In the multicenter case series by Duncan et al. (91), the median time of separation from mechanical support with ultimate return of ventricular function without transplantation was 140 hours (range 115–400 h) Prolonged periods of LVAD support in adult patients with dilated cardiomyopathy have been reported with reduction to normal in end-diastolic pressure-volume relations in some instances (95,96).

The development of pulsatile paracorporeal or implantable systems that have been used successfully in children in Europe will allow long-term support of patients presenting with profound ventricular dysfunction due to acute myocarditis (97). This approach in a larger number of patients may reveal that the majority can be supported long enough to allow return of native ventricular function, thereby avoiding transplantation.

VIII. OUTCOME

The overall survival in children with acute myocarditis who reach the hospital alive can be as high as 80% (16) and is considerably better than in adults with either myocarditis or IDC (13,98). Whether this reflects the inherently superior hemodynamic compensatory mechanisms in children or a difference in the intensity of the immune response is as yet undetermined. The impact of the introduction of mechanical support on outcome in patients with myocarditis and/or dilated cardiomyopathy is difficult to determine for a number of reasons. Reports in the medical literature are either anecdotal cases or case series with varying indications for the use of the technology and sometimes imprecise diagnosis. The largest case series is the ELSO Registry database, which reports 40–50% survival in patients in the diagnostic category myocarditis/cardiomyopathy (99). This database does not collect information on whether the exit from mechanical support is recovery of myocardial function or by way of transplantation. Undoubtedly there have been some spectacular recoveries in children with myocarditis and cardiogenic shock who have deteriorated to the point of cardiac arrest placed on ECMO or LVAD after prolonged cardiac massage, with normal neurological outcomes (16,91–93,100,101). Similar experience comes from European centers with the use of pneumatically driven BIVAD systems (97,102,103). The largest reported series is the combined experience from Toronto, Boston, and Seattle with 16 children with cardiogenic shock placed on ECMO or VAD with 12 survivors, 7 of whom had return of native ventricular function (91). Five others exited mechanical support by way of transplantation. Another remarkable feature of this series is that the duration of support was up to 10 days in one patient who regained normal function. This has implications for when the distinction between it being a definitive therapy or a bridge to transplantation is made. The situation with idiopathic cardiomyopathy is more complex. Mechanical support in this situation is primarily a bridge to transplantation, although there are occasional reports of patients being successfully weaned with return of native function (94,96). In both instances survival, both short and long term, may depend on the avoidance of the complications of organ dysfunction and sepsis.

REFERENCES

1. Bowles NE, Towbin JA. Molecular aspects of myocarditis. Curr Opin Cardiol 1998; 13(3):179–184.
2. Akhtar N, Ni J, Stromberg D, et al. Tracheal aspirate as a substrate for polymerase chain reaction detection of viral genome in childhood pneumonia and myocarditis. Circulation 1999; 99(15):2011–2018.
3. Liu P, Martino T, Opavsky MA, et al. Viral myocarditis: balance between viral infection and immune response. Can J Cardiol 1996; 12(10):935–943.
4. Martin AB, Webber S, Fricker FJ, et al. Acute myocarditis. Rapid diagnosis by PCR in children. Circulation 1994; 90(1):330–339.
5. Ni J, Bowles NE, Kim YH, et al. Viral infection of the myocardium in endocardial fibroelastosis. Molecular evidence for the role of mumps virus as an etiologic agent. Circulation 1997; 95(1):133–139.
6. Jin O, Sole MJ, Butany JW, et al. Detection of enterovirus RNA in myocardial biopsies from patients with myocarditis and cardiomyopathy using gene amplification by polymerase chain reaction. Circulation 1990; 82(1):8–16.
7. Yang D, Yu J, Luo Z, et al. Viral myocarditis: identification of five differentially expressed genes in coxsackievirus B3-infected mouse heart. Circ Res 1999; 84(6): 704–712.

8. Wiles HB, Gillette PC, Harley RA, et al. Cardiomyopathy and myocarditis in children with ventricular ectopic rhythm. J Am Coll Cardiol 1992; 20(2):359–362.
9. Noren GR, Staley NA, Bandt CM, et al. Occurrence of myocarditis in sudden death in children. J Forensic Sci 1977; 22(1):188–196.
10. Smith NM, Bourne AJ, Clapton WK, et al. The spectrum of presentation at autopsy of myocarditis in infancy and childhood. Pathology 1992; 24(3):129–131.
11. Molander N. Sudden natural death in later childhood and adolescence. Arch Dis Child 1982; 57(8):572–576.
12. Denfield SW, Garson A, Jr. Sudden death in children and young adults. Pediatr Clin North Am 1990; 37(1):215–231.
13. Mason JW, O'Connell JB, Herskowitz A, et al. A clinical trial of immunosuppressive therapy for myocarditis. The Myocarditis Treatment Trial Investigators. N Engl J Med 1995; 333(5):269–275.
14. Chan KY, Iwahara M, Benson LN, et al. Immunosuppressive therapy in the management of acute myocarditis in children: a clinical trial. J Am Coll Cardiol 1991; 17(2):458–460.
15. Drucker NA, Colan SD, Lewis AB, et al. Gamma-globulin treatment of acute myocarditis in the pediatric population. Circulation 1994; 89(1):252–257.
16. Lee KJ, McCrindle BW, Bohn DJ, et al. Clinical outcomes of acute myocarditis in childhood. Heart 1999; 82(2):226–233.
17. Mestroni L, Rocco C, Gregori D, et al. Familial dilated cardiomyopathy: evidence for genetic and phenotypic heterogeneity. Heart Muscle Disease Study Group. J Am Coll Cardiol 1999; 34(1):181–190.
18. Michels VV, Moll PP, Miller FA, et al. The frequency of familial dilated cardiomyopathy in a series of patients with idiopathic dilated cardiomyopathy. N Engl J Med 1992; 326(2):77–82.
19. Matitiau A, Perez-Atayde A, Sanders SP, et al. Infantile dilated cardiomyopathy: relation of outcome to left ventricular mechanics, hemodynamics, and histology at the time of presentation. Circulation 1994; 90(3):1310–1318.
20. Friedman RA, Moak JP, Garson A, Jr. Clinical course of idiopathic dilated cardiomyopathy in children. J Am Coll Cardiol 1991; 18(1):152–156.
21. Aretz HT, Billingham ME, Edwards WD, et al. Myocarditis. A histopathologic definition and classification. Am J Cardiovasc Pathol 1987; 1(1):3–14.
22. Wee L, Liu P, Penn L, et al. Persistence of viral genome into late stages of murine myocarditis detected by polymerase chain reaction. Circulation 1992; 86(5):1605–1614.
23. Kyu B, Matsumori A, Sato Y, et al. Cardiac persistence of cardioviral RNA detected by polymerase chain reaction in a murine model of dilated cardiomyopathy. Circulation 1992; 86(2):522–530.
24. Cronin ME, Love LA, Miller FW, et al. The natural history of encephalomyocarditis virus-induced myositis and myocarditis in mice. Viral persistence demonstrated by in situ hybridization. J Exp Med 1988; 168(5):1639–1648.
25. Bowles NE, Richardson PJ, Olsen EG, et al. Detection of Coxsackie-B-virus-specific RNA sequences in myocardial biopsy samples from patients with myocarditis and dilated cardiomyopathy. Lancet 1986; 1(8490):1120–1123.
26. Kandolf R, Ameis D, Kirschner P, et al. In situ detection of enteroviral genomes

in myocardial cells by nucleic acid hybridization: an approach to the diagnosis of viral heart disease. Proc Natl Acad Sci USA 1987; 84(17):6272–6276.
27. Why HJ, Meany BT, Richardson PJ, et al. Clinical and prognostic significance of detection of enteroviral RNA in the myocardium of patients with myocarditis or dilated cardiomyopathy. Circulation 1994; 89(6):2582–2589.
28. Godeny EK, Gauntt CJ. In situ immune autoradiographic identification of cells in heart tissues of mice with coxsackievirus B3-induced myocarditis. Am J Pathol 1987; 129(2):267–276.
29. Chow LH, Ye Y, Linder J, et al. Phenotypic analysis of infiltrating cells in human myocarditis. An immunohistochemical study in paraffin-embedded tissue. Arch Pathol Lab Med 1989; 113(12):1357–1362.
30. Molina TJ, Bachmann MF, Kundig TM, et al. Peripheral T cells in mice lacking p561ck do not express significant antiviral effector functions. J Immunol 1993; 151(2):699–706.
31. Matsumori A, Yamada T, Suzuki H, et al. Increased circulating cytokines in patients with myocarditis and cardiomyopathy. Br Heart J 1994; 72(6):561–566.
32. Yamada T, Matsumori A, Sasayama S. Therapeutic effect of anti-tumor necrosis factor-alpha antibody on the murine model of viral myocarditis induced by encephalomyocarditis virus. Circulation 1994; 89(2):846–851.
33. Habib FM, Springall DR, Davies GJ, et al. Tumour necrosis factor and inducible nitric oxide synthase in dilated cardiomyopathy. Lancet 1996; 347(9009):1151–1155.
34. Gulick T, Chung MK, Pieper SJ, et al. Interleukin 1 and tumor necrosis factor inhibit cardiac myocyte beta-adrenergic responsiveness. Proc Natl Acad Sci USA 1989; 86(17):6753–6757.
35. Finkel MS, Oddis CV, Jacob TD, et al. Negative inotropic effects of cytokines on the heart mediated by nitric oxide. Science 1992; 257(5068):387–389.
36. Brady AJ, Poole-Wilson PA, Harding SE, et al. Nitric oxide production within cardiac myocytes reduces their contractility in endotoxemia. Am J Physiol 1992; 263(6 Pt 2):H1963–1966.
37. Cobb JP, Danner RL. Nitric oxide and septic shock. JAMA 1996; 275(15):1192–1196.
38. Wang WZ, Matsumori A, Yamada T, et al. Beneficial effects of amlodipine in a murine model of congestive heart failure induced by viral myocarditis. A possible mechanism through inhibition of nitric oxide production. Circulation 1997; 95(1): 245–251.
39. Suzuki H, Matsumori A, Matoba Y, et al. Enhanced expression of superoxide dismutase messenger RNA in viral myocarditis. An SH-dependent reduction of its expression and myocardial injury. J Clin Invest 1993; 91(6):2727–2733.
40. Araki M, Kanda T, Imai S, et al. Comparative effects of losartan, captopril, and enalapril on murine acute myocarditis due to encephalomyocarditis virus. J Cardiovasc Pharmacol 1995; 26(1):61–65.
41. Rezkalla S, Kloner RA, Khatib G, et al. Effect of delayed captopril therapy on left ventricular mass and myonecrosis during acute coxsackievirus murine myocarditis. Am Heart J 1990; 120(6 Pt 1):1377–1381.
42. Rezkalla S, Kloner RA, Khatib G, et al. Beneficial effects of captopril in acute coxsackievirus B3 murine myocarditis. Circulation 1990; 81(3):1039–1046.

43. Takada H, Kishimoto C, Hiraoka Y, et al. Captopril suppresses interstitial fibrin deposition in coxsackievirus B3 myocarditis. Am J Physiol 1997; 272(1 Pt 2): H211–219.
44. Tanaka A, Matsumori A, Wang W, et al. An angiotensin II receptor antagonist reduces myocardial damage in an animal model of myocarditis. Circulation 1994; 90(4):2051–2055.
45. Tominaga M, Matsumori A, Okada I, et al. Beta-blocker treatment of dilated cardiomyopathy. Beneficial effect of carteolol in mice. Circulation 1991; 83(6):2021–2028.
46. Lee JK, Zaidi SH, Liu P, et al. A serine elastase inhibitor reduces inflammation and fibrosis and preserves cardiac function after experimentally-induced murine myocarditis. Nat Med 1998; 4(12):1383–1391.
47. Shatz A, Hiss J, Arensburg B. Myocarditis misdiagnosed as sudden infant death syndrome (SIDS). Med Sci Law 1997; 37(1):16–18.
48. Vignola PA, Aonuma K, Swaye PS, et al. Lymphocytic myocarditis presenting as unexplained ventricular arrhythmias: diagnosis with endomyocardial biopsy and response to immunosuppression. J Am Coll Cardiol 1984; 4(4):812–819.
49. Ino T, Okubo M, Akimoto K, et al. Corticosteroid therapy for ventricular tachycardia in children with silent lymphocytic myocarditis. J Pediatr 1995; 126(2):304–308.
50. Webber SA, Boyle GJ, Jaffe R, et al. Role of right ventricular endomyocardial biopsy in infants and children with suspected or possible myocarditis. Br Heart J 1994; 72(4):360–363.
51. Lim CH, Toh CC, Chia BL, et al. Stokes-Adams attacks due to acute nonspecific myocarditis. Am Heart J 1975; 90(2):172–178.
52. Camargo PR, Snitcowsky R, da Luz PL, et al. Favorable effects of immunosuppressive therapy in children with dilated cardiomyopathy and active myocarditis. Pediatr Cardiol 1995; 16(2):61–68.
53. Lauer B, Niederau C, Kuhl U, et al. Cardiac troponin T in patients with clinically suspected myocarditis. J Am Coll Cardiol 1997; 30(5):1354–1359.
54. Shanes JG, Ghali J, Billingham ME, et al. Interobserver variability in the pathologic interpretation of endomyocardial biopsy results. Circulation 1987; 75(2):401–405.
55. Hauck AJ, Kearney DL, Edwards WD. Evaluation of postmortem endomyocardial biopsy specimens from 38 patients with lymphocytic myocarditis: implications for role of sampling error. Mayo Clin Proc 1989; 64(10):1235–1245.
56. Dec GW, Jr., Palacios IF, Fallon JT, et al. Active myocarditis in the spectrum of acute dilated cardiomyopathies. Clinical features, histologic correlates, and clinical outcome. N Engl J Med 1985; 312(14):885–890.
57. Kleinert S, Weintraub RG, Wilkinson JL, et al. Myocarditis in children with dilated cardiomyopathy: incidence and outcome after dual therapy immunosuppression. J Heart Lung Transplant 1997; 16(12):1248–1254.
58. Biddle TL, Benotti JR, Creager MA, et al. Comparison of intravenous milrinone and dobutamine for congestive heart failure secondary to either ischemic or dilated cardiomyopathy. Am J Cardiol 1987; 59(15):1345–1350.
59. Eichhorn EJ, Konstam MA, Weiland DS, et al. Differential effects of milrinone and dobutamine on right ventricular preload, afterload and systolic performance in

congestive heart failure secondary to ischemic or idiopathic dilated cardiomyopathy. Am J Cardiol 1987; 60(16):1329–1333.
60. Ishiyama S, Hiroe M, Nishikawa T, et al. Nitric oxide contributes to the progression of myocardial damage in experimental autoimmune myocarditis in rats. Circulation 1997; 95(2):489–496.
61. Lewis AB, Chabot M. The effect of treatment with angiotensin-converting enzyme inhibitors on survival of pediatric patients with dilated cardiomyopathy. Pediatr Cardiol 1993; 14(1):9–12.
62. Evangelista-Masip A, Bruguera-Cortada J, Serrat-Serradell R, et al. Influence of mitral regurgitation on the response to captopril therapy for congestive heart failure caused by idiopathic dilated cardiomyopathy. Am J Cardiol 1992; 69(4): 373–376.
63. Jansson K, Hagerman I, Ostlund R, et al. The effects of metoprolol and captopril on heart rate variability in patients with idiopathic dilated cardiomyopathy. Clin Cardiol 1999; 22(6):397–402.
64. Jansson K, Dahlstrom U, Karlberg BE, et al. The circulating renin-angiotensin system during treatment with metoprolol or captopril in patients with heart failure due to non-ischaemic dilated cardiomyopathy. J Intern Med 1999; 245(5):435–443.
65. Investigators TS. Effect of enalapril on survival in patients with reduced left ventricular ejection fractions and congestive heart failure. N Engl J Med 1991; 325(5): 293–302.
66. Effects of enalapril on mortality in severe congestive heart failure. Results of the Cooperative North Scandinavian Enalapril Survival Study (CONSENSUS). N Engl J Med 1987; 316(23):1429–1435.
67. Matsumori A. Calcium channel blocker-induced protection against cardiovascular damage. Int J Cardiol 1997; 62(suppl 2):S39–46.
68. Packer M, O'Connor CM, Ghali JK, et al. Effect of amlodipine on morbidity and mortality in severe chronic heart failure. Prospective Randomized Amlodipine Survival Evaluation Study Group. N Engl J Med 1996; 335(15):1107–1114.
69. O'Connor CM, Carson PE, Miller AB, et al. Effect of amlodipine on mode of death among patients with advanced heart failure in the PRAISE trial. Prospective Randomized Amlodipine Survival Evaluation. Am J Cardiol 1998; 82(7):881–887.
70. Cesario D, Clark J, Maisel A. Beneficial effects of intermittent home administration of the inotrope/vasodilator milrinone in patients with end-stage congestive heart failure: a preliminary study. Am Heart J 1998; 135(1):121–129.
71. Brecker SJ, Xiao HB, Mbaissouroum M, et al. Effects of intravenous milrinone on left ventricular function in ischemic and idiopathic dilated cardiomyopathy. Am J Cardiol 1993; 71(2):203–209.
72. Packer M, Carver JR, Rodeheffer RJ, et al. Effect of oral milrinone on mortality in severe chronic heart failure. The PROMISE Study Research Group. N Engl J Med 1991; 325(21):1468–1475.
73. Bristow MR, Anderson FL, Port JD, et al. Differences in beta-adrenergic neuroeffector mechanisms in ischemic versus idiopathic dilated cardiomyopathy. Circulation 1991; 84(3):1024–1039.
74. Bohm M, Diet F, Feiler G, et al. Subsensitivity of the failing human heart to isopren-

aline and milrinone is related to beta-adrenoceptor downregulation. J Cardiovasc Pharmacol 1988; 12(6):726–732.
75. Limas CJ, Goldenberg IF, Limas C. Autoantibodies against beta-adrenoceptors in human idiopathic dilated cardiomyopathy. Circ Res 1989; 64(1):97–103.
76. Jansson K, Karlberg KE, Nylander E, et al. More favourable haemodynamic effects from metoprolol than from captopril in patients with dilated cardiomyopathy. Eur Heart J 1997; 18(7):1115–1121.
77. Hjalmarson A, Waagstein F. New therapeutic strategies in chronic heart failure: challenge of long-term beta-blockade. Eur Heart J 1991; 12(Suppl F):63–69.
78. Waagstein F, Bristow MR, Swedberg K, et al. Beneficial effects of metoprolol in idiopathic dilated cardiomyopathy. Metoprolol in Dilated Cardiomyopathy (MDC) Trial Study Group. Lancet 1993; 342(8885):1441–1446.
79. Shekerdemian L, Bohn D. Cardiovascular effects of mechanical ventilation. Arch Dis Child 1999; 80(5):475–480.
80. Bradley TD, Holloway RM, McLaughlin PR, et al. Cardiac output response to continuous positive airway pressure in congestive heart failure. Am Rev Respir Dis 1992; 145(2 Pt 1):377–382.
81. Naughton MT, Rahman A, Hara K, et al. Effect of continuous positive airway pressure on intrathoracic and left ventricular transmural pressures in patients with congestive heart failure. Circulation 1995; 91(6):1725–1731.
82. Tomioka N, Kishimoto C, Matsumori A, et al. Effects of prednisolone on acute viral myocarditis in mice. J Am Coll Cardiol 1986; 7(4):868–872.
83. McNamara DM, Rosenblum WD, Janosko KM, et al. Intravenous immune globulin in the therapy of myocarditis and acute cardiomyopathy. Circulation 1997; 95(11): 2476–2478.
84. Jones SR, Herskowitz A, Hutchins GM, et al. Effects of immunosuppressive therapy in biopsy-proved myocarditis and borderline myocarditis on left ventricular function. Am J Cardiol 1991; 68(4):370–376.
85. Hosenpud JD, McAnulty JH, Niles NR. Lack of objective improvement in ventricular systolic function in patients with myocarditis treated with azathioprine and prednisone. J Am Coll Cardiol 1985; 6(4):797–801.
86. Parrillo JE, Cunnion RE, Epstein SE, et al. A prospective, randomized, controlled trial of prednisone for dilated cardiomyopathy. N Engl J Med 1989; 321(16):1061–1068.
87. Gagliardi MG, Bevilacqua M, Squitieri C, et al. Dilated cardiomyopathy caused by acute myocarditis in pediatric patients: evolution of myocardial damage in a group of potential heart transpslant candidates. J Heart Lung Transplant 1993; 12(6 Pt 2):S224–229.
88. Drucker NA, Newburger JW. Viral myocarditis: diagnosis and management. Adv Pediatr 1997; 44:141–171.
89. Garg A, Shiau J, Guyatt G. The ineffectiveness of immunosuppressive therapy in lymphocytic myocarditis: an overview. Ann Intern Med 1998; 129(4):317–322.
90. Duncan BW, Hraska V, Jonas RA, et al. Mechanical circulatory support in children with cardiac disease. J Thorac Cardiovasc Surg 1999; 117(3):529–542.
91. Duncan BW, Atz AM, Bohn DJ, et al. Mechanical circulatory support for pediatric patients with acute myocarditis. Circulation 1998; 98:I–616.

92. Koenig PR, Ralston MA, Kimball TR, et al. Balloon atrial septostomy for left ventricular decompression in patients receiving extracorporeal membrane oxygenation for myocardial failure. J Pediatr 1993; 122(6):S95–99.
93. Ward KE, Tuggle DW, Gessouroun MR, et al. Transseptal decompression of the left heart during ECMO for severe myocarditis. Ann Thorac Surg 1995; 59(3):749–751.
94. Levin HR, Oz MC, Catanese KA, et al. Transient normalization of systolic and diastolic function after support with a left ventricular assist device in a patient with dilated cardiomyopathy. J Heart Lung Transplant 1996; 15(8):840–842.
95. Levin HR, Oz MC, Chen JM, et al. Reversal of chronic ventricular dilation in patients with end-stage cardiomyopathy by prolonged mechanical unloading. Circulation 1995; 91(11):2717–2720.
96. Muller J, Wallukat G, Weng YG, et al. Weaning from mechanical cardiac support in patients with idiopathic dilated cardiomyopathy. Circulation 1997; 96(2):542–549.
97. Konertz W, Hotz H, Schneider M, et al. Clinical experience with the MEDOS HIA-VAD system in infants and children: a preliminary report. Ann Thorac Surg 1997; 63(4):1138–1144.
98. Grogan M, Redfield MM, Bailey KR, et al. Long-term outcome of patients with biopsy-proved myocarditis: comparison with idiopathic dilated cardiomyopathy. J Am Coll Cardiol 1995; 26(1):80–84.
99. Tracy TF, DeLosh T, Stolar CJH. The Registry of the Extracorporeal Life Support Organization. In: Extracorporeal Cardiopulmonary Support in Critical Care. Ann Arbor, MI: The Extracorporeal Life Support Organization, 1995:251–260.
100. Meliones JN, Custer JR, Snedecor S, et al. Extracorporeal life support for cardiac assist in pediatric patients. Review of ELSO Registry data. Circulation 1991; 84(5 Suppl):III168–172.
101. Cofer BR, Warner BW, Stallion A, et al. Extracorporeal membrane oxygenation in the management of cardiac failure secondary to myocarditis. J Pediatr Surg 1993; 28(5):669–672.
102. Ishino K, Loebe M, Uhlemann F, et al. Circulatory support with paracorporeal pneumatic ventricular assist device (VAD) in infants and children. Eur J Cardiothorac Surg 1997; 11(5):965–972.
103. Stiller B, Dahnert I, Weng YG, et al. Children may survive severe myocarditis with prolonged use of biventricular assist devices. Heart 1999; 82(2):237–240.
104. Del Nido PJ, et al. Extracorporeal membrane support as a bridge to pediatric heart transplantation. Circulation 1994; 90(5 Pt 2):II66–II69.
105. Hetzer R, et al. Circulatory support with pneumatic paracorporeal ventricular assist device in infants and children. Ann Thorac Surg 1998; 66(5):1498–1506.
106. Reiss N, et al. Management of acute fulminant myocarditis using circulatory support systems. Artif Organs 1996; 20(8):964–970.
107. Konertz W, et al. Clinical experience with the MEDOS HIA-VAD system in infants and children: a preliminary report. Ann Thorac Surg 1997; 63(4):1138–1144.
108. Daily BB, et al. Pierce-Donachy pediatric VAD: progress in development. Ann Thorac Surg 1996; 61(1):437–443.

11
Long-Term Follow-Up of Children with Cardiac Disease Requiring Mechanical Circulatory Support

Andra E. Ibrahim
University of Washington School of Medicine, Seattle, Washington

Brian W. Duncan
Children's Hospital and Regional Medical Center and University of Washington School of Medicine, Seattle, Washington

I. INTRODUCTION

Mechanical circulatory support has been utilized for pediatric cardiac patients for over 20 years, yet few reports have focused on the long-term follow-up of these critically ill children. Because surviving children may be left with significant physical or neurological abnormalities, it is imperative that long-term outcomes of these children are continuously evaluated in order to confirm that this heroic therapy is worthwhile. Whether poor outcomes are the result of the treatment given or the underlying disease has been difficult to determine. By definition, these children were not expected to survive without mechanical support; thus, a true control group with which to compare outcomes does not exist. Because extracorporeal membrane oxygenation (ECMO) has been more widely used for neonates with respiratory failure, long-term follow-up studies are available for this population. In this chapter, the results of long-term outcome studies of pediatric cardiac patients who received mechanical circulatory support will be reviewed, supplemented by information from outcome studies of survivors of ECMO for respiratory failure.

II. SURVIVAL AND GENERAL HEALTH

The indication for implementing mechanical circulatory support is often based on individual institutional criteria that predict the likelihood of survival without mechanical circulatory support to be less than 20%. Because of this poor prognosis, mechanical circulatory support has been accepted as one of the final options available for these critically ill children. Most reports have documented survival–to–hospital-discharge rates for children with heart disease who receive mechanical circulatory support ranging from 25 to 75% (1–7). In these children who survive to hospital discharge, long-term survival is excellent and ranges from 83 to 94% (6,8–10). At Children's Hospital, Boston, 40% of children with heart disease who required mechanical circulatory support with either ECMO or ventricular assist device (VAD) survived to hospital discharge (1). The long-term survival of these hospital survivors was over 90% for both ECMO- and VAD-supported patients over a median duration of follow-up of 42 months (Fig. 1) (11). Based on these results, it can be expected that the majority of children who receive mechanical circulatory support for cardiac disease and survive to hospital

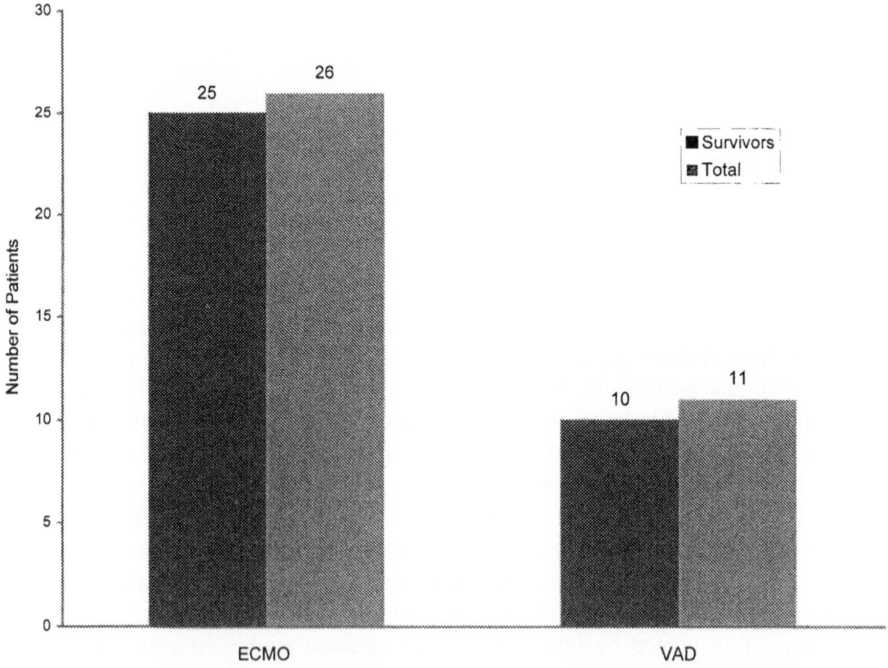

Fig. 1 Long-term survivors for ECMO and VAD compared to total number of children who survived to hospital discharge. (From Ref. 11.)

discharge will be long-term survivors. This supports the hypothesis that many of these critically ill children have reversible causes of cardiopulmonary failure, such as pulmonary hypertension or postcardiotomy failure, and if successfully supported acutely, many will survive.

As part of our study of the children with heart disease who survived ECMO or VAD, we conducted a parental questionnaire regarding general health and quality-of-life issues. Eighty percent of the parents of these surviving children reported their children's overall health as good to excellent (11). In regard to their physical growth, the median height in the ECMO-supported group was at the 28th percentile (range 10–97) and 32nd percentile in the VAD-supported group (range 1–53) (Fig. 2). The median weight in the ECMO-supported patients was at the 36th percentile (range 15–97) and in the VAD supported patients at the 44th percentile (range 1–95).

The survival-to-discharge rate for neonates who require ECMO support for respiratory failure is higher (approximately 75–87%) than the hospital survival for ECMO-supported children with cardiac disease (7,12–17). However, long-term outcome after hospital discharge is similar for the two groups, with 77–

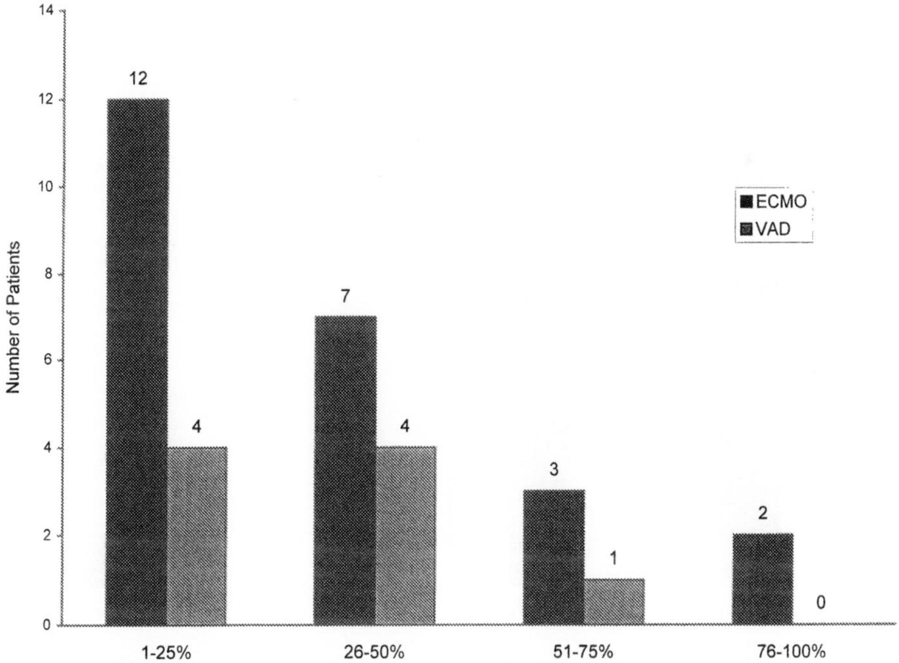

Fig. 2 Percentile height as described by standardized growth curves in long-term survivors of ECMO compared to VAD.

97% of the neonatal respiratory failure patients surviving long-term after hospital discharge (15,16,18). Long-term ECMO survivors with respiratory failure are also often small for their age. Small stature, determined using standardized growth curves for height and weight, has been found to occur in nearly 30% of these patients as well (16,17).

III. CARDIAC FUNCTION

Children with cardiac disease who require mechanical circulatory support frequently experience remarkable recovery of myocardial function. Excellent recovery of cardiac function with a normal exercise capacity was found to occur in 86% of children who survived ECMO for cardiopulmonary failure (5). Others have reported that 94% of ECMO survivors have excellent exercise capacity and are classified as New York Heart Association functional Class I (8). Our experience is consistent with these reports in that 95% of ECMO-supported patients

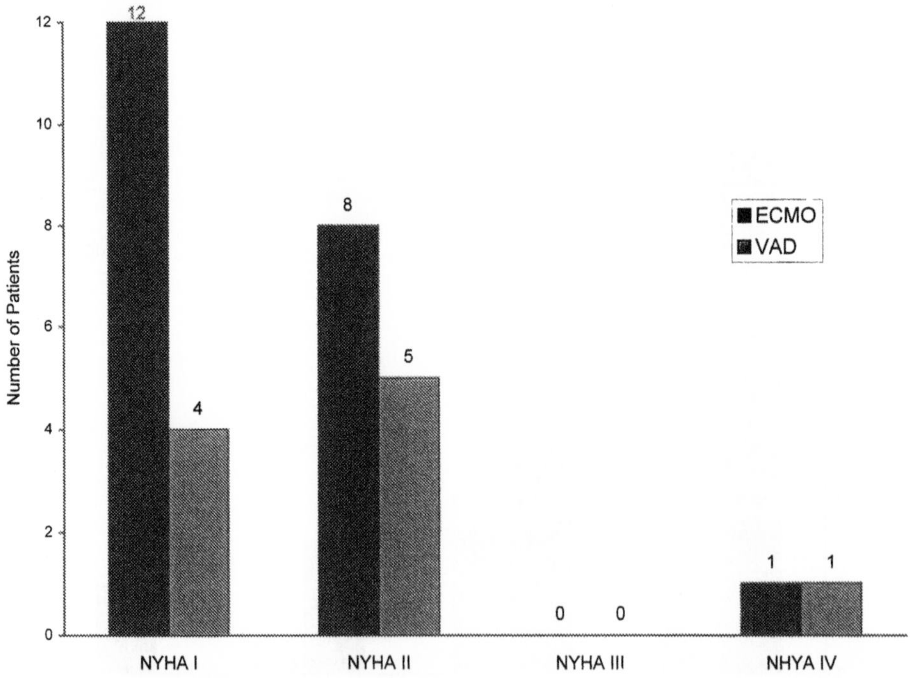

Fig. 3 New York Heart Association (NYHA) cardiac functional status of long-term survivors of ECMO and VAD.

Table 1 Residual Cardiac Lesions by Echocardiography in Long-Term Survivors of Mechanical Circulatory Support with ECMO or VAD

	ECMO (N = 23)	VAD (N = 10)
Normal left ventricular function	18	9
Depressed left ventricular function	0	1
Moderate/severe mitral regurgitation	0	2
Depressed right ventricular function	2	0
Severe tricuspid regurgitation	1	0
Right ventricular outflow tract obstruction	2	0
Moderate/severe pulmonic regurgitation	4	1
Residual ventricular septal defect	3	0
Pulmonary hypertension	0	1

Source: Ref. 11.

and 90% of VAD-supported patients were in NYHA Class I or Class II during long-term follow-up (Fig. 3). All ECMO-supported patients for whom an assessment of left ventricular function was available demonstrated normal ventricular function, while 9 of 10 VAD-supported patients had normal ventricular function after more than 3 years of follow-up (11) (Table 1).

Although recovery of myocardial function may be anticipated, further cardiac surgery has been required for some survivors of pediatric cardiac ECMO (5). Many of the significant residual cardiac lesions represent the long-term sequelae of primary corrective or palliative procedures such as homograft degeneration and pulmonic regurgitation secondary to transannular patching of the right ventricular outflow tract. From our review, 84% of the ECMO-supported patients and 70% of the VAD-supported patients remain free of further cardiac procedures (mean follow-up 42 months) (11).

IV. ASSOCIATED MEDICAL CONDITIONS

Although the survivors of mechanical circulatory support may demonstrate significant improvement in their underlying cardiopulmonary disease, these children often have associated medical conditions that contribute to their morbidity. Reactive airway disease, gastroesophageal reflux, and feeding problems were common among the long-term survivors of ECMO and VAD that we reviewed (11). Respiratory infection was the most common indication for hospital readmission in the

ECMO group, and noncardiac surgery was the most common indication in the VAD group.

V. NEUROLOGICAL OUTCOMES

A. Neurological Outcomes Prior to Hospital Discharge

The most worrisome consequence of critical illness requiring mechanical circulatory support is the possibility of significant neurological and developmental abnormalities. Because critically ill children who are treated with conventional therapy instead of mechanical circulatory support are also susceptible to neurodevelopmental abnormalities, the occurrence of neurodevelopmental abnormalities cannot be fully attributed to mode of therapy. The incidence of neurological injury in pediatric cardiac ECMO survivors varies widely among available reports due to differences in neurological testing, variations in the definition of injury, and the fact that most studies include only a small number of patients. Neurological injury seen in ECMO-supported children is multifactorial due to intracranial hemorrhage, anoxic injury, and possibly the effects of unilateral carotid artery ligation. A spectrum of the manifestations of neurological injury exists that includes developmental delay, motor deficits, seizure disorders, and abnormalities in cognitive functioning.

From our experience, in-hospital neurological complications occurred in significantly more ECMO-supported patients than VAD-supported patients (31% vs. 13%, respectively; $p = 0.042$) (1). We found intracranial hemorrhage, seizures, and cerebral infarction to be the three most common neurological complications comprising 36, 23, and 18% of all central nervous system complications, respectively. Possible explanations for poorer neurological outcomes in ECMO-supported patients include the use of ECMO in neonates with more severe coexisting disease. Sixty percent of the ECMO-supported group were neonates compared with the VAD-supported patients, where only 10% of patients were neonates. Other explanations for poorer neurological outcomes after ECMO support relate to differences in the components and maintenance of the circuit. The presence of an oxygenator in the ECMO circuit and longer tubing compared to VAD increase the likelihood of air or particulate embolic events. In addition, levels of anticoagulation that are required for ECMO are generally higher than those employed for VAD, increasing the risks of intracranial hemorrhage. In our experience, in-hospital neurological complications were independent of presupport cardiac arrest, the use of carotid cannulation, or the performance of carotid reconstruction in patients who underwent neck cannulation (1).

B. Neurological Outcomes During Long-Term Follow-Up

Of various reports describing long-term neurological outcome in ECMO survivors with congenital heart disease, the incidence of neurological impairment varies from 0 to 56% (9,19–21). The trends that we observed during hospitalization persisted during the period of follow-up, with 59% of ECMO survivors and 20% of VAD survivors demonstrating moderate to severe neurological impairment during long-term follow-up (11) (Fig. 4). The impairment demonstrated by these children was variable and included delay in attaining developmental milestones, gross motor abnormalities (cerebral palsy, hemiplegia), sensory deficits (cortical blindness, deafness), and learning disabilities.

This experience was further analyzed to determine which factors present during the initial hospitalization when mechanical circulatory support was utilized were associated with poor long-term neurological outcomes. Factors that were found to be associated with poor outcomes included low bodyweight and the use of circulatory arrest during cardiac surgery prior to the institution of mechanical circulatory support (Table 2). Small size (low bodyweight) at the time of support was significantly associated with adverse, long-term neurological outcomes in both ECMO- and VAD-supported patients. Neonates and infants may be at higher risk for neurological complications due to increased susceptibility to intracranial hemorrhage as well as greater complexity of their underlying cardiac disease. The association of neurological impairment with the use of hypo-

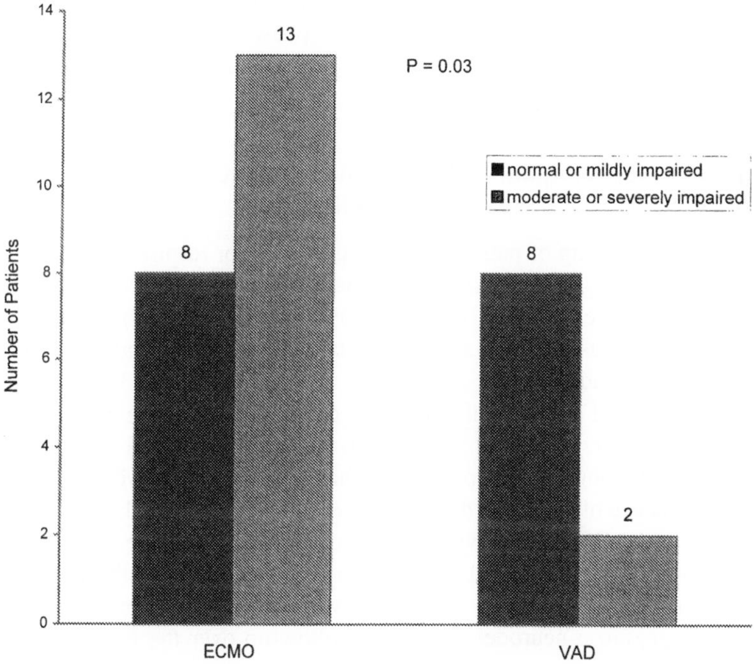

Fig. 4 Neurological impairment of long-term survivors of ECMO compared to VAD.

Table 2 Clinical Parameters at the Time of ECMO or VAD Support Associated with Long-Term Adverse Neurological Outcomes

	No neurological impairment	Neurological impairment	*p*-value
Weight	6.5 kg (range 3.4–71 kg)	4.1 kg (range 2.4–15.6 kg)	0.01
Circulatory arrest	5/17 used circulatory arrest	11/15 used circulatory arrest	0.03

Source: Ref. 11.

thermic circulatory arrest during cardiac surgery in this analysis is consistent with reports that have demonstrated the adverse impact of circulatory arrest on subsequent neurocognitive development (22,23).

Factors that were not associated with poor long-term neurological outcomes included in-hospital neurological complications during the initial hospitalization, neck cannulation, carotid reconstruction after ECMO, and the need for cardiopulmonary resuscitation (CPR) prior to support (11). This lack of association with in-hospital neurological complications supports the observation that patients suffering neurological injury during hospitalization may recover without sequelae, while other long-term neurological problems may only become apparent as the child grows older. These results further underscore the difficulties in predicting the extent of neurological injury during the acute phase of care in these children and the necessity of long-term follow-up to assess ultimate neurological status.

C. Long-Term Neurological Outcomes After ECMO Support for Neonatal Respiratory Failure

During long-term follow-up of patients surviving ECMO for respiratory failure, the incidence of neurological abnormality including motor deficits and seizure disorders has been reported to range from 13 to 45% (13,15–17,24–27). Developmental abnormality [measured by Bayley's Mental Developmental Index (MDI) and the Psychomotor Index (PDI)] has ranged from 10 to 29% (13,15,27,43) (Fig. 5). The presence of cerebral infarction and chronic lung disease have been identified as risk factors leading to abnormal neurodevelopmental outcomes (24,28). Infants with congenital diaphragmatic hernia requiring ECMO support have a higher incidence of cognitive delay compared to infants with other diagnoses (29). Nevertheless, ECMO survivors of respiratory failure do quite well overall as mean scores on the MDI and PDI have been found to be in the normal range (13,15,24). Since the majority of children with disabilities were identified by one year of age, close neurodevelopmental follow-up over the first year of life is clearly indicated.

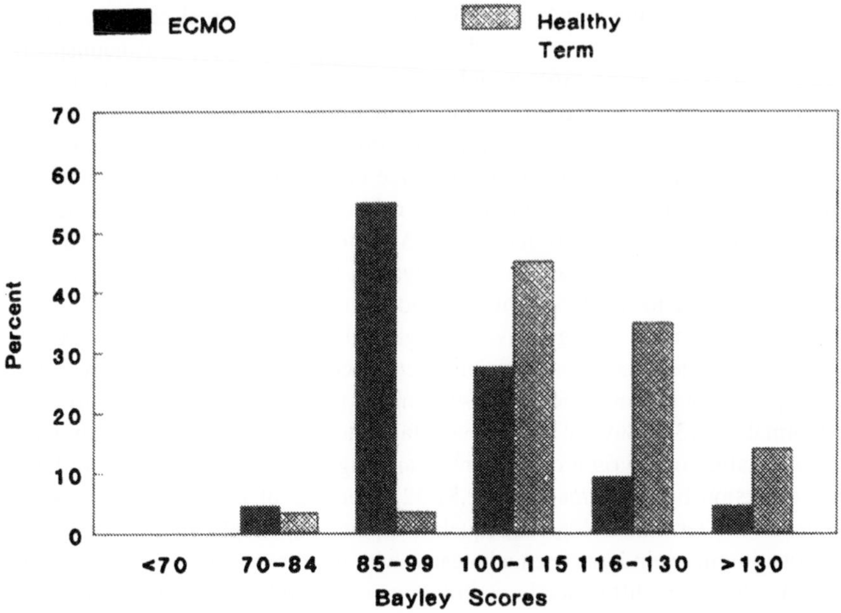

Fig. 5 The distribution of 24-month Bayley's Mental Developmental Index scores for all survivors of ECMO compared to healthy term infants. (From Ref. 43.)

D. Neurosensory Hearing Loss

Critical illness has been associated with a high incidence of delayed-onset high-frequency neurosensory hearing loss, thus frequent and complete audiological testing by a certified audiologist is recommended. Hearing loss has been reported to occur in 3–21% of survivors of severe respiratory illness, which may be due to metabolic disturbances and exposure to ototoxic drugs (16,24,41,42). No relationship has been found between the treatment modality (ECMO vs. conventional ventilation) and hearing loss in these children (28). Fifteen percent of ECMO survivors with respiratory failure have been reported to demonstrate speech and language difficulties when formally tested (16).

E. The Influence of Carotid Artery Ligation or Repair on Neurological Outcome After ECMO

Neck cannulation for ECMO employing the carotid artery and internal jugular vein has raised concerns regarding the long-term impact on neurological outcomes in these children. Unilateral carotid artery ligation is known to alter cerebral blood flow as the vertebrobasilar and contralateral internal carotid systems become the main sources of reperfusion of the ipsilateral cerebral hemisphere via the circle of Willis (36). Simultaneous systemic heparizination at a time when cerebral blood flow is altered may increase the risk for intracranial hemorrhage. The lack of association between carotid cannulation and neurological outcomes after ECMO support that we have observed is in agreement with the majority of the literature examining the role of carotid cannulation or reconstruction for children who require ECMO for respiratory failure. Adverse effects of right common carotid artery ligation have been suggested by ipsilateral hemispheric focal abnormalities found on head computed tomography, neuromotor abnormalities suggestive of right-sided brain injury, and increased slowing over the right hemisphere on electroencephalogram (37). However, follow-up has not demonstrated adverse clinical outcomes corresponding to these abnormalities (38). Several reports have failed to demonstrate an association between ligation of the right carotid artery and jugular vein and a consistent lateralizing lesion by neuroimaging (12,31,32). Because of the theoretical risk for serious long-term neurological sequelae, repair of the right carotid artery and internal jugular vein have been advocated with good results (20). However, others have found no difference in neurological outcome between patients who underwent carotid artery reconstruction compared with those managed with carotid ligation (39,40).

F. Predicting Poor Neurological Outcome After Mechanical Circulatory Support

Numerous techniques have been developed in an attempt to predict the long-term neurological outcome of children who require ECMO. Neuroimaging studies including computed tomography, cranial ultrasound, and magnetic resonance imaging have been evaluated for their capability to predict long-term neurological outcome in children who require ECMO for respiratory failure. Neuroimaging as a predictor of neurocognitive outcome has produced variable results. Both intracerebral hemorrhage (30) and nonhemorrhagic abnormalities (31) detected on neuroimaging studies have been associated with delayed development in ECMO survivors (Fig. 6). A moderate or severe neuroimaging abnormality (intracranial hemorrhage, cerebral infarction, or other abnormalities) obtained at the time of discharge from the neonatal intensive care unit has also been associated with delayed development in ECMO survivors (28). Although mean neuroimaging scores were found to be significantly worse in survivors with delayed development, the sensitivity and specificity of normal neuroimaging findings predicting normal outcome were only 65% and 63%, respectively, suggesting that outcome cannot be accurately predicted in individual patients (31). The finding of enlarged cerebrospinal fluid spaces by neuroimaging has been associated with lower MDI

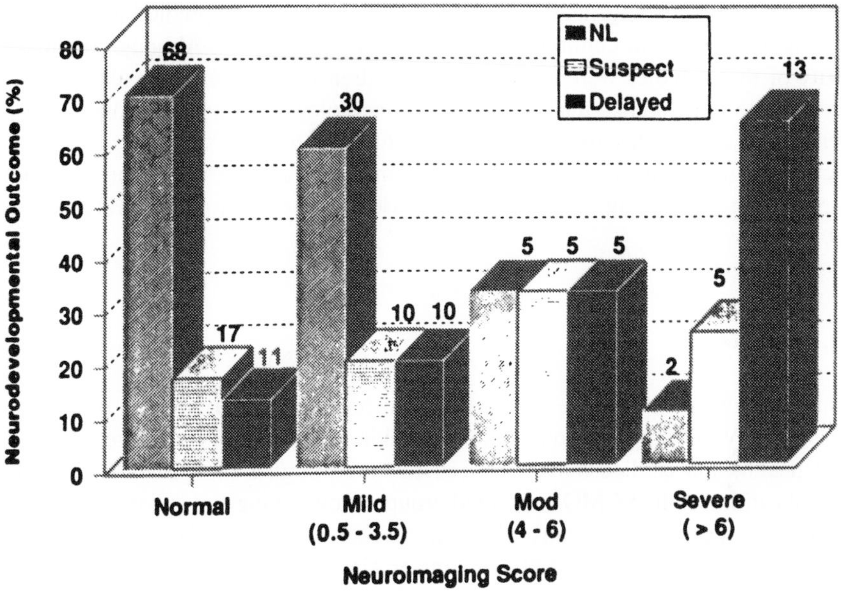

Fig. 6 Degree of abnormality of neuroimaging in neonates treated with ECMO is related to neurodevelopmental outcome (NL = normal development; mod = moderate). (From Ref. 31.)

and PDI scores at 6 and 12 months (32). The absence of intracranial hemorrhage, cerebral infarction, or cerebral atrophy by ultrasound or magnetic resonance imaging has been correlated with normal short-term neurodevelopmental outcomes (33). Conversely, others reports have found that computed tomography and electroencephalography during the neonatal period showed no relationship to developmental scores or neurological examination at one year of age (15). Pathology detected by head ultrasound may indicate neurological injury, however, studies have demonstrated that a normal head ultrasound does not exclude the possibility of significant ischemic injury to the brain (34).

Clinical factors at the time of initiation of ECMO support have also been used to predict the incidence of neurological injury. In children who require ECMO for respiratory failure, the presence of low birthweight, sepsis, congenital diaphragmatic hernia, and persistent pulmonary hypertension have been associated with a higher incidence of delayed development. Low serial plasma lactate concentrations ($\leq$15 mmol/L) before the initiation of ECMO or the first 12 hours of ECMO were predictive of favorable outcomes as measured by the Bayley Scales of Infant Development (35).

The above findings underline the difficulty in accurately predicting the neurological outcomes of children surviving mechanical support. Although the majority of these studies were performed in children with respiratory failure, they corroborate our findings that the short-term neurological status of pediatric patients with cardiac disease requiring mechanical circulatory support is not predictive of their ultimate neurological outcomes. Clearly, these patients require careful long-term follow-up with ongoing assessment of their neurodevelopmental status.

VI. SUMMARY

Children with heart disease who survive to hospital discharge after requiring ECMO or VAD support demonstrate favorable long-term survival, overall general health, and cardiac outcomes. The relatively higher rates of neurological complications in the ECMO-supported group are disturbing and appear to be due to multiple causes in critically ill children. These results may be improved by modifications in ECMO that utilize simpler circuits requiring less anticoagulation. This discussion further underscores the difficulties in predicting the extent of neurological injury during the acute phases of care in these children and the necessity of long-term follow-up to assess ultimate neurological status.

REFERENCES

1. Duncan BW, Hraska V, Jonas RA, Wessel DL, Del Nido PJ, Laussen PC, Mayer JE, LaPierre RA, Wilson JM. Mechanical circulatory support in children with cardiac disease. J Thorac Cardiovasc Surg 1999; 117:529–542.
2. Black MD, Coles JG, Williams WG, Rebeyka IM, Trusler GA, Bohn D, Gruenwald C, Freedom RM. Determinants of success in pediatric cardiac patients undergoing extracorporeal membrane oxygenation. Ann Thorac Surg 1995; 60:133–138.
3. Walters HL, Hakimi M, Rice MD, Lyons JM, Whittlesey GC, Klein MD. Pediatric cardiac surgical ECMO: multivariate analysis of risk factors for hospital death. Ann Thorac Surg 1995; 60:329–337.
4. Anderson HL, Attorri RJ, Custer JR, Chapman RA, Bartlett RH. Extracorporeal membrane oxygenation for pediatric cardiopulmonary failure. J Thorac Cardiovasc Surg 1990; 99:1011–1021.
5. Ziomek S, Harrell JE, Fasules JW, Faulkner SC, Chipman CW, Moss M, Frazier E, Van Devanter SH. Extracorporeal membrane oxygenation for cardiac failure after congenital heart operation. Ann Thorac Surg 1992; 54:861–868.
6. Dalton HJ, Siewers RD, Fuhrman BP, Del Nido P, Thompson AE, Shaver MG, Dowhy M. Extracorporeal membrane oxygenation for cardiac rescue in children with severe myocardial dysfunction. Critical Care Med 1993; 21:1020–1028.

7. Tracy TF, DeLosh T, Bartlett RH. Extracorporeal Life Support Organization 1994. ASAIO 1994; 40:1017–1019.
8. Raithel SC, Pennington G, Boegner E, Fiore A, Weber TR: Extracorporeal membrane oxygenation in children after cardiac surgery. Circulation 1992; 86(suppl II): II-305–II-310.
9. Rogers AJ, Trento A, Siewers RD, Griffith BP, Hardesty RL, Pahl E, Beerman LB, Fricker FJ, Fischer DR. Extracorporeal membrane oxygenation for postcardiotomy cardiogenic shock in children. Ann Thorac Surg 1989; 47:903–906.
10. Kanter KR, Pennington G, Weber TR, Zambie MA, Braun P, Martychenko V. Extracorporeal membrane oxygenation for postoperative cardiac support in children. J Thorac Cardiovasc Surg 1987; 93:27–35.
11. Ibrahim AE, Duncan BW, Blume ED, Jonas RA. Long-term follow-up of pediatric cardiac patients requiring mechanical circulatory support. Ann Thorac Surg 2000; 69:186–192.
12. Glass P, Miller M, Short B. Morbidity for survivors of extracorporeal membrane oxygenation: neurodevelopmental outcome at 1 year of age. Pediatrics 1989; 83:72–78.
13. Walsh-Sukys MC, Bauer RE, Cornell DJ, Friedman HG, Stork EK, Hack M. Severe respiratory failure in neonates: mortality and morbidity rates and neurodevelopmental outcomes. J Pediatr 1994; 125:104–110.
14. Stolar CJH, Snedecor SM, Bartlett RH. Extracorporeal membrane oxygenation and neonatal respiratory failure: experience from the extracorporeal life support organization. J Pediatr Surg 1991; 26:563–571.
15. Flusser H, Dodge NN, Engle WE, Garg BP, West KW. Neurodevelopmental outcome and respiratory morbidity for extracorporeal membrane oxygenation survivors at 1 year of age. J Perinatol 1993; XIII:266–271.
16. Schumacher RE, Palmer TW, Roloff DW, LaClaire PA, Bartlett RH. Follow-up of infants treated with extracorporeal membrane oxygenation for newborn respiratory failure. Pediatrics 1991; 87:451–457.
17. Towne BH, Lott IT, Hicks DA, Healey T. Long-term follow-up of infants and children treated with extracorporeal membrane oxygenation (ECMO): a preliminary report. J Pediatr Surg 1985; 20:410–414.
18. Field DJ, Group UCET. UK collaborative randomised trial of neonatal extracorporeal membrane oxygenation. Lancet 1996; 348:75–82.
19. Klein MD, Shaheen KW, Whittlesey GC, Pinsky WW, Arciniegas E. Extracorporeal membrane oxygenation for the circulatory support of children after repair of congenital heart disease. J Thorac Cardiovasc Surg 1990; 100:498–505.
20. Weinhaus L, Canter C, Noetzel M, McAlister W, Spray TL. Extracorporeal membrane oxygenation for circulatory support after repair of congenital heart defects. Ann Thorac Surg 1989; 48:206–212.
21. Delius RE, Bove EL, Meliones JN, Custer JR, Moler FW, Crowley D, Amirikia A, Behrendt DM, Bartlett RH. Use of extracorporeal life support in patients with congenital heart disease. Crit Care Med 1992; 20:1216–1222.
22. Newberger JW, Jonas RA, Wernovsky G, Wypij D, Hickey PR, Kuban KCK, Farrell DM, et al. Developmental and neurologic status of children after heart surgery with hypothermic circulatory arrest or low-flow cardiopulmonary bypass. N Engl J Med 1995; 332:549–555.

23. Bellinger DC, Jonas RA, Rappaport LA, Wypij D, Wernovsky G, Kuban KC, Barnes PD, Holmes GL, Hickey PR, et al. Developmental and neurologic status of children after heart surgery with hypothermic circulatory arrest or low-flow cardiopulmonary bypass. N Engl J Med 1995; 332:349–355.
24. Hofkosh D, Thompson AE, Nozza RJ, Kemp SS, Bowen A, Feldman HM. Ten years of extracorporeal membrane oxygenation: neurodevelopmental outcome. Pediatrics 1991; 87:549–555.
25. Krummel TM, Greenfield LJ, Kirkpatrick BV, Mueller DG, Kerkering KW, Ormazabal M, Myer EC, Barnes RW, Salzberg AM. The early evaluation of survivors after extracorporeal membrane oxygenation for neonatal pulmonary failure. J Pediatr Surg 1984; 19:585–590.
26. Kotagal S, Weber TR, Keenan W, Vogler C, Cross J, Narawong D. Neurological outcome following extracorporeal membrane oxygenation for severe newborn respiratory failure. Child Neurol Soc suppl: 393 (Abstract).
27. Andrews AF, Nixon CA, Cilley RE, Roloff DW, Bartlett RH. One- to three-year outcome for 14 neonatal survivors of extracorporeal membrane oxygenation. Pediatrics 1986; 78:692–698.
28. Vaucher YE, Dudell GG, Bejar R, Gist K. Predictors of early childhood outcome in candidates for extracorporeal membrane oxygenation. J Pediatr 1996; 128:109–117.
29. Stolar CJH, Crisafi MA, Driscoll YT: Neurocognitive outcome for neonates treated with extracorporeal membrane oxygenation: Are infants with congenital diaphragmatic hernia different? J Pediatric Surg 1995; 30:366–372.
30. Dela Cruz TV, Stewart DL, Winston SJ, Weatherman KS, Phelps JL, Mendoza JC. Risk factors for intracranial hemorrhage in the extracorporeal membrane oxygenation patient. J Perinatol 1997; 17:18–23.
31. Bulas DI, Glass P, O'Donnell RM, Taylor GA, Short BL, Vezina GL. Neonates treated with ECMO: predictive value of early CT and US neuroimaging findings on short-term neurodevelopmental outcome. Radiology 1995; 195:407–412.
32. Lago P, Rebsamen S, Clancy RR, Pinto-Martin J, Kessler A, Zimmerman R, Schmelling D, Bernbaum J, Gerdes M, D'Agostino JA, Baumgart S. MRI, MRA, and neurodevelopmental outcome following neonatal ECMO. Pediatr Neurol 1995; 12:294–304.
33. Griffin MP, Minifee PK, Landry SH, Allison PL, Swischuk LE, Zwischenberger JB. Neurodevelopmental outcome in neonates after extracorporeal membrane oxygenation: cranial magnetic resonance imaging and ultrasonography correlation. J Pediatr Surg 1992; 27:33–35.
34. Lazar EL, Abramson SJ, Weinstein S, Stolar CJH. Neuroimaging of brain injury in neonates treated with extracorporeal membrane oxygenation: lessons learned from serial examinations. J Pediatr Surg 1994; 29:186–191.
35. Cheung P-Y, Robertson CMT, Finer NN. Plasma lactate as a predictor of early childhood neurodevelopmental outcome of neonates with severe hypoxaemia requiring extracorporeal membrane oxygenation. Arch Dis Child 1996; 74:F47–F50.
36. Raju TNK, Kim SY, Meller JL, Srinivasan G, Ghai V, Reyes H. Circle of Willis blood velocity and flow direction after common carotid artery ligation for neonatal extracorporeal membrane oxygenation. Pediatrics 1989; 83:343–347.

37. Schumacher RE, Barks JDE, Johnston MV, Donn SM, Scher MS, Roloff DW, Bartlett RH. Right-sided brain lesions in infants following extracorporeal membrane oxygenation. Pediatrics 1988; 82:155–161.
38. von Allmen D, Ryckman FC. Cardiac arrest in the ECMO candidate. J Pediatr Surg 1991; 26:143–146.
39. McGahren ED, Mallik K, Rodgers SBM. Neurological outcome is diminished in survivors of congenital diaphragmatic hernia requiring extracorporeal membrane oxygenation. J Pediatr Surg 1997; 32:1216–1220.
40. Baumgart S, Streletz LJ, Needleman L, Merton DA, Wolfson PJ, Desai SA, McKee LM, Desai H, Spitzer AR, Graziani LJ. Right common carotid artery reconstruction after extracorporeal membrane oxygenation: Vascular imaging, cerebral circulation, electroencephalographic, and neurodevelopmental correlates to recovery. J Pediatrics 1994; 125:295–304.
41. Glass P, Wagner AE, Papero PH, Rajasingham SR, Civitello LA, Kjaer MS, Coffman CE, Getson PR, Short BL: Neurodevelopmental status at age five years of neonates treated with extracorporeal membrane oxygenation. J Pediatrics 1995; 127: 447–457.
42. Glass P, Bulas DI, Wagner AE, Rajasingham SR, Civitello LA, Papero PH, Coffman CE, Short BL. Severity of brain injury following neonatal extracorporeal membrane oxygenation and outcome at age 5 years. Dev Med Child Neurol 1997; 39:441–448.
43. Wildin SR, Landry SH, Zwischenberger JB. Prospective, controlled study of developmental outcome in survivors of extracorporeal membrane oxygenation: the first 24 months. Pediatrics 1994; 93:404–408.

12

The Use of Mechanical Circulatory Support in Pediatric Cardiac Transplantation

Emile A. Bacha, Leslie Smoot, and Pedro J. del Nido
Children's Hospital and Harvard Medical School, Boston, Massachusetts

Patricia O'Brien
Children's Hospital, Boston, Massachusetts

I. INTRODUCTION

The most common indication for mechanical circulatory support in children is for contractile dysfunction following reconstructive cardiac surgery. More recently, however, with the expanded use of cardiac transplantation in patients with congenital heart defects, there is a growing experience with mechanical support of children awaiting transplantation (1). Similarly, due to the encouraging short- and long-term results with the use of extracorporeal membrane oxygenation (ECMO) in children following cardiac arrest, there is increasing experience with ECMO support for posttransplant patients having severe graft dysfunction from rejection (2). We have established a program for mechanical circulatory support in children as a bridge to transplantation and for "rescue" therapy in cases of severe rejection and hemodynamic instability. Based on previous observations, we have developed criteria defining indications for support and criteria for decision making in the management of circulatory support. In this report we describe our methods of management of circulatory support, indications for use as bridge to transplant or as "rescue" therapy posttransplant, and results from 1990 to the present.

II. MECHANICAL SUPPORT AS A BRIDGE TO TRANSPLANTATION

In this category two patient groups can be identified, which require different assessment and management. The largest group consists of children who develop severe contractile dysfunction following reconstructive cardiac surgery and show little if any recovery of contractile function early on. The second group is composed of children with cardiomyopathy who are already considered candidates for transplantation but who have further hemodynamic deterioration due to either contractile dysfunction or arrhythmia and require mechanical circulatory support. Although there are important similarities among the two groups, management of mechanical support, types of complications, and their management are sufficiently different that separate consideration is warranted.

A. Postcardiotomy Circulatory Support

1. Indications for Support

Although this group is the most heterogeneous with respect to anatomical defects and etiology of low cardiac output, approach to management of support and decision making regarding indications for transplantation is relatively uniform. The decision as to whether to support with mechanical assistance usually has already been made, and the critical decisions remaining include whether the child is or remains a candidate for transplantation and the technique of support that will minimize complications and is suitable for long-term support. As with any patient requiring mechanical circulatory support after reconstructive surgery, an immediate and thorough evaluation of the cause for low cardiac output must be made since a significant number may have potentially correctable residual defects as the etiology of low output. This type of evaluation is also helpful in determining whether the child is a candidate for long-term support and/or transplantation. Frequently, complete evaluation requires echocardiography and diagnostic cardiac catheterization to determine the presence or absence of important hemodynamic residual or previously undetected defects. This is particularly important in cases where cardiac contractile function appears adequate but attempts at weaning off circulatory support fail. If found, repair of the residual defect remains the best option in spite of the potential technical difficulty in effecting complete repair.

2. Techniques of Support

Available methods of mechanical circulatory support in children are limited due to a number factors. Distensibility of the thoracic aorta and limited ability to adjust proper timing of balloon inflation have limited the use of intra-aortic balloon counterpulsation (IABP) in children. Furthermore, since the etiology of dysfunction is rarely coronary obstruction, augmenting coronary flow is rarely helpful. Balloon deflation in early systole can potentially augment ventricular ejection, but to a limited extent in children. For these reasons, IABP has a very limited role in circulatory assistance as a bridge to transplantation in children and very few reports exist of this method having been used successfully (3).

The two most commonly used techniques of pretransplant circulatory support in children have been ECMO and, in cases where lung function is adequate and pulmonary resistance relatively low, ventricular assistance with a centrifugal pump (1,4–7). In Europe, where there is access to a pneumatically driven pediatric-size pulsatile device, long-term support with such a device has also been used successfully in children pretransplant (8,9). The majority of experience in North America, however, is with veno-arterial ECMO. This is due primarily to the ready availability of roller-pump systems in pediatric cardiac centers and the frequent use of ECMO for respiratory support in neonates, resulting in familiarity with its use.

ECMO for long-term (>7 days) support, however, requires a different management strategy than ECMO for respiratory support. To avoid complications with hemorrhage, mediastinal infection, and compression of cardiac structures, choice of cannula, cannulation site, and cannula position are important. Thin-walled flexible cannulas are now available that, due to their favorable outer- to inner-diameter ratio, facilitate pump flow and venous return, allow greater choice of cannulation site, and can be tunneled subcutaneously, permitting more secure closure of the mediastinum.

Postcardiotomy transmediastinal cannulation has the advantages of ready access for venous and arterial cannulation sites, faster access in an emergency, and the possibility of addition of vents for left atrial or ventricular decompression. Potential disadvantages include increased mediastinal bleeding, usually due to mediastinal dissection, higher likelihood of a poorly sealed mediastinal wound, increased risk of infection, poor cannula position (particularly the atrial cannula, which can compress coronary arteries as the sternum comes together, pushing the venous cannula medially). Cannulation via neck vessel avoids these potential complications, but access usually requires a new incision (supraclavicular or groin). Venous cannula position is harder to judge, and poor venous return from the cannula tip not being in the right atrium can be a significant problem and usually requires carotid artery and jugular vein ligation, which may increase the risk of neurological injury. Femoral artery cannulation is rarely used in infants due to the small size of the groin vessels. Even in older children, limb ischemia frequently requires cannulation of the distal femoral artery via a side port from the arterial cannula to prevent irreversible ischemic injury. Femoral venous cannulation can also be complicated by the need for long cannulas to reach the right atrium in order to achieve adequate venous return.

Unlike ECMO for respiratory failure, mechanical support for cardiac dysfunction requires decompression of the ventricles to prevent further damage from overdistention. For the right ventricle right atrial decompression with the venous cannula is usually sufficient. However, for the left ventricle, atrial decompression is frequently insufficient particularly if aortic regurgitation is present, necessitating cannulation of the left ventricle by positioning a cannula across the mitral valve.

Ventricular assist devices are usually utilized in cases of unilateral ventricular dysfunction and rarely for biventricular dysfunction in children. Examples include left ventricular (LV) dysfunction from anomalous origin of the left coronary from the pulmonary artery and right coronary ostial injury at the time of aorto-septoplasty for LV outflow obstruction. Right ventricular dysfunction due to elevated pulmonary vascular resistance will be discussed later in the section on posttransplant mechanical circulatory support. Cannulation is almost always via sternotomy incision, and most commonly, atrial cannulation is used for inflow and direct aortic cannulation, without use of a synthetic graft, for arterial outflow.

Anticoagulation is used in all patients with heparin infusion maintaining activated clotting time (ACT) between 180 to 220 seconds. Lower ACT can be accepted if bleeding is significant with increased risk of thrombus formation in the oxygenator or at the cannulation sites. Platelet transfusions are given to maintain the total platelet count greater than 100,000/mL. Administration of clotting factors with fresh frozen plasma or cryoprecipitate is also used in conjunction with platelet administration when excessive bleeding is observed from the cannula sites or when there is a decreasing need for heparin to maintain anticoagulation, indicating consumption of clotting factors. If ventricular function is recovering and bleeding is problematic, we have found that infusion of antifibrinolytic agents is effective in reducing bleeding temporarily. We have been hesitant, however, to use antifibrinolytic agents in patients with severe ventricular dysfunction or where a prosthesis has been inserted due to the potential for thrombus formation.

Pulmonary edema from left atrial hypertension in patients with severe left ventricular dysfunction is a frequent complication that can be avoided if detected and treated early. In any patient with severe ventricular dysfunction where LV ejection is minimal, decompression should be considered. Signs of left ventricular dilatation, elevated left atrial or capillary wedge pressures (>12–15 mmHg), or a change in lung compliance should be considered an indication for LV decompression. If direct access to mediastinal structures is not available, creation of an interatrial communication in the catheterization laboratory by transseptal puncture and balloon dilatation or insertion of a long sheathe via femoral vein, connected to the venous return line, can be effective in decompressing the left atrium.

Infectious complication risk increases over time, and the majority of children on support with an open mediastinal wound develop bacteremia within 7–10 days. Although we use antibiotic prophylaxis to cover *Staphylococcus aureus*, broad-spectrum prophylactic antibiotic therapy is best avoided since selection for resistant organisms or fungal infections can occur. Antiseptic solutions to keep the mediastinum clean and topical antibiotic ointment are routinely used at our institution. When sepsis is suspected, preemptive use of broad-spectrum antibiotics covering potential pathogens (gram-positive cocci and gram-negatives, including *Pseudomonas*) is frequently employed. Positive cultures without signs of sepsis are usually treated by observation and repeat cultures and are not an absolute contraindication to transplantation if an organ becomes available. If hemodynamic instability or increased third space loss is observed, then antibiotics are started covering likely pathogens pending positive identification of the organism. In this case, transplantation is delayed until a clear response to antibiotic therapy is observed.

3. *Indications for Transplantation*

The decision to list a child who is on mechanical circulatory support for heart transplantation is usually complex involving many factors, including assessment of end-organ function, detailed cardiac evaluation to look for residual defects, investigation of alternative cardiac procedures, and evaluation of recovery of cardiac contractile function, along with the standard criteria for transplantation.

If a thorough search for residual cardiac defects has been performed and evaluation of end-organ function including neurological status does not demonstrate irreversible injury, then assessment of the degree of contractile recovery should be made. In our experience as well as that of others (1,6,8), in the children that were able to be weaned from circulatory support, the majority showed significant recovery of contractile function within 48–72 hours after initiating mechanical support. In children supported by ECMO or centrifugal pump, this is usually evident by the observation of pulsatility on the arterial line tracing. If minimal or no recovery of contractile function is observed after 2–3 days of support, then consideration should be given to placing the child on the transplant waiting list. Other criteria for heart transplantation should also be considered, such as the presence of pulmonary hypertension, irreversible neurological injury, or contraindication to chronic immune suppressive therapy.

4. *Complications*

The most frequent complications seen in children on mechanical circulatory support for postcardiotomy contractile dysfunction include bleeding, infection, and, if left ventricular distention is left untreated, pulmonary edema. The timing of onset and degree of bleeding is in large part dependent on the timing of initiation of support with respect to the cardiac procedure and whether reopening the sternotomy incision was required for cannulation. Fresh incisions or recent dissection of healing incisions results in bleeding that is difficult to control in patients receiving continuous heparin infusion. The rate of blood loss can be minimized by careful hemostasis after cannulation, particularly reinforcement of cannulation sites; if possible, cannulation via neck or groin vessels if mechanical support is initiated after the sternal incision has been closed; keeping platelet counts and clotting factor levels optimal; and permitting the activated clotting times to fall to 160–180 seconds. Although significant bleeding occurs in nearly all children, particularly the longer the support run continues, if attention is paid to controlling the potential sources of blood loss in combination with adequate replacement of platelet and clotting factors, rarely should bleeding be a cause for discontinuation of support prior to transplantation.

Sepsis is also a frequent complication of circulatory support with the incidence increasing the longer the child is on mechanical support. Gram-positive organisms are more commonly seen in younger patients, whereas gram-negative or enteric bacteremia is seen more commonly in older children. Positive cultures obtained from the circuit should be repeated with peripheral blood cultures since contamination of the sample is a frequent problem in samples obtained from sites in the circuit that are accessed repeatedly. Clinical signs of sepsis are usually evident by hemodynamic instability with hypotension while on support and third space fluid retention. Transplantation should be delayed in cases where signs of sepsis are evident but can be considered early after starting antibiotic therapy if there is improvement in hemodynamic stability. In such cases, delay in starting steroid and/or azathioprine therapy following transplantation should be considered until sepsis is well controlled.

End-organ dysfunction occurring while on mechanical support is rare in the absence of sepsis or inadequate perfusion flow rate. For this reason, aggressive management of sepsis and careful attention to cannula size and position is imperative in the management of children undergoing circulatory support as a bridge to transplantation.

B. Hemodynamic Instability in Children Awaiting Transplant

1. Indications for Support

Rapidly progressive deterioration of cardiac function or onset of potentially malignant ventricular arrhythmia is a well-known feature of end-stage cardiomyopathy. Administration of intravenous inotropic therapy is frequently effective in temporarily improving contractile function. However, eventually this treatment becomes ineffective, whereby patients require higher doses or cannot be weaned from inotropic support. In such cases, consideration should be given to mechanical circulatory support prior to significant end-organ damage. In cases where the onset of illness is rapid and cardiac function deteriorates rapidly, such as with viral myocarditis, mechanical circulatory support can be very effective in maintaining organ perfusion while cardiac function recovers or, if no recovery is seen, while awaiting transplantation (2).

Ventricular arrhythmia can also complicate end-stage cardiomyopathy, and in cases where recurrent or poorly controlled ventricular tachycardia is seen, urgent initiation of mechanical circulatory support may be required. In such cases, ventricular decompression may also make control of the arrhythmia with medications easier to manage since the negative inotropic effects of many of these drugs is no longer important if full cardiac support is achieved, such as with ECMO or biventricular assist devices.

Another much smaller group of patients is the group with congenital heart defects that are deemed inoperable and are awaiting transplantation. Although in the majority of these children options for conventional procedures do exist, the treating institution may opt for transplantation due to the high risk (short or long term) of conventional surgery. The indications for mechanical circulatory support while awaiting transplantation in this group are frequently limited to resuscitation from hemodynamic decompensation. Application of mechanical support in young infants listed for heart transplant has been reported, but few of these children survived to transplantation (10). In this report, the group of infants receiving mechanical circulatory support included children with hypoplastic left heart syndrome or an equivalent single ventricle lesion. Management of this group is particularly difficult due to the presence of a patent arterial duct in the face of falling pulmonary resistance, resulting in pulmonary overcirculation and limited systemic perfusion.

2. Techniques of Support

The method of cannulation in children who have not had a recent sternotomy is most commonly through neck vessels and, in older children, through the femoral vessels. Adequate venous decompression must be assured when inserting the cannula through a site remote from the right atrium. This is more frequently a problem with femoral vein cannulation due to the short length of the small ECMO cannulas available.

In spite of decompressing the right heart, left ventricular distention is a frequent problem due to the inability of the left ventricle to pump against the pressure generated by the mechanical pump. For this reason, inotropic support should not be discontinued after initiating circulatory support unless there is evidence that the left ventricle is capable of ejecting against systemic resistance. This may be evident by the presence of pulsatility on the arterial line tracing and should be confirmed by echocardiography. If an interatrial communication is present and of adequate size, left atrial decompression may be accomplished by the single venous cannula. In cases where left atrial distention is observed, creation or enlargement of the interatrial communication can be achieved in the catheterization laboratory. In rare cases with very poor left ventricular function or when aortic regurgitation is present, direct left ventricular decompression may be necessary by placement of a sheath across the atrial septum and mitral valve and connecting the sheath to the venous return line.

3. Complications

The types of complications seen in this group of children is similar to those seen in postcardiotomy patients with the exception that bleeding is less common early during the run. Bleeding at the cannulation site or from nasal intubation occurs frequently after 5–7 days of support. Pulmonary edema from left ventricular and left atrial distention is also an important potential complication in this group. As discussed in the previous section, early recognition and treatment is usually effective in preventing lung damage. Early in our experience we found that once pulmonary edema has developed, recovery of lung function on ECMO may take several days and frequently lags behind radiographic improvement. In one case, ECMO support was required in a child for 3 days after transplantation due to respiratory dysfunction and hypoxia (4). Sepsis is also less frequent early in this group compared to the postcardiotomy patients, primarily due to the absence of open wound sites. Late during the run, however, sepsis risk is the same as in the postcardiotomy patients.

III. POSTTRANSPLANT CARDIAC SUPPORT

Requirement for mechanical circulatory support in children posttransplantation is uncommon, but indications can be divided into the group that exhibit early graft dysfunction and those that have hemodynamic decompensation late, usually due to severe graft rejection. The techniques of support are the same as described for postcardiotomy children or children with cardiomyopathy and hemodynamic decompensation. Transsternal cannulation is used most often when graft dysfunction is seen early and peripheral cannulation via neck or femoral vessel when graft decompensation occurs late. In patients requiring circulatory support soon after transplantation, as with children requiring postcardiotomy support, a thorough evaluation of the etiology of graft dysfunction is imperative to achieve optimal results. If technical problems are detected with the implantation or residual defects are present, these should be corrected. This latter complication is most often seen in children having transplantation for treatment of congenital heart defects. Frequently anatomical distortion or unusual anatomy makes connection to the donor heart chambers difficult. Treatment of peripheral pulmonary artery stenosis should also be undertaken particularly if right ventricular dysfunction is suspected. It is unwise to assume that early graft dysfunction or right ventricular failure is due to poor preservation techniques during explant or transport or to hyperacute rejection. Although these complications do occur, they are uncommon, and this diagnosis should be made only after an exhaustive search for other causes or ventricular dysfunction.

A. Circulatory Support for Graft Failure

In the uncommon circumstance that poor myocardial preservation or coronary air emboli are the cause of ventricular dysfunction, recovery of contractile function is seen frequently after 3–5 days, even in cases where little contractile activity is seen initially. It is therefore worthwhile, in this group, to consider mechanical circulatory support early, prior to prolonged use of high-dose inotropic support, which may further damage the myocardium. Multiple attempts at weaning off bypass with increasing doses of inotropic drugs may result in converting a reversible injury to an irreversible one.

The management of circulatory support in this group of patients is the same as for the postcardiotomy group except that immune suppressive therapy must be initiated at some point after transplantation. Most of these patients have already received bolus steroids on bypass during the transplant procedure, and in some centers azathioprine and/or cyclosporin are administered before or during surgery. Continuation of immune suppression is best deferred until end-organ function, and specifically renal function can be assessed. In cases where renal function is not impaired, cyclosporin or tacrolimus may be started within 12 or 24 hours after transplantation with careful monitoring of effects of renal function. Often steroid therapy is withheld until discontinuation of mechanical support and sternal closure is accomplished or imminent.

B. Graft Right Ventricular Failure

Right ventricular (RV) dysfunction is one of the more common causes of low cardiac output in children immediately following heart transplantation. Elevated pulmonary vascular resistance and a right ventricle unprepared for the high afterload is a frequent mechanism for RV dysfunction. However, other causes should be ruled out prior to invoking this mechanism. Donor pulmonary artery distortion, recipient pulmonary artery or pulmonary vein stenosis, air emboli into the right coronary, or tricuspid regurgitation from donor right atrial distortion should be ruled out as well. These latter causes can be corrected if recognized, and although mechanical support may still be required briefly, recovery of RV function usually occurs within a few days.

In cases where elevated pulmonary vascular resistance is the cause of RV dysfunction, mechanical circulatory support alone may not be successful and other adjunct treatments should be initiated. If a positive response in pulmonary resistance to high inspired oxygen or nitric oxide therapy was noted pretransplant, then this should be initiated early and continued briefly even after weaning off circulatory support. Right ventricular ''training'' by gradual weaning from circulatory support may be attempted but is usually difficult due to our limited ability to quantify right ventricular contractile function. Too rapid a weaning may further damage the right ventricle resulting in irreversible injury. For these reasons, RV ''training,'' unlike the experience with left ventricle, is rarely successful.

C. Circulatory Support for Severe Rejection

Based on the generally good outcome in children placed on mechanical circulatory support for sudden unexpected cardiac arrest, several centers have begun using rapid response institution of ECMO therapy in transplant patients having severe low cardiac output or cardiac arrest due to severe rejection (1,6,7). The justification has been that the rejection episode is usually reversible with aggressive immune suppression therapy and that recovery of graft function to previous levels can usually be expected.

Management of circulatory support in this group is similar to that of children with cardiomyopathy awaiting heart transplantation with the exception that immune suppression therapy is the main treatment that will permit successful discontinuation of mechanical support. Usually a combination of pulse steroid therapy and antilymphocyte therapy is undertaken. Careful monitoring of renal function during circulatory support is important since impaired renal function can significantly complicate the management of maintenance rejection therapy with cyclosporin or tacrolimus.

IV. RESULTS

Experience with mechanical circulatory support in children pre– or post–cardiac transplantation is limited in most transplant centers (4–7). This is due in part to the relatively small overall number of children listed for transplantation compared to adults and the limitations inherent in the types of support devices available for children. Many centers are hesitant to initiate mechanical support with ECMO or centrifugal pump due to the high incidence of complications and the limited time that mechanical support can be maintained without significant complications.

Our experience with centrifugal pump for ventricular assistance and ECMO pre- and posttransplant includes a total of 20 patients from September 1990 to July 1999. During this time period 71 heart transplants were performed at Children's Hospital. Thirteen children had mechanical support pretransplant, 2 of

Table 1 Results with Mechanical Support and Heart Transplant in Children

Pretransplant support:		13pts.	*Posttransplant support*:		9pts.
VAD-3pts.			VAD-4pts.		
ECMO-10pts.			ECMO-5pts.		
Survival:	*early*	*late*	Survival:	*early*	*late*
	9/13 (69%)	8/13 (62%)		4/9 (44%)	2/9 (22%)

VAD = Ventricular assist device; ECMO = extracorporeal membrane oxygenation.

whom also required support posttransplant. Nine children were placed on mechanical support posttransplant, including the 2 who where supported pretransplant. The type of mechanical support device and results are shown in Table 1.

Nine patients (69%) who were supported pretransplant survived mechanical support and received a transplant and survived to discharge from the hospital. One of the initial survivors died within 6 months after transplantation for an overall long-term survival of 62%. This result is similar and slightly better than previous reports with similar cohort of patients (4,6,7). The small number and heterogeneity of the patients precludes statistical analysis of risk factors, however, it is likely that increased experience, earlier initiation of support, and improved patient selection may further improve these results.

In contrast with the encouraging results with mechanical support pretransplant, posttransplant circulatory support had very limited impact on survival. Of the nine children supported posttransplant, only four could be weaned from support, and two of these died within one year after circulatory support. In this group it is important to differentiate the patients who required support for early graft dysfunction from those placed on mechanical assistance late after transplantation. In the early graft dysfunction group, delay in initiating support, inadequate ventricular decompression, and fixed elevated pulmonary vascular resistance were significant contributing factors for worse outcome. These factors may be significantly reduced with early recognition of graft dysfunction, particularly RV failure, initiation of mechanical support prior to or instead of high-dose inotropic support in patients with severe low cardiac output, and, if responsive, use of selective pulmonary vasodilators such as nitric oxide.

V. CONCLUSIONS

Mechanical circulatory support can play an important role in the management of heart transplant patients, both as a bridge to transplantation and for posttransplant support in cases of early graft dysfunction or severe rejection. The available systems for children are limited, and in North America ECMO or ventricular assist with a centrifugal pump remain the most commonly used techniques. Postcardiotomy mechanical support pretransplant is still the most common indication, and mechanical support for early graft dysfunction is a close second. The early results in the former group is encouraging, with over 50% of the children being successfully weaned from support and surviving long term. Results with mechanical support for graft dysfunction either early after transplantation or late due to severe rejection are not as good. The reasons for this finding are multiple and include our inability to recognize and treat the causes of RV dysfunction early after transplantation and the difficulty in managing immune suppression therapy in children with recurrent episodes of severe rejection.

REFERENCES

1. Duncan BW, Hraska V, Jonas RA, Wessel DL, del Nido PJ, Laussen PC, Mayer JE, Lapierre RA, Wilson JM. Mechanical circulatory support in children with cardiac disease. J Thorac Cardiovasc Surg 1999; 117:529–542.
2. del Nido PJ, Dalton HJ, Thompson AE, Siewers RD. Extracorporeal membrane oxygenator rescue in children during cardiac arrest after cardiac surgery. Circulation 1992; 86:II300–304.
3. Park JK, Hsu DT, Gersony WM. Intraaortic balloon pump management of refractory congestive heart failure in children. Pediatr Card 1993; 14:19–22.
4. del Nido PJ, Armitage JM, Fricker FJ, Shaver M, Cipriani L, Dayal G, Park SC, Siewers RD. Extracorporeal membrane oxygenation support as a bridge to pediatric heart transplantation. Circulation 1994; 90:II66–II69.
5. Delius RE, Zwischenberger JB, Cilley R, Behrendt DM, Bove EL, Deeb M, Crowley D, Heidelberger KP, Bartlett RH. Prolonged extracorporeal support of pediatric and adolescent cardiac transplant patients. Ann Thorac Surg 1990; 50:791–795 (updated in Ann Thorac Surg 1998; 65:877–878).
6. Galantowicz ME, Stolar CJ. Extracorporeal membrane oxygenation for perioperative support in pediatric heart transplantation. J Thorac Cardiovasc Surg 1991; 102:148–151.
7. Whyte RI, Deeb GM, McCurry KR, Anderson HL, Bolling SF, Bartlett RH. Extracorporeal life support after heart or lung transplantation. Ann Thorac Surg 1994; 58:754–759.
8. Ishino K, Weng Y, Alexi-Meskishvili V, Loebe M, Uhlemann F, Lange PE, Hetzer R. Extracorporeal membrane oxygenation as a bridge to cardiac transplantation in children. Artif Organs 1996; 20:728–732.
9. Sidiropoulos A, Hotz H, Konertz W. Pediatric circulatory support. J Heart Lung Transplant 1998; 17:1172–1176.
10. Morrow WR. Naftel D, Chinnock R, Canter C, Boucek M, Zales V, McGiffin DC, Kirklin JK. Outcome of listing for heart transplantation in infants younger than six months: predictors of death and interval to transplantation. J Heart Lung Transplant 1997; 16:1255–1265.

13

The Use of Extracorporeal Membrane Oxygenation for Cardiac Support in Children with Noncardiac Disease

Caroline Killick and Allan Goldman
Great Ormond Street Hospital for Children, London, England

I. INTRODUCTION

Extracorporeal membrane oxygenation (ECMO) is a well-established treatment for cardiorespiratory failure in the neonatal and paediatric population. The majority of pediatric patients supported with ECMO have isolated respiratory failure secondary to pneumonia and acute lung injury and can be supported by venovenous ECMO.

The need for extracorporeal circulatory support in noncardiac neonatal and pediatric patients usually arises as a result of septic shock. This chapter therefore focuses on this scenario.

Septic shock is a life-threatening yet potentially reversible disease fulfilling the major criteria for ECMO. Venoarterial ECMO can provide circulatory support in refractory shock when the myocardium fails, in a similar fashion to perioperative support given to children following surgery for congenital heart disease. Shock is often associated with multiorgan failure, and ECMO may help to restore tissue perfusion and reverse pulmonary hypertension, a common occurrence in neonatal and pediatric sepsis.

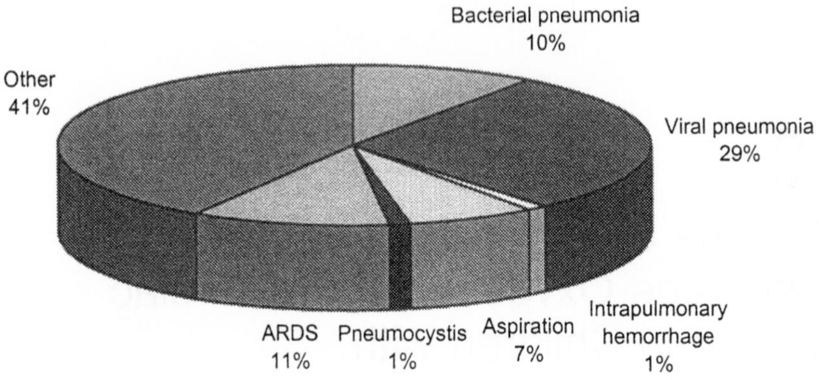

Fig. 1 Data from ELSO registry, 1986–1998 (n = 1631).

II. CARDIOVASCULAR DISTURBANCES IN SEPTIC SHOCK

In septic shock, inadequate tissue perfusion with impaired cellular respiration results from a complex interplay of several pathophysiological mechanisms, including hypovolemic, distributive, and cardiogenic shock (1,2). The initial hemodynamic disturbance is dominated by massive vasodilation and capillary leak of plasma into the extravascular space. Administration of fluid during this phase can lead to a transient improvement in intravascular volume with a fall in systemic vascular resistance, accompanied by a normal or increased cardiac output and tachycardia.

As septic shock progresses, this hyperdynamic state is complicated by right and left ventricular dysfunction with decreased ejection fraction and dilatation of the ventricles. Volume loading in this circumstance can lead to overdistension of the ventricle beyond the optimal point on the Frank-Starling curve with reduced left ventricular stroke work (3). The most convincing explanation for the myocardial dysfunction observed in sepsis is that of a circulating myocardial depressant substance. Experiments using human serum incubated with rat myocardial cell preparations show that serum from healthy volunteers does not affect rat myocardial cell contraction, whereas that from patients with septic shock produces a significant decrease in the extent and velocity of shortening (4). This substance has not yet been isolated.

III. INFLAMMATORY MEDIATORS

The pathophysiology of sepsis is thought to evolve from a complex cascade of events triggered by the release of exotoxins, endotoxins, and endogenous in-

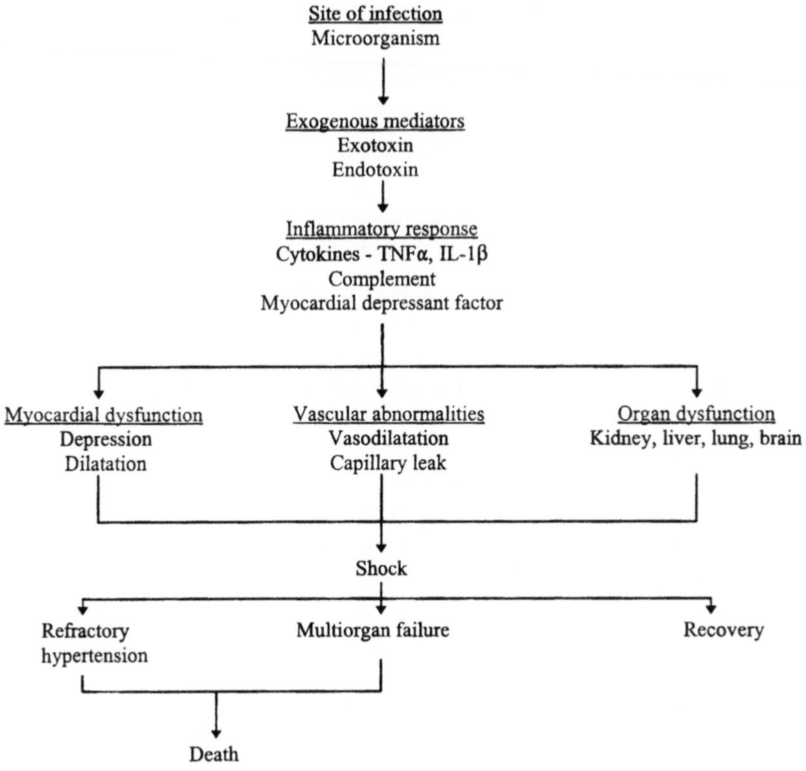

Fig. 2 Cascade of events in septic shock.

flammatory mediators. Tumor necrosis factor (TNFα) produced by monocytes and macrophages, as well as other endogenous cytokines, such as interleukin (IL)-1β and IL-6, have been implicated in multiorgan failure and depression of myocardial function (5,6). Figure 2 shows the cascade of events and pathogenesis of septic shock.

From a therapeutic point of view, several promising agents designed to diminish the production or effects of pro-inflammatory cytokines, particularly TNFα and IL-1β, have been studied with little effect on outcome (7). Recent studies have questioned this approach and hypothesized that damage is not necessarily the result of excess pro-inflammatory cytokines but rather due to an imbalance between pro- and anti-inflammatory cytokines (8). Promising strategies aimed at manipulating the systemic inflammatory response have not, however, been shown to significantly improve outcome in human beings (9,10).

IV. TREATMENT STRATEGIES IN SEPTIC SHOCK

Current treatment in septic shock is directed at three main steps in the pathogenesis of the septic process.

1. Eradication of infection by the early use of appropriate antimicrobial therapy
2. Modulating the systemic inflammatory response (discussed earlier)
3. Support of vital organ function in specialized intensive care units

Conventional management of critically ill patients with septic shock remains the domain of the intensive care staff in ensuring vital end organ perfusion and function. In the early phase of the disease process, the focus is on providing optimal fluid management to restore intravascular volume and maintaining ventricular filling at the optimal point on the Frank-Starling curve. In pediatric practice the challenge is to accurately assess left atrial filling and adequacy of cardiac output to meet the high metabolic demands.

Central venous pressure monitoring is an unreliable indicator of left heart filling, and Swan-Ganz catheters are rarely used in children. Our practice therefore is to use a combination of clinical, echocardiographic, and biochemical markers. Echocardiography can be a useful tool in assessing left atrial filling and ventricular function. Serially measured biochemical markers such as serum lactate and pH are helpful in assessing adequacy of tissue perfusion.

Vasoactive drugs should be chosen according to the primary pathophysiological process contributing to the patient's state of shock. In the early vasodilatory phase, most authors recommend the aggressive use of a systemic vasoconstrictor agent such as noradrenaline. As shock progresses, inotropic drugs such as dopamine, dobutamine, and adrenaline with β-adrenergic effects are needed. If the myocardium fails despite appropriate support with high doses of inotropes, vasopressors, and optimal intravascular fluid filling, the use of ECMO might be considered.

Although not a curative treatment, ECMO is able to support both cardiac and pulmonary function, allowing these compromised organs time to rest and recover while maintaining oxygenated blood flow to other vital organs. ECMO is, however, costly, invasive, and requires anticoagulation and the use of large volumes of blood products. It places septic patients at higher risk of intracerebral hemorrhage due to underlying coagulopathy. It should therefore be reserved for patients who have failed conventional treatment and have a high predicted mortality.

V. INDICATIONS FOR ECMO

There are no established criteria for the use of ECMO in septic shock. There are no indices similar to the alveolar-arterial oxygen gradient and oxygenation index

(OI) used in patients with respiratory failure to predict impending death. Indications for ECMO in this group are therefore similar to that for cardiac support after congenital heart surgery:-

- Progressive hypotension with signs of worsening end organ perfusion (lactic acidosis, renal or other organ failure) despite adequate fluid resuscitation and high dose inotropic support (epinephrine/norepinephrine doses of the order of 1 mcg/kg/min).
- A potentially reversible disease process

VI. EXCLUSIONS

Factors excluding the use of ECMO include (a) recent cerebral haemorrhage or irreversible brain injury and (b) prolonged cardiac arrest requiring CPR for more than 5 minutes.

VII. TIMING OF REFERRAL FOR ECMO

We encourage early discussion and/or referral of ventilated septicemic patients on moderate doses of epinephrine or norepinephrine, particularly if the patient remains hemodynamically labile with rapidly increasing inotropic requirements. Children with meningococcal disease who have a high Glasgow meningococcal septicemia prognostic score also warrant early discussion and referral (11).

VIII. PRACTICALITIES

Veno-arterial ECMO is established in routine fashion with cannulation of neck vessels. It is crucial to ensure that the largest venous drainage cannula that can be safely inserted is used, in anticipation of high flow requirements. High flows (150–200%) are often required to meet the increased metabolic demands of the septic patient, and to achieve this excellent venous drainage is required. Initial flows of 150 mL/kg in infants <10 kg or 3 L/m^2 in children >10 kg should be employed. If this cannot be achieved with a single venous cannula, an additional drainage cannula, usually inserted in the femoral vein, may be required.

Flows are adjusted according to routine criteria to achieve adequate systemic blood pressures and good perfusion using standard parameters of end-organ perfusion such as lactate, pH, urine output and mixed venous oxygen saturations >65%. In most cases inotropic support can be rapidly weaned once ECMO is established. In some cases it may be necessary to continue vasoconstrictor agents in the first 48 hours following cannulation to maintain adequate blood pressure, although prolonged requirement for vasopressor support on ECMO is an ominous sign.

An aggressive policy for optimizing hemostasis with clotting factor replacement minimizes the risk of intracerebral bleeding. Our aim is to keep the activated clotting times (ACT) 1½–2 times normal (160–180 seconds measured on a Hemotech device), platelet count at 120,000–150,000/dL and fibrinogen at 200 mg/dL.

IX. CONTROVERSIES

In patients with purpura fulminans on ECMO, the use of vasodilator and antiplatelet aggregator agents such as prostacyclin (PGI_2) as well as thrombolytic drugs such as tissue-type plasminogen activator (alteplase, TPA) remains controversial due to concerns about intracerebral hemorrhage as well as a lack of objective evidence demonstrating efficacy. We elect to use low-dose PGI_2 in such patients on ECMO.

The routine use of hemofiltration in septic patients is another area of controversy. Previous studies have shown that while cytokines and other inflammatory mediators are removed by hemofiltration, the serum levels are unchanged. Hemofiltration does, however, allow a more liberal use of blood products to correct coagulopathies and more rapid correction of fluid balance and electrolyte abnormalities. Our policy is to use hemofiltration in all patients with septic shock on ECMO.

Levels of antithrombin III, protein C, and protein S have been demonstrated to be low in patients with meningococcal disease. Replacement of these factors has not definitely been shown to improve survival, but it seems reasonable to use fresh frozen plasma as the fluid expander in these particular patients.

X. ACUTE RESPIRATORY DISTRESS SYNDROME

Ventilation should be reduced to routine respiratory rest settings in patients with associated acute respiratory distress syndrome (ARDS) on ECMO (i.e., high PEEP and low FiO_2). In children with sepsis who do not have ARDS, we typically use low-pressure, low-FiO_2 ventilation sufficient to maintain lung volume.

XI. WEANING

Myocardial recovery is heralded by the return of the pulse wave on the arterial trace, improvement in ventricular function on echocardiographic examination, and normal perfusion on low ECMO flows with moderate doses of inotropes.

We perform routine echocardiographic assessments of cardiac function every 48 hours on low ECMO flow (<50%) to assess ventricular recovery.

If ventricular function appears good, patients progress to a trial of weaning on moderate inotropic support. Adequacy of organ perfusion is assessed with the patient separated from the circuit by clamping the ECMO cannulae, and if the patient remains stable for one hour decannulation is performed. The vessels are reconstructed if surgically feasible.

XII. PATIENT OUTCOME

There are a limited number of papers on this subject. Most published literature on the use of ECMO for patients with septicemia comes from the neonatal population. According to the ELSO registry, 2,124 of 13,708 neonatal cases (15%) have pneumonia or sepsis as the primary diagnosis. Neonatal sepsis may, however, be difficult to distinguish clinically from other disorders making up the spectrum of persistent pulmonary hypertension of the newborn (PPHN). It may rapidly progress to shock with hypotension, leukopenia, and bleeding diathesis. Neonatal sepsis can also cause PPHN with all its clinical sequelae.

McCune and colleagues were the first to report, in 1990, their experience of ECMO in neonatal sepsis (12). Ten of the 100 babies in their series had documented septic shock with an overall predicted mortality rate well in excess of 80%. All of the babies survived, although they required significantly longer ventilatory support and had a higher incidence of chronic lung disease than the nonseptic babies. They also had a higher incidence of intracranial haemorrhage compared with the nonseptic infants treated with ECMO (40% vs. 26%). This was probably due to preexisting coagulopathy.

Hocker and colleagues compared the infants treated at their center with overwhelming group B *Streptococcus* infection before the advent of ECMO with those treated later with ECMO (13). Neonates managed on ECMO were shown to have an improved survival compared with those managed conventionally (87% vs. 58%). This study is limited by the use of historical controls with all its inherent problems.

Meyer and colleagues reviewed all 1060 babies on the ELSO registry between 1987 and 1993 with a primary diagnosis of sepsis (14). Survival was seen to be lower in the infants with sepsis (77% vs. 82%) compared with infants receiving ECMO for noninfective causes. The septic babies also had a higher incidence of seizures, cerebral infarct, and hemorrhage and required hemofiltration more frequently than the nonseptic neonatal ECMO patients. The overall incidence of intracerebral hemorrhage in the septic patients was 25% compared to 11% for the nonseptic patients.

Beca and Butt in 1994 were the first to report on the use of ECMO for septic shock in the pediatric population (15). They described nine children, mean age 12 years (range 2–15) who received ECMO for septic shock with positive blood cultures. Causative organisms were *Streptococcus pneumoniae* in three patients, *Staphylococcus aureus* in two patients, and one case each of *Neisseria meningitis*, mycoplasma, pertussis, and parainfluenza. All had evidence of multiorgan failure with increasing hypotension and acidosis despite high-dose inotropic support. Most also had severe respiratory failure, hepatic dysfunction, renal failure, and disseminated intravascular coagulation. ECMO was continued for a median duration of 34 hours (range 17–79). Five of nine (60%) survived. Of the four children who died, ECMO was withdrawn in two because of brain death, one patient died from fulminant hepatic and myocardial failure, and the fourth patient died from progressive lung damage with staphylococcal abscesses. Follow-up of the five survivors at 12–36 months revealed that all were leading functionally normal lives, although one who had had an intracerebral hemorrhage had evidence of a mild hemiplegia.

We recently reviewed all patients treated with ECMO for severe meningococcal disease in the United Kingdom and Australia between 1989 and 1997 (16). Twelve cases were identified, aged from 4 months to 18 years. Seven patients required extracorporeal cardiac support for septic shock and five ECMO for respiratory support due to ARDS. The predicted mortality for the patients with shock was 81–88% based on Pediatric Risk of Mortality (PRISM) and Glasgow Meningococcal Septicemia Prognostic Score (GMSPS). All had multiorgan failure. Six of the 12 patients required cardiopulmonary resuscitation before ECMO, and the other 6 were deteriorating despite maximal conventional therapy. The median duration of ECMO was 76 hours. Four of the seven patients with shock and four of the five with ARDS survived. Six of the eight survivors are leading functionally normal lives at one year. One patient has mild hemiplegia and mild visual impairment from a vitreous hemorrhage, and one lost all fingers due to gangrene before ECMO. Of the four patients who died, ECLS was discontinued in two patients because of brain death and in the other two because of severe limb ischemia requiring four-limb amputation.

There have not, however, been any randomized controlled trials examining the role of ECMO in any group of patients with septic shock. A randomized controlled trial of ECMO in such patients would be difficult because of the problems in standardizing selection criteria, the small number of patients, and the ethical question of randomizing patients at a point near death.

XIII. CONCLUSION

There are several encouraging reports in the literature suggesting that ECMO may have a role in managing patients with septic shock refractory to maximal conventional treatment and that ECMO should be considered in such patients. Intensive care and emergency room staff need to be aware of the potential role of ECMO in these patients and of the indications to initiate early communication and/or referral to a center capable of implementing ECMO.

REFERENCES

1. Parillo JE. Pathogenetic mechanisms of septic shock. N Engl J Med 1993; 328: 1471–1477.
2. Parker MM. Pathophysiology of cardiovascular dysfunction in septic shock. New Horizons 1998; 6:130–138.
3. Parker MM, Shelhamer JH, Bacharach SL, et al. Profound but reversible myocardial depression in patients with septic shock. Ann Intern Med 1984; 100:483–490.
4. Parrillo JE, Burch C, Shelhamer JH, et al. A circulating myocardial depressant substance in humans with septic shock. J Clin Invest 1985; 76:1539–1553.
5. Suffredini AF, Fromm RE, Parker MM, et al. The cardiovascular response of normal humans to the administration of endotoxin. N Engl J Med 1989; 321:280–287.
6. Kumar A, Thota V, Dee L, et al. Tumor necrosis factor a and interleukin 1B are responsible for in vitro myocardial cell depression induced by human septic shock serum. J Exp Med 1996; 183:949–958.
7. Zeni F, Freeman B, Natanson C. Anti-inflammatory therapies to treat sepsis and septic shock: a reassessment (editorial comment). Crit Care Med 1997; 25:1095–1100.
8. Docke WD, Randow F, Syrbe U, et al. Monocyte deactivation in septic patients: restoration by IFN-gamma treatment. Nat Med 1997; 3:678–681.
9. Heyderman R. Sepsis and intravascular thrombosis. Arch Dis Child 1993; 68:621–625.
10. Gidelman LA, Pizov R, Sprung CL. New therapeutic approaches in sepsis: a critical review. Int Care Med 1995; 21:S269–272.
11. Thomson AP, Sills JA, Hart A. Validation of the Glasgow meningococcal septicaemia prognostic score: a 10 year retrospective study. Crit Care Med 1991; 19:26–28.
12. McCune S, Short BL, Miller MK, et al. Extracorporeal membrane oxygenation therapy in neonates with septic shock. J Ped Surg 1990; 25:479–482.
13. Hocker JR, Simpson PM, Rabalais MD, et al. Extracorporeal membrane oxygenation and early-onset group B streptococcal sepsis. Pediatrics 1992; 89:1–4.
14. Meyer DM, Jessen ME, ELSO. Results of extracorporeal membrane oxygenation in neonates with sepsis. J Thorac Cardiovasc Surg 1995; 109:419–427.
15. Beca J, Butt W. Extracorporeal membrane oxygenation for refractory septic shock in children. Pediatrics 1994; 93:726–729.
16. Goldman AP, Kerr SJ, Butt W, et al. Extracorporeal support for intractable cardiorespiratory failure due to meningococcal disease. Lancet 1997; 349:466–469.

14

The Use of Extracorporeal Membrane Oxygenation for Perioperative Support in Pediatric Lung Transplantation Patients

Jill Ibrahim, Eric N. Mendeloff, and Charles B. Huddleston
St. Louis Children's Hospital and Washington University School of Medicine, St. Louis, Missouri

Lung transplantation emerged as a modality to treat end-stage lung disease in the 1980s. Early in this experience, extracorporeal membrane oxygenation (ECMO) was attempted as a support measure in those patients in whom all other attempts at stabilization had proven inadequate. At that time, the need for ECMO was (and is in some centers) considered to be a contraindication to lung transplantation due to the dismal survival rates of patients transplanted during ECMO support (1). Additionally, lung transplantation and its concomitant immunosuppression has been considered a contraindication to posttransplant ECMO support (2). However, at the present time, ECMO provides the only effective means of "mechanical support" for the patient dying from pulmonary failure, on the basis of parenchymal or pulmonary vascular disease.

Unfortunately, ECMO provides reliable support for only a limited time period. In that sense, the "mechanical support" technology for failing lungs lags behind what has been developed for the failing heart (ventricular assist devices) or kidneys (dialysis), where mechanical support may be provided for months.

Most of the previously reported information regarding ECMO and lung transplantation concerns adult patients. While this provides a useful background, the experience in this group of patients may not be appropriately applied to children. This is particularly true in infants, where the waiting time for donor organs is shorter and the disease processes are different than in adults. In this chapter we will review both the available literature as well as our own experience with ECMO in the context of pediatric lung transplantation.

I. ECMO USE IN THE PRE–LUNG TRANSPLANT SETTING

One potential use for ECMO in patients with end-stage lung disease is as a ''bridge'' to transplantation. This generally occurs in one of two situations: an infant (usually neonate) with respiratory failure of unknown cause who is too ill to tolerate a diagnostic procedure, or a child with a known diagnosis who is deteriorating due to the primary disease process or an intercurrent illness (e.g., pneumonia). The issues that arise when ECMO is considered for these patients are:

1. Is it likely the patient will wean from ECMO?
2. Is lung transplantation an option?
3. What is the anticipated waiting time for donor lungs?

The likelihood of successful weaning from ECMO is primarily diagnosis-dependent. Time and space preclude a complete catalog of diagnoses for which lung transplantation in infants and children has been applied (3,4). Therefore we will confine the discussion to a few diagnoses from our own experience.

Primary pulmonary hypertension (PPH) and persistent pulmonary hypertension of the newborn (PPHN) have occasionally produced such severe hemodynamic instability that ECMO is required. ECMO in this situation has proven a very effective therapy (5). Despite this, there are many treatment options available for PPH or PPHN that should be exhausted prior to the institution of ECMO support, although circumstances occasionally dictate otherwise. These options include inotropic support, mechanical ventilation with adequate sedation and neuromuscular blockade, inhaled nitric oxide (6,7), intravenous prostacyclin (8), and creation of an atrial septal defect (9). Once ECMO is initiated, most of these measures should be applied to optimize the likelihood of weaning from ECMO support.

Surfactant protein B (SP-B) deficiency results in severe respiratory failure immediately after birth. It is a rare, recessively inherited disorder of surfactant production for which there is no available treatment. It is not unusual for an infant to be placed on ECMO within 24 hours of birth under the assumption that the diagnosis is something more typical, such as meconium aspiration. The correct diagnosis is made by either genetic testing or staining of pulmonary lavage fluid for surfactant protein B. In virtually every case referred to our institution,

ECMO has been successfully weaned (or avoided completely) with the use of high-frequency oscillating ventilation in conjunction with neuromuscular blockade (10).

Pulmonary alveolar capillary dysplasia is a rare congenital anomaly of lung development in which there is malalignment of the airway and vascular bed in the lung parenchyma. There is no effective conventional treatment; therefore lung transplantation is the only means of therapy. The lung disease is so severe that virtually all infants will require ECMO, and there is essentially no possibility of weaning ECMO in this disease process (11).

Congenital pulmonary vein stenosis may present with varying degrees of involvement of the pulmonary veins. The process may be isolated to one vein at the veno-atrial junction or may involve diffuse narrowing throughout the pulmonary veins in both lungs. This causes severe pulmonary hypertension that, unlike primary pulmonary hypertension, does not respond to medical therapy. Deteriorating patients may be temporarily palliated with balloon dilation and stent placement, and occasional patients may have anatomy suitable for radical pulmonary venoplasty. However, those with the diffuse form of this disease who require ECMO will likely be unable to be weaned (12).

It is not uncommon for a patient with congenital diaphragmatic hernia to require ECMO during the course of therapy. This is related to inadequate volume of lung tissue with associated pulmonary hypertension. There are no accurate predictors of the ability to wean from ECMO in this circumstance (13,14). In general, those who can be successfully weaned will progressively improve over time from a pulmonary standpoint and will not require lung transplantation. However, for those unable to wean, lung transplantation remains the only treatment (15). Unfortunately, by the time this determination is made, there usually has been considerable time spent on ECMO.

Complications while on ECMO are common and may create a situation unfavorable for transplantation. Bleeding is a frequent complication because of the need for anticoagulation and clotting factor consumption within the circuit. Heparin-bonded circuits have reduced these risks somewhat and are appropriately applied to patients who are likely to be on ECMO for an extended period of time. Intracranial hemorrhage is the most common bleeding complication that precludes transplantation. Two additional ECMO complications that are contraindications to transplantation include sepsis (16) and renal insufficiency.

The anticipated waiting time for donor organs should play a key role in the decision to use ECMO as a "bridge" to lung transplantation. There is a correlation between time on ECMO and significant complications that factors into this decision. The average waiting time from listing to transplantation varies widely in children and is primarily related to age and body weight. In infants less than 6 months of age, the waiting time has been the shortest in our experience, averaging 34 days. Adolescents compete with adults and wait an average of

Table 1 Characteristics of Patients Placed on ECMO Prior to Lung Transplantation

Patient no.	Age (y)	Diagnosis	Prior Tx/Surgery	Transplant procedure	Days of ECMO pre-Tx	Outcome
Patients transplanted while on ECMO						
1	2.0	Scimitar syndrome, pulmonary hypertension, hypoplastic R lung, tracheal stenosis	Repair of scimitar syndrome, R pneumonectomy, tracheal stenosis repair	SLT (donor RLL)	7	Required ECMO post-tx due to graft failure, expired one week post-tx
2	0.1	DILV, TGA, CoA, CDH	None	HLT	19	ECMO post-tx for pulmonary hypertension for 6 days; renal failure; expired 2 months post-tx due to intracerebral hemorrhage
3	0.5	CAVC, PVS, pulmonary hypertension	Repair CAVC, lung tx, MV repair	RE-tx; BLT	16	Expired 14 weeks post-tx due to MSOF
4	0.1	CDH	Repair CDH	BLT	11	Expired 2 weeks post-tx due to MSOF
5	10.0	Pulmonary fibrosis, nephrotic syndrome	Kidney tx, lung tx	Re-tx; BLT	1	Expired 2 weeks post-tx due to graft failure and MSOF
6	1.5	PDA, pulmonary hypertension	None	BLT	13	Expired 8 weeks post-tx due to PTLD
7	0.3	PVS, pulmonary hypertension	None	BLT (donor lower lobes)	26	Alive and well, 5 years

Patients weaned from ECMO prior to transplant						
8	0.2	SP-B deficiency	None	BLT (donor lower lobes)	6	Alive and well, 5 years
9	0.2	SP-B deficiency	None	BLT	7	Alive and well, 5.5 years
10	0.2	CIP	None	BLT	10	Expired 9 months post-tx, unknown cause
11	0.3	CIP	None	BLT	7	Alive and well, 1.5 years
12	0.2	SP-B deficiency	None	BLT	5	Expired 3 months post-tx due to liver failure
13	0.4	Pulmonary hypertension	None	BLT	8	Alive and well, 9 months
Patients who died on ECMO awaiting transplant						
14	0.1	Pulmonary hypertension	None	N/A	15	Expired with ECMO wean, sepsis and renal failure
15	0.1	Pulmonary ACD	None	N/A	19	CVA, expired with ECMO wean
16	0.1	SP-B deficiency	None	N/A	18	IVH, expired with ECMO wean
17	0.1	Pulmonary hypertension	None	N/A	5	Expired, cardiac arrest 3 weeks following ECMO decannulation

ACD = Alveolar-capillary dysplasia; BLT = bilateral lung transplant; CAVC = complete atrioventricular canal; CDH = congenital diaphragmatic hernia; CIP = chronic interstitial pneumonitis; CoA = coarctation of the aorta; CVA = cerebral vascular accident; DILV = double inlet left ventricle; HLT = heart-lung transplant; MSOF = multisystem organ failure; MV = mitral valve; PDA = patent ductus arteriosus; PTLD = posttransplant lymphoproliferative disease; PVS = pulmonary vein stenosis; RLL = right lower lobe; SLT = single lung transplant; SP-B = surfactant protein B; TGV = transposition of the great vessels; Tx = transplant.

nearly one year. It is obviously impractical to keep an older child on ECMO for months, recognizing that there are case reports documenting ECMO courses for greater than 2 months without significant complications. However, in a small infant it is not unreasonable to anticipate an offer for donor lungs during a 3- to 4-week ECMO course. Likewise, an older child who has already been listed for several months before deteriorating also has a reasonable probability of an organ offer. In certain cases one needs to be more flexible in donor acceptability as well. For example, in small infants and children, lobar transplantation from larger donors is a viable option (17,18).

The experience reported in the literature regarding lung transplantation while on ECMO is limited mainly to adults. Early reports were discouraging, with no survivors (19,20). In 1985, the Toronto lung transplant group described a patient with paraquat poisoning who was supported before the initial transplant as well as prior to retransplantation for graft failure (21). He was weaned from ECMO in both cases but died 2 months following the last course of ECMO. Jurmann et al. reported a series of five adults supported by ECMO prior to lung transplantation (22). Three of these patients demonstrated long-term survival.

At our institution a total of 174 pediatric lung transplants have been performed in an 8-year period beginning in 1990. Twenty-five (14%) of these patients required ECMO at some time prior to or following transplantation. Of these, 7 patients were transplanted while on ECMO. The characteristics of these patients are outlined in Table 1. Primary diagnoses in this subset of patients are varied and often complex in nature. Five patients demonstrated early survival and were successfully decannulated, but only one achieved long-term survival.

Six additional patients were placed on ECMO during their course but were decannulated prior to transplantation. Four of these six are long-term survivors, and they are also characterized in Table 1. Clearly this subgroup of patients has demonstrated the best survival advantage.

Finally, four patients were placed on ECMO prior to transplantation but were unable to be weaned, eventually developing complications that precluded transplantation. All were removed from the transplant list, withdrawn from ECMO support, and expired immediately thereafter. Three of the four developed an intracranial hemorrhage, and the other developed sepsis. The average time on ECMO for these four patients was 18 days; the average time on ECMO in the transplanted group was 13 days.

In summary, 17 patients were placed on ECMO prior to transplantation. Four died prior to transplantation from complications of ECMO and 5 (29%) are long-term survivors. Therefore, it is possible for good outcomes to result from an aggressive approach in isolated patients. The ideal patient is actually one in whom it is possible to wean ECMO prior to lung transplantation through the implementation of an aggressive medical approach when possible. One must recognize, however, that there are only limited data available on which to draw conclusions or make recommendations. We continue to maintain an aggressive posture for small infants in whom we have significant experience in ECMO management and for whom the waiting time for organs is relatively short.

II. ECMO FOR POST–LUNG TRANSPLANT SUPPORT

Donor lung function is abnormal in 13–35% of posttransplant patients (23) and is responsible for approximately 25% of early deaths (24). This abnormal function is referred to as reperfusion injury, primary graft failure, reimplantation response, donor lung dysfunction, or early graft dysfunction. All refer to the inability of the graft to maintain adequate oxygenation and ventilation in the posttransplant setting. Hallmarks of early graft dysfunction include increased oxygen requirements as evidenced by decreasing PaO_2/FiO_2 ratio, progressive increases in ventilator settings, early chest x-ray findings of pan-lobar infiltrates (Fig. 1), increased pulmonary artery pressures, decreased pulmonary compliance, and alveolar damage on lung biopsy. Clinically, the picture is one of severe pulmonary edema. Occasionally this phenomenon occurs in the operating room within minutes of reperfusion.

The exact nature of the injury is speculative and likely multifactorial. Contributing factors include surgical trauma, blood and blood product transfusions, donor lung ischemia, adequacy of graft preservation, denervation, and lymphatic disruption (25). Recipient factors may also involve the release of toxic inflammatory mediators by neutrophils accumulating in the graft as well as acute rejection. One must also rule out technical problems including stenosis or kinking of pulmonary veins obstructing pulmonary venous return, pulmonary artery stenosis, and airway dehiscence. We perform bronchoscopy and perfusion scans in the first 12 hours posttransplant to exclude these possibilities. Transesophageal echocardiography is very helpful in evaluating pulmonary venous return (26) and is now used routinely both in the operating room and the intensive care unit.

The role of ECMO in this setting is not just to salvage the patient by providing a viable level of oxygenation, but also to prevent further injury to the fragile newly transplanted lung from barotrauma and oxygen toxicity. However, this has to be balanced against the potential pitfalls of bleeding and infection encountered with ECMO.

Another potential problem in this group of patients relates to pulmonary blood flow and blood supply to the bronchial anastomosis. The lung transplant procedure disrupts the bronchial arteries so that circulation to the bronchial anastomosis is supplied from retrograde flow via collaterals originating from the pulmonary arterial system. Veno-arterial ECMO reduces pulmonary artery blood

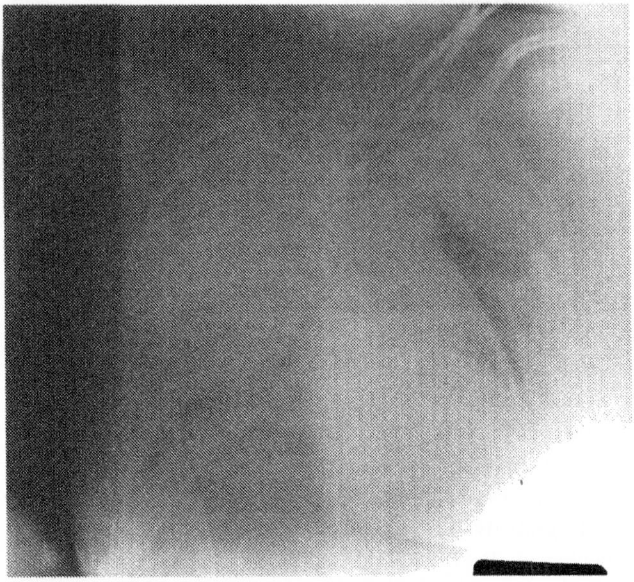

(a)

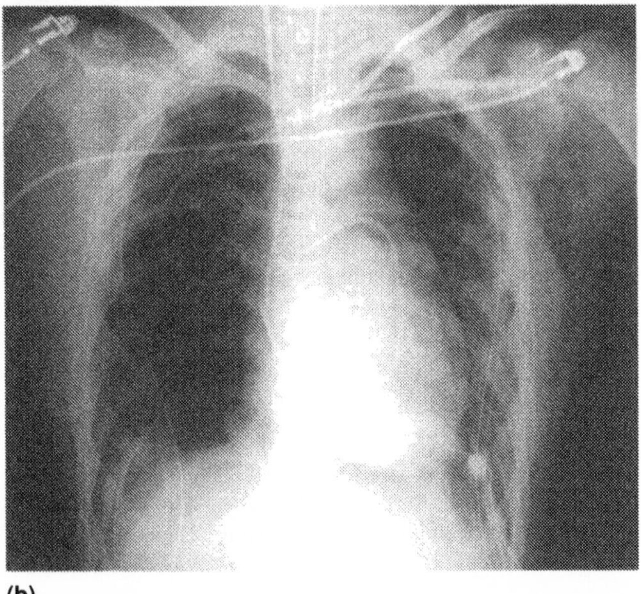

(b)

Fig. 1 (a) Chest radiograph of a 14-year-old male with early graft dysfunction/reperfusion injury immediately after bilateral lung transplantation. (b) The same patient after 4 days on ECMO at the time of decannulation. This patient was cannulated through the chest incision, however, the cannulae are radiolucent and therefore not seen.

flow significantly and may result in relative ischemia to the bronchial anastomosis, leading to breakdown and dehiscence. Fortunately, we have not yet seen this complication in our transplant population.

Alternatively, excessive bleeding occurring following lung transplantation is a very common complication and almost always results in the need for reexploration as well as the use of multiple blood products.

The experience with ECMO post–lung transplantation in the literature is varied and scant. The University of Michigan reported a series of four adults who were supported in the early postoperative period (<14 days) (27). Two of these cases were considered to be secondary to early graft dysfunction (reperfusion injury), one was rejection-mediated, and one secondary to both rejection and infection. Both patients cannulated on the day of transplant incurred significant bleeding complications. Three of the four were weaned from ECMO, but only one patient survived to hospital discharge. The University of Pittsburgh reported a series of eight adults requiring ECMO support the day of transplantation (<10 hours posttransplant) for early graft dysfunction (28). Seven of the eight were successfully weaned from ECMO, and six patients survived to discharge. This series, however, excluded patients placed on ECMO secondary to surgical or technical complications at the vascular or bronchial anastomoses, infection, or acute rejection. Of the seven patients excluded for these reasons, there were no survivors (29). This difference suggests that ECMO is efficacious in the treatment of early graft dysfunction that is secondary to reperfusion injury but not for other causes of respiratory failure following lung transplantation. Unfortunately, it is often difficult to identify the cause of the problem when lungs are failing immediately following transplantation. The above authors suggest that early institution of ECMO may reduce injury to the lung by reducing barotrauma and oxygen toxicity.

At Barnes Hospital/Washington University, 11 adult patients have been supported by ECMO in the early posttransplant period. Three of these patients expired while on ECMO, 2 were "bridged" to retransplantation, and 6 were successfully weaned from ECMO without retransplantation. A total of 7 patients (64%) survived to hospital discharge.

At our institution we have placed 16 patients on ECMO following lung transplantation. The characteristics of these patients are detailed in Table 2. Ten of these patients were placed on ECMO less than one week following transplant, with the majority requiring ECMO immediately for reperfusion injury. Three patients were retransplanted, and all 3 expired. In fact, only 2 of the 16 patients (13%) placed on ECMO at our institution following lung transplantation survived. Many of these patients were in critical condition prior to their transplant; 5 were on ECMO and 7 were mechanically ventilated in the intensive care unit. Thus, our results with ECMO in the post–lung transplant setting are not good and can be described as successful only occasionally in rescuing a patient.

Table 2 Characteristics of Patients Requiring Posttransplant ECMO

Patient no.	Age (y)	Diagnosis	Etiology of graft failure	Transplant procedure	Days of EDMO post-Tx	POD # placed on ECMO	Outcome
Patients requiring early posttransplant ECMO							
1	2.0	Scimitar syndrome, pulmonary hypertension, hypoplastic R lung, tracheal stenosis	Reperfusion injury	SLT (donor RLL)	6	0	Expired from graft failure, hemorrhage, renal failure on ECMO
2	0.1	DILV, TGV, CoA, CDH	Pulmonary hypertension, ?donor related	HLT	6	0	Expired from IVH 2 months after ECMO decannulation
3	0.5	CAVC, PVS, pulmonary hypertension	Reperfusion injury	Re-tx, BLT	8	0	Expired from MSOF 14 weeks after ECMO decannulation
4	0.1	CDH	Reperfusion injury	BLT	14	0	Expired from MSOF on ECMO
5	1.8	Pulmonary hypertension, BPD, s/p inadvertent LPA ligation	Reperfusion injury	BLT	4	0	Alive and well, 8 yrs post-tx
6	0.3	ToF/pulmonary atresia, tiny PAs	Reperfusion injury	BLT, ToF repair, RV-PA homograft	9	0	Expired from graft failure, myocardial failure, IVH on ECMO
7	0.3	Pulmonary vein stenosis	LPA occlusion, reperfusion injury	BLT	9	0	Expired from MSOF on ECMO
8	14.0	Primary pulmonary hypertension	Reperfusion injury, small donor lungs	BLT	4	0	Alive and well, 14 months post-tx

9	13.0	ARDS	Reperfusion injury	SLT (left)	6	0	Expired from hemorrhage and graft failure on ECMO
10	18.0	CF, IgA nephropathy	Infection (aspergillosis)	Re-tx, BLT	2	6	Expired from aspergillosis on ECMO
11	4.0	JRA, pulmonary fibrosis	Unknown, possible antibody-mediated rejection	BLT	1	7	Expired from graft failure, hemorrhage, post-tx day 10
12	13.0	CF	Reperfusion injury	BLT (living related donors)	2	7	Expired following ECMO wean and retransplantation from sepsis
13	10.0	Pulmonary fibrosis, nephrotic syndrome, s/p kidney transplant	Unknown, possible antibody-mediated rejection	BLT	1	7	Expired following retransplantation from graft failure
Patients requiring late posttransplant ECMO							
14	1.6	Primary pulmonary hypertension	Graft failure and parainfluenza pneumonia	BLT	8	25	Expired from graft failure and hemorrhage on ECMO
15	0.3	Surfactant protein B deficiency	Infection (adenovirus)	BLT	5	35	Expired following ECMO decannulation from adenovirus infection
16	0.2	ToF/Pulmonary atresia, tiny MAPCAs	Infection (adenovirus)	HLT	10	43	Expired from adenovirus infection on ECMO

ARDS = Adult respiratory distress syndrome; BLT = bilateral lung transplant; BPD = bronchopulmonary dysplasia; CDH = congenital diaphragmatic hernia; CF = cystic fibrosis; CoA = coarctation of the aorta; DILV = double-inlet left ventricle; HLT = heart-lung transplant; JRA = juvenile rheumatoid arthritis; MAPCA = multiple aorto-pulmonary collaterals; MSOF = multisystem organ failure; PA = pulmonary arteries; SLT = single lung transplant; TGV = transposition of the great vessels; ToF = tetralogy of Fallot.

Both of the survivors in our group were placed on ECMO early, within 2 hours of their transplant, and only two patients could even be weaned from ECMO if initiated any time after the first posttransplant day. These results are in stark contrast with those seen in the adult series reported above. The reasons for this discrepancy are not clear, but they may relate to the severity of illness leading up to the transplant.

The need for ECMO support ''late'' (>7 days) following lung transplantation differs from that required ''early'' (<7 days) in terms of underlying cause. In most cases infection and/or rejection are the culprits in the ''late'' setting, whereas reperfusion injury or preservation problems are implicated ''early'' posttransplant. Glassman et al. reported their experience with six patients placed on ECMO at >8 days posttransplant, all of whom had either rejection or infection (29); there were no survivors. Jurmann et al. reported one patient who developed pulmonary failure secondary to bacterial pneumonia of the graft and was placed on ECMO posttransplant day 11; this patient was retransplanted the same day and has achieved long-term survival (22). There are other individual case reports in the literature regarding post–lung transplant ECMO (29). In our pediatric experience, six patients were placed on ECMO at least one week posttransplant. Only one was secondary to reperfusion injury, which had gradually progressed since the time of transplantation. These patients are also characterized in Table 2. Two patients required late ECMO for presumed antibody mediated rejection. Although conclusive evidence of rejection was not obtained in these patients, both had immunological disorders that could make the diagnosis more likely, as no other etiology was found. However, both cases were refractory to aggressive immunosuppression including plasmapheresis. All six patients who required ECMO at 7 days or later ultimately died, and only one was able to be successfully weaned from ECMO support.

Thus, despite the fact that we view rejection and infection as eminently treatable conditions in transplant patients, ECMO continues to have a very poor prognosis in both the adult and pediatric age groups when used for these indications. Notably, infections with *Adenovirus* are notoriously difficult to treat, as are invasive *Aspergillus* infections. In summary, the decision to use ECMO in the late transplantation period remains one to be made on a case-by-case basis at this time.

III. TECHNICAL CONSIDERATIONS

The basic management of ECMO in the setting of lung transplantation is similar to ECMO for other conditions and is covered elsewhere in this book. Additionally, preferences vary somewhat from institution to institution and therefore will not be covered in this chapter. There are some considerations however, that are unique to these patients that may affect the approach taken when placing a patient on ECMO. For patients on ECMO as a "bridge" to transplant, the anticipated time on ECMO would be longer than for the usual patient placed on ECMO for respiratory distress or following cardiac surgery. Therefore, one might be inclined to use a heparin-bonded circuit to decrease the need for anticoagulation seen in the use of a standard circuit.

Furthermore, use of a veno-venous approach (as opposed to veno-arterial) may be indicated. Veno-venous cannulation is possible only when cardiac and circulatory support is not an issue. This is not an option in patients with a significant cardiopulmonary diagnosis (e.g., congenital heart disease or pulmonary hypertension with right heart failure).

Having said this, the literature is not fully supportive of the purported benefits of veno-venous ECMO over veno-arterial ECMO. Klein et al. reported their experience with both veno-arterial and veno-venous ECMO in newborns with respiratory failure (30). Of 11 patients treated with veno-venous ECMO, 3 needed conversions to veno-arterial ECMO because of worsening hemodynamics. Survival was 10 of 11 in the veno-venous group and 11 of 16 in the veno-arterial group. The authors attribute this survival difference to the overall poorer condition of the patients placed on veno-arterial support at the initiation of ECMO. When a large infant population (643 pairs) was retrospectively matched for the degree of respiratory and hemodynamic failure, no survival advantage or difference in the incidence of intracranial hemorrhage was noted with veno-venous ECMO (31).

In veno-venous ECMO the right atrium is cannulated through the right internal jugular vein for venous drainage, and arterialized blood is returned to the venous system through the right common femoral vein. Disadvantages to this method include a longer time necessary for cannula placement, maintaining the groin wound site (sterility, breakdown), persistent leg swelling with impaired venous return, increased incidence of cannula kinking, and increased hemolysis. Some of these problems may be circumvented by a double lumen venous cannula, which serves both drainage and return functions. These cannulae are available in sizes suitable for infants as well as older children. Veno-arterial ECMO in the pretransplant setting is done in the standard fashion using internal jugular vein and common carotid artery for infants and young children and the femoral vessels for teenagers.

If a patient is unable to be weaned from cardiopulmonary bypass while in the operating room, then the arterial and venous cannulae are left in place (central cannulation) and the cannulae are brought out through the chest incision. For those patients who develop severe graft dysfunction in the early posttransplant period ($<$7 days), central cannulation through the chest incision may be preferred. This permits accuracy in cannulae placement as well as the ability to perform an open lung biopsy for diagnostic reasons at the time of cannulation.

When graft failure occurs outside of the operating room, again veno-venous cannulation is an option. However, in this setting, veno-venous ECMO may promote more pulmonary edema, as the entire cardiac output remains traversing the pulmonary bed. Yet veno-arterial ECMO reduces the amount of pulmonary blood flow. This may result in anaerobic conditions in the lungs (32), which has been postulated as contributing to the ischemia of the bronchial anastomosis, as collateral flow is diminished. These considerations must be weighed when choosing the method of cannulation.

In the late postoperative period (>7 days) cannulation through the chest incision is no longer a preferred option, mainly because of bleeding complications incurred from the unavoidable lysing of chest adhesions. During this period either veno-arterial ECMO placed through the neck vessels or percutaneous peripheral cannulation via the femoral vessels (in children >10 years of age) are the best options.

IV. CONCLUSIONS

In examining this diverse population of children, what remains very clear is that the results achieved utilizing ECMO in the perioperative lung transplant patient are not very encouraging. However, as the field of lung transplantation expands, so will the use of this technology in this setting, for it is usually the only means of rescue support available to these patients. With the likely increased use of ECMO, we will be able to draw further conclusions regarding its efficacy.

What we can conclude from this preliminary data is that patients who are able to be weaned from ECMO prior to lung transplantation clearly have improved survival rates. Therefore, once the decision has been made to proceed to transplantation, every possible measure should be used to enhance the probability of weaning these patients from ECMO, including high-frequency ventilation, nitric oxide, inotropic support, and even toxic oxygen levels when necessary.

As has been shown in the pediatric cardiac transplant population, ECMO is more effective in lung transplant patients when it is needed in the acute period and less effective in late graft dysfunction due to rejection or infection (33). However, at the time a patient has undergone lung transplantation, a substantial amount of resources, both financial and emotional, has been invested in the child's care. In this setting it is extremely difficult to withhold an additional escalation of support when the cause for the patient's decline is often not known at the time when ECMO becomes necessary. One always hopes the nature of the injury is reversible, although clearly that is not always the case. The difficulty lies in the uncertainty, and while ECMO may be a life-saving measure in a select few of these patients, we know that the prognosis for most is poor. The consideration of all of these factors is required when using ECMO as perioperative support in lung transplantation.

REFERENCES

1. Slaughter MS, Nielsen K, Bolman RM 3rd. Extracorporeal membrane oxygenation after lung or heart-lung transplantation. ASAIO J 1993; 39(3):M453–456.
2. Mair P, Balogh D. Anaesthetic and intensive are considerations for patients undergoing heart of lung transplantation. Acta Anaesthesiol Scan Suppl 1997; 111:78–79.
3. Bridges ND, Mallory GB, Huddleston CB, Canter CE, Sweet SC, Spray TL. Lung transplantation in children and young adults with cardiovascular disease. Ann Thorac Surg 1995; 59:813–821.
4. Starnes VA, Oyer PE, Bernstein D, Baum D, Gamberg P, Miller J, Shumway NE. Heart, heart-lung, and lung transplantation in the first year of life. Ann Thorac Surg 1992; 53:306–310.
5. O'Rourke PP, Crone RK, Vacanti JP, et al. Extracorporeal membrane oxygenation and conventional medical therapy in neonates with persistent pulmonary hypertension of the newborn: a prospective randomized study. Pediatrics 1989; 84:957–963.
6. Roberts JD, Fineman, JR, Morin FC 3rd, Shaul PW, Rimar S, Schreiber MD, Polin RA, Zwass MS, Zayek MM, Gross I, Heymann MA, Zapol WM. Inhaled nitric oxide and persistent pulmonary hypertension of the newborn. The Inhaled Nitric Oxide Study Group. N Engl J Med 1997; 336(9):605–610.
7. Inhaled Nitric Oxide Study Group. Inhaled nitric oxide in full-term and nearly full-term infants with hypoxic respiratory failure. N Engl J Med 1997; 336(9):597–604.
8. Barst RJ, Maislin G, Fishman AP. Vasodilator therapy for primary pulmonary hypertension in children. Circulation 1999; 99:1197–1208.
9. Sandoval J, Gaspar J, Pulido T, Bautista E, Martinez-Guerra ML, Zeballos M, Palomar A, Gomez A. Graded balloon dilation atrial septostomy in severe primary pulmonary hypertension: a therapeutic alternative for patients nonresponsive to vasodilator treatment. J Am Coll Cardiol 1998; 32(2):297–304.
10. Hamvas A, Nogee LM, Mallory GB, Spray TL, Huddleston CB, August A, Dehner LP, DeMello DE, Moxley M, Nelson R, Cole FS, Colten HR. Lung transplantation for treatment of infants with surfactant protein B deficiency. J Pediatr 1997; 130(2):231–239.
11. Steinhorn RH, Cox PN, Fineman JR, Finer NN, Rosenberg EM, Silver MM, Tyebkhan J, Zwass MS, Morin FC 3rd. Inhaled nitric oxide enhances oxygenation but not survival in infants with alveolar capillary dysplasia. J Pediatr 1997; 130(3):417–422.
12. Sun CJ, Doyle T, Ringel RE. Pulmonary vein stenosis. Hum Pathol 1995; 26(8): 880–886.
13. Steimle CN, Meric F, Hirschl RB, et al. Effect of extracorporeal life support on survival when applied to all patients with congenital diaphragmatic hernia. J Pediatr Surg 1994; 29:997–1001.
14. Stolar C, Dillon P, Reyes C. Selective use of extracorporeal membrane oxygenation in the management of congenital diaphragmatic hernia. J Pediatr Surg 1988; 23: 207–211.
15. Langer J. Congenital diaphragmatic hernia. Chest Surg Clin North Am 1998; 8(2): 300–314.
16. Meyer DM, Jessen ME, Eberhart RC. Neonatal extracorporeal membrane oxygenation complicated by sepsi. Extracorporeal Life Support Organization. Ann Thorac Surg 1995; 59(4):975–980.
17. Crombleholme TM, Adzick NS, Hardy K, et al. Pulmonary lobar transplantation in

neonatal swine: a model for treatment of congenital diaphragmatic hernia. J Pediatr Surg 1990; 25:11–18.

18. Van Meurs K, Rhine WD, Benitz WE, Shochat SJ, Hartman GE, Sheehan AM, Starnes VA. Lobar lung transplantation as a treatment for congenital diaphragmatic hernia. J Pediatr Surg 1994; 29(12):1557–1560.
19. Veith FJ. Lung transplantation. Surg Clin North Am 1978; 58:357–364.
20. Nelems JM, Diffin J, Glynn MFX, Brebner J, Scott AA, Cooper JD. Extracorporeal membrane oxygenator support for human lung transplantation. J Thorac Cardiovasc Surg 1978; 76(1):28–32.
21. The Toronto Lung Transplant Group: Sequential bilateral lung transplantation for paraquat poisoning. J Thorac Cardiovasc Surg 1984; 89:734–742.
22. Jurmann MJ, Schaefers HJ, Demertzis S, Haverich A, Wahlers T, Borst HG. Emergency lung transplantation after extracorporeal membrane oxygenation. ASAIO 1993; M448–M552.
23. Christie JD, Bavaria JE, Palevsky HI, Litzky L, Blumenthal NP, Kaiser LR, Kotloff RM. Primary graft failure following lung transplantation. Chest 1998; 114(1):51–60.
24. Hosenspud JD, Bennett LE, Keck BM, Fiol B, Novick Rj. THe registry of the international society for heart and lung transplantation: fourteenth official report—1997. J Heart Lung Transplant 1997; 16(7):691–712.
25. Prop J, Ehrie MG, Crapo JD, Nieuwenhuis P, Widevuur RH. Reimplantation response in isografted rat lungs: analysis of causal factors. J Thorac Cardiovasc Surg 1984; 87:702–711.
26. Leibowitz DW, Smith CR, Michler RE, Ginsburg M, Schulman LL, et al. Incidence of pulmonary vein complications after lung transplantation: a prospective transesophageal echocardiographic study. J Am Coll Cardiol 1994; 24(3):671–675.
27. Whyte RI, Deeb GM, McCurry KR, Anderson HL 3rd, Bolling SF, Bartlett RH. Extracorporeal life support after heart or lung transplantation. Ann Thorac Surg 1994; 58:754–759.
28. Zenati MS, Pham SM, Keenan RJ, Griffith BP. Extracorporeal membrane oxygenation for lung transplant recipients with primary severe donor lung dysfunction. Transplant Int 1996; 9:227–230.
29. Glassman LR, Keenan RJ, Fabrizio MC, Sonett JR, Bierman MI, Pham SM, Griffith BP. Extracorporeal membrane oxygenation as an adjunct for primary graft failure in adult lung transplant recipients. J Thorac Cardiovasc Surg 1995; 110(3):723–726.
30. Klein MD, Andrews AF, Wesley JR, Toomasian J, Nixon C, Roloff D, Bartlett RH. Venovenous perfusion in ECMO for newborn respiratory insufficiency. A clinical comparison with venoarterial perfusion. Ann Surg 1985; 201(4):520–526.
31. Gauger PG, Hirschl RB, Delosh TN, Dechert RE, Tracy T, Bartlett RH. A matched pairs analysis of venoarterial and venovenous extracorporeal life support in neonatal respiratory failure. ASAIO J 1995; 41(3):M573–M579.
32. Lee KH, Rico P, Boujoukos AJ, Keenan RJ, Pinsky MR. Measurement of lung oxygen consumption in a patient after double-lung transplant. J Thorac Cardiovasc Surg 1995; 110(6):1764–1765.
33. Galantowicz ME, Stolar CJ. Extracorporeal membrane oxygenation for perioperative support in pediatric heart transplantation. J Thorac Cardiovasc Surg 1991; 102(1): 148–151.

15

The Use of the HeartMate Left Ventricular Assist Device in Children

David N. Helman, Mehmet C. Oz, and Mark E. Galantowicz
Columbia-Presbyterian Medical Center and College of Physicians and Surgeons of Columbia University, New York, New York

I. INTRODUCTION

Although long-term implantable left ventricular assist devices (LVADs) designed specifically for small patients are not yet widely available, a subset of the pediatric patient population can be supported with currently available long-term devices. We have utilized the TCI HeartMate LVAD (Thermo Cardiosystems, Inc., Woburn, MA) in pediatric patients in need of long-term cardiac support since 1993. Although the HeartMate LVAD was designed for adults, it is possible to use this U.S. Food and Drug Administration (FDA)–approved device as a life-sustaining measure in smaller pediatric patients with the use of innovative techniques to account for the discrepancy between device and patient size. The HeartMate LVAD has been a vital first step towards the eventual solution of the problem of pediatric patients in need of long-term mechanical cardiac support. Pediatric patients have been successfully supported with this device, which facilitates discharge home and resumption of normal activities with the device in place while awaiting heart transplantation.

II. HEARTMATE LVAD

The HeartMate LVAD consists of a titanium housing containing a flexible, textured polyurethane diaphragm attached to a pusher plate (1). The device incorporates two porcine valves and Dacron inflow and outflow grafts. Movement of the pusher plate generates a pulsatile flow with a maximum stroke volume of approximately 85 mL and maximum pump flow of approximately 10 L/min. Implantation can be performed in the pre- or intraperitoneal position (2). The inflow cannula of the device is inserted in the apex of the left ventricle, and the outflow graft is anastomosed to the right lateral aspect of the ascending aorta (Fig. 1). Although the original version of the HeartMate was pneumatically driven, the newer vented-electric (VE) version is our device of choice. The VE HeartMate is powered by a wearable battery pack providing a 6-hour period of freedom from recharging that allows for patient mobility,

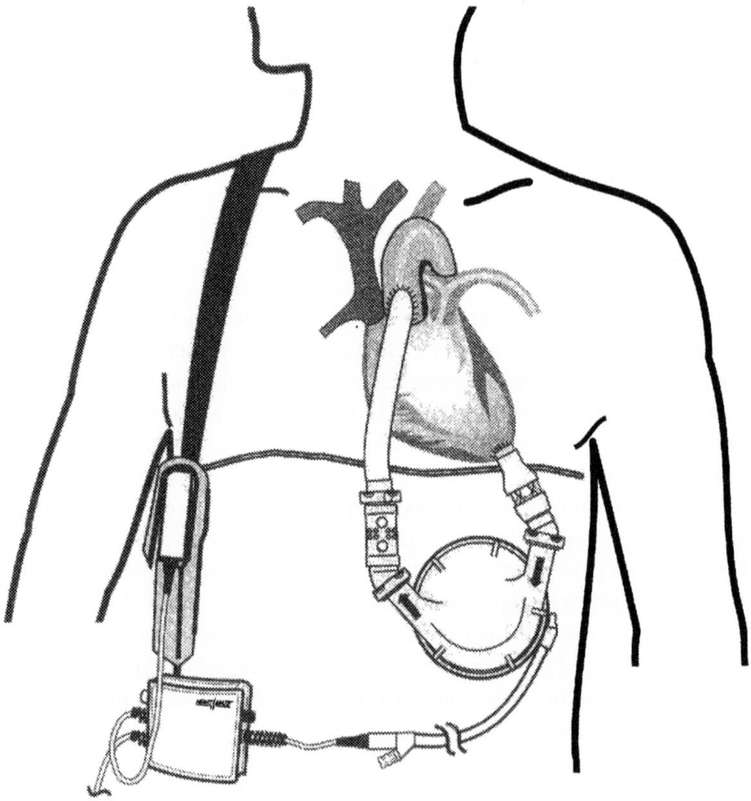

Fig. 1 Schematic diagram of HeartMate LVAD. (Courtesy of Thermo Cardiosystems, Inc., Woburn, MA.)

facilitating rehabilitation and discharge home with the device in place. A single drive line exits the skin and provides electrical connections as well as an emergency backup pumping capability. The HeartMate LVAD does not require systemic anticoagulation due to blood contacting surfaces that have been textured to affect the formation of a pseudo-intima reducing thrombogenicity (3,4).

The HeartMate LVAD was specifically designed for patients with body surface areas (BSA) greater than 1.5 m^2, thus limiting its utility for pediatric patients and small adults (5). The patient size constraint is partially a result of the need to generate flows greater than 3 L/min to reduce the risk of thrombus formation. Device fit issues include anastomoses to the left ventricle and ascending aorta as well as positioning and fit of the device itself in the preperitoneal space of the left upper quadrant of the abdomen. Intra-abdominal device placement in pediatric patients is complicated by the fact that the costal angle is narrower in children than in adults. In addition, the anterior-posterior dimension of the abdomen in pediatric patients can make it challenging to place the device in this position without causing compression of intra-abdominal organs, twisting of the inflow connector, or abdominal wall necrosis. The smallest patient implanted with a TCI LVAD to date was a child with a BSA of 1.2 m^2 (R. B. Silverstein, personal communication).

The HeartMate VE LVAD was approved in 1998 by FDA for use as a long-term bridge to transplantation. Over 1500 HeartMate LVADs have been implanted worldwide, and of these 40 have been implanted in patients less than 21 years old (J. Heatley, personal communication). Of 40 patients supported with this device, 26 (65%) went on to transplant, one (3%) had the device explanted without subsequent transplantation, 9 (23%) expired prior to transplantation, and 4 (10%) are still being supported with the device.

III. GOALS OF LONG-TERM LVAD SUPPORT

The vast majority of patients, both adult and pediatric, who have been supported with TCI LVADs had the devices implanted with eventual transplantation as the goal. There does appear to be a small subset of patients, approximately 10%, with end-stage heart failure in whom recovery of native myocardial function during LVAD support may occur to the point where LVAD explanation without subsequent heart transplantation is possible. Work at our institution regarding the use of exercise testing as an evaluation of myocardial recovery during LVAD support is ongoing (6). What remains to be identified are reliable indicators of sustainable myocardial recovery that could be used to guide decisions regarding LVAD explantation versus transplantation. While the number of patients suitable for LVAD explant will likely grow with the development of innovative treatments for end-stage heart failure, at present, the majority of long-term LVADs are implanted as bridges to transplantation.

In this setting, LVAD use helps to preserve the scarce resource of pediatric donor hearts and also allows for stabilization of the patient prior to heart transplantation. The preservation of end-organ function along with nutritional support and rehabilitation has the effect of transferring the risks associated with a surgical procedure in a critically ill patient from the heart transplantation procedure to the LVAD implantation procedure, thus minimizing the risk of a failed heart transplant squandering a precious donor heart.

IV. MECHANICAL CARDIAC ASSIST STRATEGY IN PEDIATRIC PATIENTS

We have stratified pediatric patients in need of mechanical cardiac support into three categories based on body size. The smallest patient in whom we have implanted a TCI LVAD was a child with a BSA of 1.4 m^2.

For patients with a BSA of less than 1.0 m^2 in need of cardiac support, we have used Medtronic Bio-Medicus centrifugal pumps (Bio-Medicus, Eden Prarie, MN). Although not FDA approved for this use, we have employed this device in critically ill patients with no other options (7,8). These devices are extracorporeal pumps and are limited to temporary support. Bio-Medicus pumps have been used in the smallest patients for temporary support but have limitations due to the requirement for continuous monitoring and adjustment by a perfusionist. Heparin-bonded circuits, which may reduce the level of necessary anticoagulation and may decrease bleeding and inflammation, have been used in centrifugal pump circuits (9).

In general, patients with BSAs ranging from 1.0 to 1.5 m^2 have been supported with the ABIOMED BVS 5000 pulsatile pump (ABIOMED, Inc., Danvers, MA) (8). This extracorporeal, pulsatile device provides temporary ventricular support but does not require the same degree of 24-hour-per-day perfusionist monitoring required with extracorporeal centrifugal pumps and has cannulas designed for postcardiotomy use. The ABIOMED device requires a minimum flow of 2 L/min to prevent clotting, thus imposing a minimum limit on patient BSA of approximately 1.0 m^2 (8). Our smallest patient successfully supported with an ABIOMED BVS 5000 was a girl with a BSA of 1.06 m^2 in need of biventricular support. This device utilizes a sutured outflow graft anastomosis to the aorta when used as an LVAD that reduces the problems of bleeding when compared to the pursestring aortic cannulation technique that is utilized with the Bio-Medicus centrifugal pump.

V. PEDIATRIC HEARTMATE IMPLANTATION TECHNIQUES

Following the administration of the serine protease inhibitor aprotinin (Bayer, West Haven, CT) to reduce hemorrhage and inflammation with subsequent right heart failure (10), cardiopulmonary bypass is instituted and the left ventricle is vented through the apex. The HeartMate LVAD is implanted in a pocket made in the preperitoneal space of the left upper quadrant of the abdomen, ideally before systemic heparinization. The LVAD is implanted without the use of cardioplegia or aortic cross-clamping. The LVAD inflow cuff is sutured to the apex of the left ventricle taking wide bites of myocardium with pledgetted 2-O coated, braided polyester sutures. Care is taken to tie the sutures gently since this is a low-pressure connection, due to decompression by the LVAD, and bleeding is unlikely unless the sutures pull through the muscle. The LVAD outflow graft is sewn to the right lateral aspect of the ascending aorta. When the inflow and outflow anastomoses are completed, LVAD pumping is begun and the patient is placed in steep Trendelenburg position during weaning from cardiopulmonary bypass to reduce the risk of air embolism.

In order to facilitate placement of the TCI LVAD in smaller patients, we have utilized a prosthetic polytetrafluoroethylene graft to close the fascial layers of the abdominal wound over the device. We believe this technique also reduces the likelihood of wound dehiscence (Fig. 2) (11).

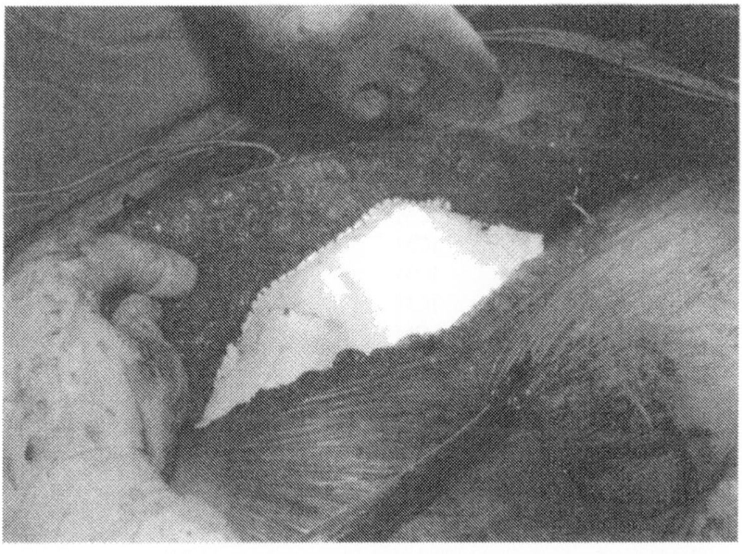

Fig. 2 Prosthetic graft fascial closure of abdomen following LVAD implantation.

VI. EXPERIENCE WITH PEDIATRIC HEARTMATE LVADs

At our institution we implanted 13 HeartMate LVADs in patients less than 21 years old from 1993 to 1998 (Table 1). One of the patients received two devices. Two of the implanted devices were the early pneumatic version, and 11 were of the vented-electric type.

Eight of our pediatric patients supported with long-term LVADs were male and 4 were female. The average age of these patients was 16 years (range: 11–20). The average weight was 67 kg (range: 48–91) with heights averaging 174 cm (range: 153–191). Average BSA was 1.8 m^2 (range: 1.4–2.2).

The etiology of heart failure in these patients was idiopathic in 10 (83%), viral myocarditis in 1 (8%), and Ebstein's anomaly in 1 (8%). Patients were selected for long-term LVAD implantation if they were eligible for heart transplantation and showed evidence of end-organ failure. We have previously reported a screening scale that incorporates factors predictive of successful LVAD implantation (12). Factors with a high relative risk for unsuccessful LVAD placement were (1) oliguria, (2) ventilator dependence, (3) reoperation status, (4) elevated central venous pressure, and (5) elevated prothrombin time. Timely LVAD insertion prevents irreversible deterioration of end-organ function and facilitates postoperative recovery, especially with pediatric patients who are able to withstand end-stage heart failure longer prior to sudden hemodynamic collapse.

Table 1 Clinical Characteristics of Pediatric HeartMate LVAD Patients

Patient no.	Age (y)	BSA (m^2)	Diagnosis	LVAD support (days)	Outcome
1	20	1.8	ICM	23	Expired
2	13	1.4	ICM	22	Transplant
3	18	2.0	ICM	186	Explant
4	16	1.7	ICM	208	Transplant
5	19	1.9	ICM	283	Transplant
6a	11	1.6	ICM	397	Explant
6b	14	1.7	ICM	89	Transplant
7	14	2.0	ICM	3	Expired
8	14	1.6	ICM	89	Transplant
9	18	2.2	Viral CM	148	Transplant
10	17	1.7	ICM	138	Transplant
11	12	1.8	ICM	11	Expired
12	18	1.9	Congenital	0	Transplant

Note: Patient 6a and 6b are the same patient, who received two different LVADs.
CM = Cardiomyopathy; ICM = idiopathic cardiomyopathy.

Average duration of LVAD support was 123 days with a range of zero to 397 days (median = 89 days). One patient could not be supported with the device due to a congenitally small left ventricle that prohibited the generation of adequate flows. This patient underwent a successful emergent heart transplantation.

Of the 13 TCI LVADs implanted, 8 resulted in successful bridging to transplantation. Two of the LVADs were explanted without subsequent heart transplantation, and 3 patients expired with their LVAD in place. One of the patients undergoing explantation had a sudden deterioration in cardiac function 3 months following LVAD explantation in the setting of a viral illness and expired. The other patient in whom an LVAD was explanted experienced a gradual diminution in myocardial function over a 6-month period requiring implantation of a second LVAD and was successfully supported to transplantation.

Bleeding complications occur quite frequently in patients receiving ventricular assist devices. In the 13 LVAD implantations in our pediatric patients, there were 2 early and 1 late reoperations for hemorrhage. The early reoperations were for mediastinal hemorrhage, while the late reoperation was to repair a hole in the LVAD outflow graft (10). Blood or device infections occurred in 4 patients (31%). Despite the absence of systemic anticoagulation, there was only one thromboembolic event in a noninfected patient, which consisted of a small retinal artery embolism that resulted in a transient ischemic attack with no residual deficit.

Three deaths occurred in the patients during the period of LVAD support. One death was due to an air embolism that occurred during repositioning of the LVAD inflow connector. One patient expired of sepsis and multiple organ system failure. One patient developed pulmonary and cerebral infarcts in the setting of sepsis.

VII. EARLY POST-LVAD IMPLANTATION MANAGEMENT

In addition to the utilization of aprotinin intraoperatively to reduce postoperative bleeding, we have adopted several postoperative strategies specific to LVAD implantation. We occasionally leave the chest open in the immediate postoperative period to allow for early identification of hemorrhage. Leaving the chest open early also has the salutary benefit of decreasing mechanical compression of the right ventricle. Subsequent closure of the chest is facilitated by a reduction in swelling of the spleen and liver as venous congestion is improved by the LVAD.

Right heart failure following LVAD implantation was treated with the pulmonary vasodilator, inhaled nitric oxide (NO) (13). In this series of 13 LVADs, 11 were implanted during the time period during which we were using NO. Of these 11 cases, NO was used postoperatively in 3 patients (27%). Vasodilatory hypotension occurs frequently in the early postoperative period following LVAD implantation and we have used intravenous arginine vasopressin (AVP) (Parke-Davis, Morris Plains, NJ) in this setting (14). Twelve of the 13 LVAD implantations in this series took place after we first began using AVP for vasodilatory shock. Of these 12 cases, AVP was used in 5 (42%).

VIII. LATE POST-LVAD IMPLANTATION MANAGEMENT

Once the patient has been stabilized with the LVAD device, the primary objective is physical rehabilitation while awaiting heart transplantation. A significant benefit of the wearable vented-electric HeartMate device is the possibility of discharge home from the hospital with the device (15). Outpatient LVAD support in pediatric patients allows for obvious psychological benefits as well as for an opportunity to resume normal activities prior to transplantation. Seven of the eight patients eligible for discharge from the hospital with VE devices were supported successfully at home. None of these patients expired during outpatient LVAD support. Device malfunctions were minor and were handled by the patient's family members. Patients were able to return to school and recreational activities such as skating, bicycling, and snowboarding during LVAD support.

IX. FUTURE OF LVADs IN PEDIATRIC PATIENTS

While the TCI HeartMate can provide long-term cardiac support for larger pediatric patients, limitations imposed by its minimal flow requirement and dimensions prohibit its use in all pediatric patients. A number of axial pumps currently at various stages of development are significantly smaller and, thus, more applicable to pediatric patients than presently available pulsatile LVADs. ABIOMED is in the preclinical evaluation phase of a pneumatic pump designed to generate flows of 1.5–3.5 L/min in patients with BSAs ranging from 0.6 to 1.4 m^2 (R.T.V. Kung, personal communication). TCI is currently developing the HeartMate II, which is an axial pump that will weigh approximately one pound and have a diameter of 1.25 inches with the ability to pump from 2 to 10 L/min (R.B. Silverstein, personal communication). The development of this and other smaller pumps will undoubtedly expand the current capabilities of life-sustaining mechanical cardiac support devices for the full spectrum of pediatric patients.

REFERENCES

1. Argenziano M, Oz MC, Rose EA. The continuing evolution of mechanical ventricular assistance. Curr Problems Surg 1997; 34:317–386.

2. Poirier VL. The HeartMate left ventricular assist system: worldwide clinical results. Eur J Cardio-Thorac Surg 1997; 11(suppl):S39–S44.
3. Dasse KA, Chipman SD, Sherman CN, Levine AH, Frazier OH. Clinical experience with textured blood contacting surfaces in ventricular assist devices. ASAIO Trans 1987; 33:418–425.
4. Rose EA, Levin HR, Oz MC, Frazier OH, Macmanus Q, Burton NA, et al. Artificial circulatory support with textured interior surfaces. A counterintuitive approach to minimizing thromboembolism. Circulation 1994; 90:II87–II91.
5. Oz MC, Rose EA, Levin HR. Selection criteria for placement of left ventricular assist devices. Am Heart J 1995; 129:173–177.
6. Mancini DM, Beniaminovitz A, Levin H, Catanese K, Flannery M, DiTullio M, et al. Low incidence of myocardial recovery after left ventricular assist device implantation in patients with chronic heart failure. Circulation 1998; 98:2383–2389.
7. Williams MR, Quaegebeur JM, Hsu DT, Addonizio LJ, Kichuk MR, Oz MC. Biventricular assist device as a bridge to transplantation in a pediatric patient. Ann Thorac Surg 1996; 62:578–580.
8. Ashton RC, Oz MC, Michler RE, Champsaur G, Catanese KA, Hsu DT, et al. Left ventricular assist device options in pediatric patients. ASAIO J 1995; 41:M277–M280.
9. Aldea GS, Doursounian M, O'Gara P, Treanor P, Shapira OM, Lazar HL, et al. Heparin-bonded circuits with a reduced anticoagulation protocol in primary CABG: a prospective, randomized study. Ann Thorac Surg 1996; 62:410–418.
10. Goldstein DJ, Seldomridge JA, Chen JM, Catanese KA, DeRosa CM, Weinberg, et al. Use of aprotinin in LVAD recipients reduces blood loss, blood use, and perioperative mortality. Ann Thorac Surg 1995; 59:1063–1067.
11. Oz MC, Goldstein DJ, Rose EA. Preperitoneal placement of ventricular assist devices: an illustrated stepwise approach. J Cardiac Surg 1995; 10:288–294.
12. Oz MC, Goldstein DJ, Pepino P, Weinberg AD, Thompson SM, Catanese KA, et al. Screening scale predicts patients successfully receiving long-term implantable left ventricular assist devices. Circulation 1995; 92:II169–II173.
13. Argenziano M, Choudhri AF, Moazami N, Rose EA, Smith CR, Levin HR, et al. Randomized, double-blind trial of inhaled nitric oxide in LVAD recipients with pulmonary hypertension. Ann Thorac Surg 1998; 65:340–345.
14. Argenziano M, Choudhri AF, Oz MC, Rose EA, Smith CR, Landry DW. A prospective randomized trial of arginine vasopressin in the treatment of vasodilatory shock after left ventricular assist device placement. Circulation 1997; 96:II-286–II-290.
15. Catanese KA, Goldstein DJ, Williams DL, Foray AT, Illick CD, Gardocki, et al. Outpatient left ventricular assist device support: a destination rather than a bridge. Ann Thorac Surg 1996; 62:646–652.

16

Clinical Applications in Children of the MEDOS Ventricular Assist Device

Wolfgang F. Konertz
Charité, Humboldt University, Berlin, Germany

I. INTRODUCTION

Mechanical circulatory support in infants and children is still evolving. The need for cardiac assist in pediatric patients may be growing because increasingly complex forms of congenital heart disease are amenable to surgery today. In addition, the success of pediatric cardiac transplantation and the existing donor scarcity stress the need for support systems covering the wide demands of pediatric patients. The MEDOS ventricular assist device (VAD) permits support of small babies, children, and adults by offering a variety of different-sized pumps that can be matched to the needs of every patient.

II. DESCRIPTION

Sufficient hemodynamic support by cardiac assist systems has the potential to prevent multiple organ failure. Cardiac unloading with increased coronary artery circulation may restore depleted energy sources, which aids in recovery of the heart. The system should be able to support systemic circulation adequately for several days or weeks to serve as a bridge to transplantation. To meet these requirements the MEDOS VAD pneumatic driven paracorporeal system was developed by Reul and coworkers at the Helmholtz Institute Aachen (1) and the Medos Medizintechnik GmbH, a company for innovative cardiovascular medical products.

A. Ventricles

The MEDOS VAD ventricles are the result of a long-term development at the Helmholtz Institute for Biomedical Engineering. A central goal during development was to provide a device that met the requirements of a broad spectrum of patient sizes. The application of modern engineering technologies established a manufacturing process that produced ventricles that were effective and flexible with a high level of reliability and user-friendliness. Ventricles from 9 to 80 mL stroke volume are available, meeting the demands of nearly every clinical situation.

Under consideration of the medical requirements for VADs, the application of advanced engineering technologies including CAD design, FEM stress analysis, NC milling, and plastics technology resulted in a high-performance ventricle (2–4).

Design of the pump housing was aimed toward providing a completely transparent pump made of polyurethane. In a clinical situation this allows visual control of the ventricles, valves, and inlet/outlet connectors. Fluid dynamics and flow properties of the ventricles provide optimal washout. The multilayer diaphragm is constructed to achieve uniform stress distribution, and the diaphragm-housing junction is seamless to lower thrombogenicity.

The MEDOS VAD is equipped with two tri-leaflet polyurethane valves with optimized stress distribution and excellent flow characteristics (Fig. 1). They permit rapid opening and closing, which results in minimal energy loss, minimal pressure drop, and low leakage. They are noiseless and the sinus portion is adjusted to minimize thrombotic events.

The concept of ventricles available in different sizes provides optimum washout of the pumps regardless of patient size. This minimizes the potential for

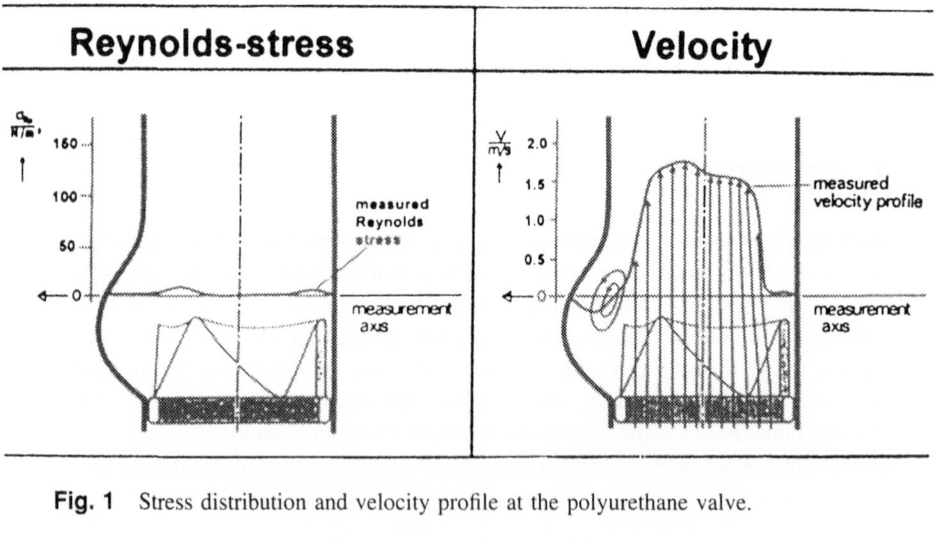

Fig. 1 Stress distribution and velocity profile at the polyurethane valve.

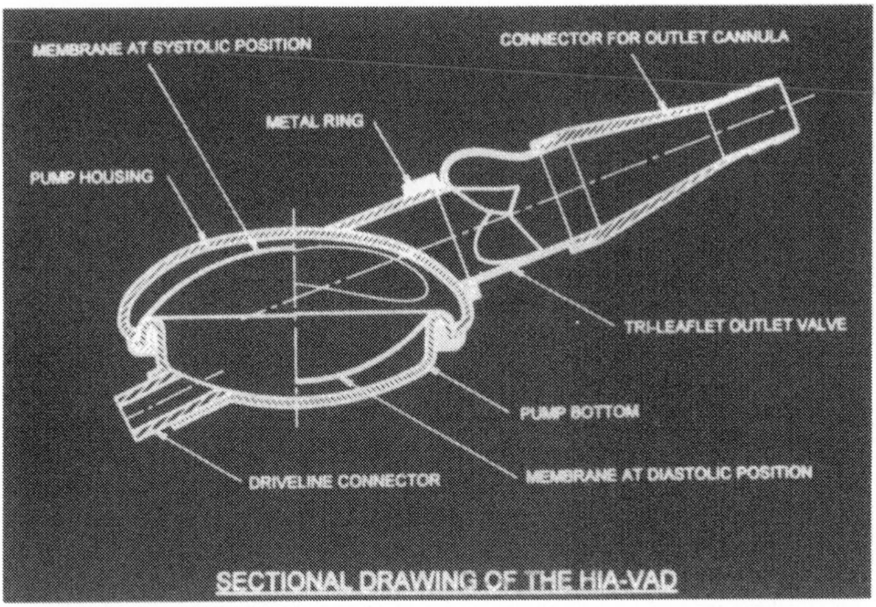

Fig. 2 Cross-sectional view of the Medos ventricle.

thrombotic complications. The MEDOS VAD is available with stroke volumes of 10, 25, 60, and 80 mL for left-ventricular and with 10% reduced stroke volumes for each size for right-ventricular support. A cross-sectional view of the complete ventricle is shown in Fig. 2. The configuration of the system with eight sizes of pumps and three valve sizes is shown in Table 1. The ventricle, the valves, and both cannulae can be coated with heparin, which provides stable biocompatible and antithrombotic surfaces for long-term use.

Table 1 Configuration of the MEDOS VAD System

Patient	Stroke volume (mL)	Valve size (mm)
Large adult patient, left	80	21
Large adult patient, right	72	21
Adult, left	60	21
Adult, right	54	21
Children, left	25	16
Children, right	22.5	16
Infant, left	10	12
Infant, right	9	12

B. Drive System

The MEDOS pneumatic driver is a stand-alone system comprised of a control and pressure unit. This state-of-the-art technology was designed specifically for the MEDOS VAD. The main characteristics of the driver are:

System flexibility that allows left, right, and biventricular pumping mode of the 10, 25, 60 and 80 mL MEDOS VAD
Smooth systolic and diastolic operation mode (physiological dp/dt) due to linear servovalves
Complete adjustability of heart rate, blood pressure and systolic range for each pump size (Table 2)
In case of stationary operation, an external pressure and vacuum supply to be used as an alternative to the internal one

The complete pneumatic driver with the power supply unit and the control unit is shown in Fig. 3. The power supply unit contains a battery and compressor, which allows operation of the system for at least 1 hour off any external power/pressure/vacuum supply.

The system is activated and operated with the control unit which allows for synchronous and asynchronous modes of operation. The user is guided by a menu-driven system on the touch screen monitor with four different displays

Display #1: VAD selection
Display #2: VAD-parameter adjustment
Display #3: ECG-triggering
Display #4: Setting of parameter limits

A comprehensive alarm system provides protection against malfunction and faults. Figures 4–7 show examples of the user-system dialog for operation of this system. Continuous recording of pump operation data and displayed alarms are possible via a PC interface. Safety features, such as automatic activation of

Table 2 Technical Data of the Drive Unit

Parameter	Adjustable range
Pulse rate	60–180 9.0/10 mL VAD
	60–150 22.5/25 mL VAD
	60–120 54.0/60 mL VAD
	60–100 72.0/80 mL VAD
Pressure	
systolic	50–300 mmHg
diastolic	−1 to 99 mmHg
Systolic time setting range	20–50%

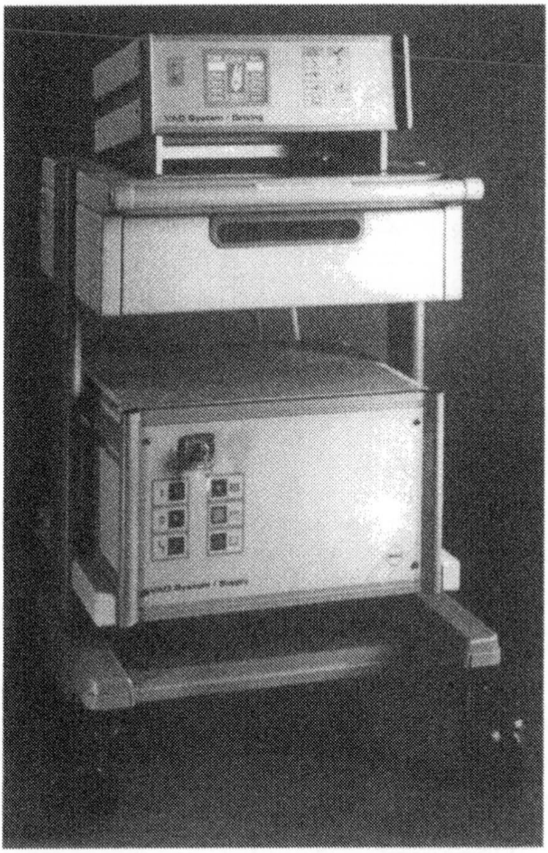

Fig. 3 The MEDOS VAD drive unit. The control unit (top) with interactive touch screen monitor and the power supply unit (bottom).

the internal compressor in case of external pressure supply disconnection or failure, add to the reliability of the system. In case of ac power failure, the internal battery is activated automatically.

C. Cannulas

Cannulas of the appropriate size are available for each ventricle. The atrial inlet cannula has a wide bore and is wire reinforced and bendable at the tip, which allows optimal positioning within the chest (Fig. 8). An inlet cannula for left ventricular apical access is also available. The outlet cannula has a vascular graft

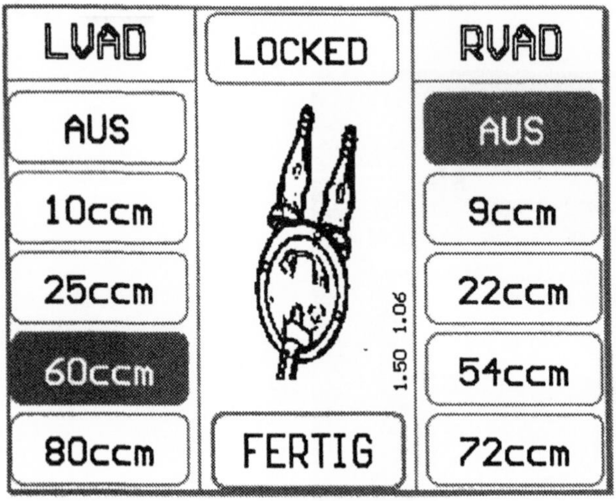

Fig. 4 Display #1: VAD selection, type, and size. When the MEDOS driving system is switched on, display #1 always appears first. It serves for the selection of LVAD, RVAD or both. When the proper size for the present application is selected, press ''FERTIG'' (READY). The screen then automatically switches to display #2.

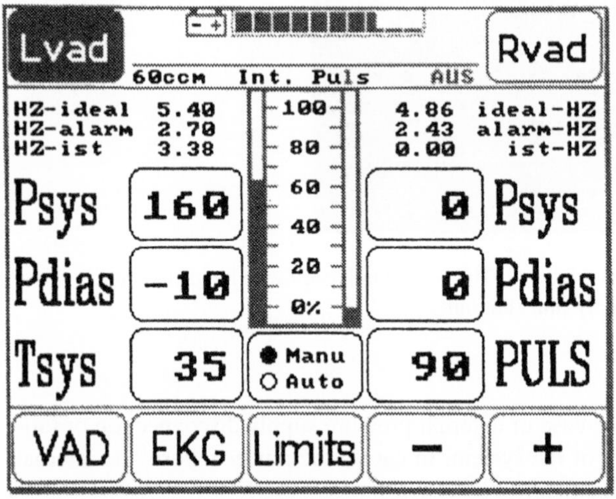

Fig. 5 Display #2 VAD parameter adjustment. This display serves for the adjustment of the pump parameters. It is preset to starting values of Psys = 120 mmHg, Pdias = −5 mmHg, systolic duration of 35%, and a starting pulse rate of 40 bpm. All these parameters can be varied by touching the appropriate window and subsequently touching the ''+'' or ''−'' field. When the parameters are properly selected, touch the ''VAD'' switch left on the screen. The pump is now in a fixed frequency mode. By touching the ''EKG'' (ECG) window, display #3 appears.

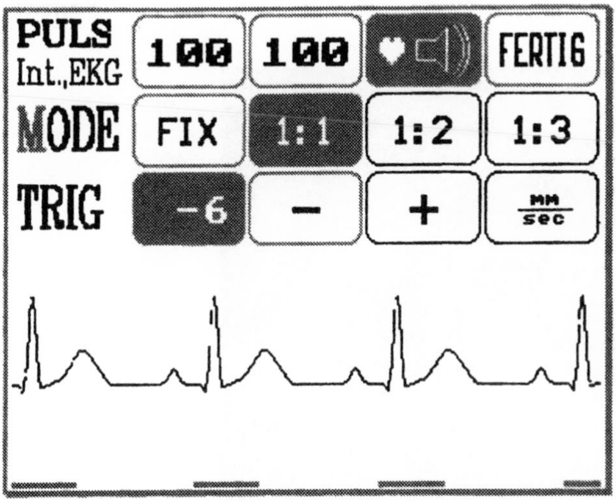

Fig. 6 Display #3: ECG triggering: Within this display it is possible to switch between fixed frequency mode or 1 : 1, 1 : 2, 1 : 3 ECG triggering. The patient ECG heart rate appears in the upper panel, second window. At the same time the ECG tracing is displayed on the lower half of the display and the pump delay with respect to the R-wave can be varied by touching the "+" or "−" windows. By touching "FERTIG" (READY) the screen is returned to display 2. When "LIMITS" of display #2 is pressed, display #4 appears.

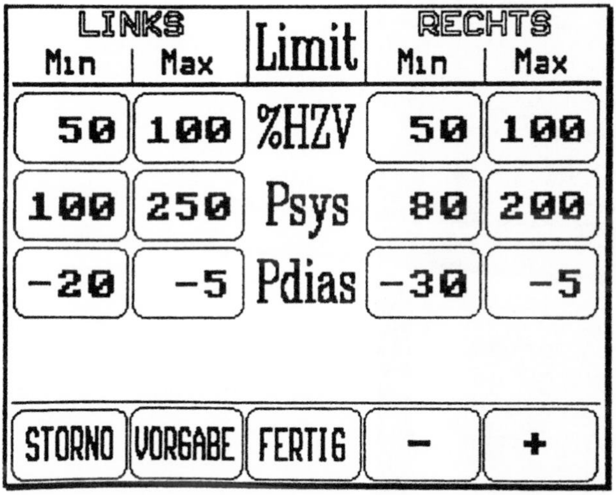

Fig. 7 Display #4: Setting of parameter limits: this display serves for setting the upper and lower pressure limits. If these limits are exceeded the drive unit sounds an alarm signal. Also, the minimum value of the "HZV" (pump output) can be set to a preselected value less than 100%. When the pump output falls below this preset minimum, a system alarm is heard. By touching the window "FERTIG" (READY), the screen again returns to display #2.

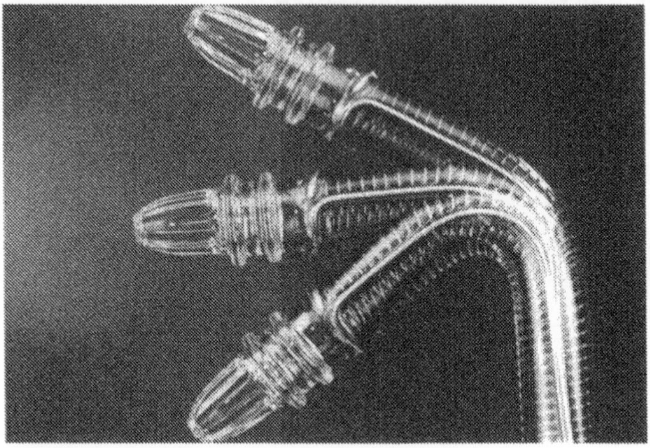

Fig. 8 Inlet (venous) cannula for the MEDOS VAD.

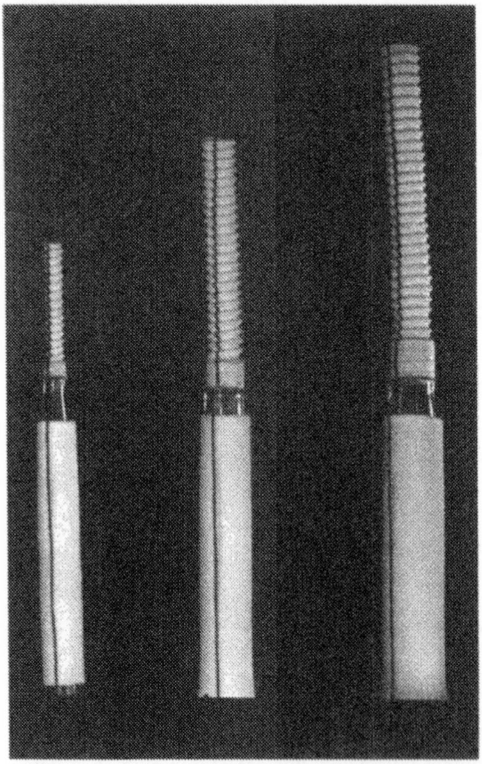

Fig. 9 Outlet (arterial) cannula for the MEDOS VAD.

at the tip that can be trimmed and sewn to the appropriate artery (Fig. 9). The middle part of any cannula is covered with Dacron felt to permit rapid ingrowth of host tissue and sealing of the skin at the cannula insertion site.

III. EXPERIMENTAL EVALUATION

The pump has been evaluated thoroughly in vitro and in vivo. In vitro evaluation was performed on engineering issues and design perfection (2–4). The newly developed polyurethane valves were also subject to intensive study (5). Animal experiments led to further design improvements, which ultimately led to the device for clinical use (6). Extensive testing was also performed at the University of Groningen, Netherlands, and at the University of Leuven, Belgium (7–9). Further animal experiments with left and biventricular support were performed by Waldenberger (10). This elegant experimental model of left heart failure due to severe stunning demonstrated that in the presence of any increase in pulmonary vascular resistance, biventricular support gives far better results than left ventricular support alone.

IV. CLINICAL APPLICATION

The MEDOS-VAD has been in clinical use in Germany since 1994. The first clinical use in February 1994 in an adult by Sievers and coworkers (11) was followed by the first pediatric use as a bridge to transplant in March 1994 at the Charité, Berlin. The five day pump run was terminated after an adequate donor heart was identified and successful cardiac transplantation was performed. As of the end of 1998 the MEDOS-VAD has been used in 359 patients at 53 institutions, with nearly 20% of this experience comprised of pediatric applications.

A. Intention to Treat and Indications

Principally, mechanical circulatory support can be used to provide recovery from cardiac failure or surgical trauma or as bridge to transplant in terminally failing hearts.

As more centers perform human heart transplantation, the long-standing problem of shortages of donor hearts appears to be getting worse. Acute cardiac decompensation in patients waiting for an acceptable donor is not infrequent. As demonstrated by VAD and total artificial heart implantations, several systems are suitable for circulatory support in patients awaiting heart transplantation. However, due to the lack of reliable systems in appropriate sizes, their use in infants and children has been limited.

In the clinical setting of a patient who cannot be weaned from cardiopulmonary bypass, mechanical circulatory assist may be considered after adequacy of the repair is confirmed and residual stenoses or shunts are ruled out. If there is potential for recovery, prompt establishment of circulatory support may be helpful in this situation. Nonsurgical cardiogenic shock or heart failure are situations that may occur in children during the course of acute myocarditis, after chemotherapy with cardiotoxic drugs, in the course of neuromuscular disorders, or after severe cardiac trauma. These conditions possess the potential for recovery and are appropriate indications for mechanical circulatory assist. In our series we utilized mechanical circulatory support as a bridge to transplantation in three patients. Nine additional patients were supported for anticipated recovery of reversibly damaged hearts.

Current indications for circulatory assist in children are heart failure after surgery for congenital heart disease and temporary support in patients with cardiomyopathy or acute myocarditis. Until recently only extracorporeal membrane oxygenation (ECMO) was utilized in children, with rather unsatisfying results in instances where ventricular support was needed. Postoperative support has been the most frequent reason for mechanical circulatory support in our series and most others (12–17). The majority of patients have had open-heart surgery or cardiac transplantation and could not be weaned from the heart-lung machine due to severe right or left ventricular dysfunction. Contraindications to mechanical circulatory support include multiple organ failure, severe coagulopathy, intracranial hemorrhage, neurological impairment, and sepsis. These describe situations in which open-heart surgery is normally not performed, so that most children after open-heart surgery meet criteria for mechanical circulatory support. A subset of patients have had low cardiac output or cardiac arrest in the intensive care unit following successful weaning from cardiopulmonary bypass. In such patients, technical failure of the operation should be ruled out, which may only be possible after stabilization with mechanical circulatory support. Two of 12 patients treated with the MEDOS VAD in our series fall into this group. Patients in which mechanical circulatory support is used as bridge to transplantation should meet institutional criteria for transplantation. Other factors such as body size or blood group, which may have an impact on the timely availability of a donor heart, must be taken into account. With the MEDOS VAD, Scheld and coworkers (18) successfuly bridged an infant over 14 days to cardiac transplantation.

B. Modes of Support

The MEDOS VAD provides univentricular and biventricular support. Most often, even in the presence of right ventricular (RV) failure, left ventricular (LV) unloading with LV decompression and circulatory improvement may alleviate right ventricular dysfunction. An isolated LVAD was used in 5 out of 12 patients in our unit. Unlike in adults, where right ventricular failure may complicate left ventricular support, this did not occur in any of our pediatric LVAD patients. Three patients required right ventricular support, and one patient required biventricular support. A unique subset of patients, that we encountered in our series were three patients after failed Norwood. ''Univentricular support'' proved to be enormously difficult because little is known regarding issues such as optimal cannula placement or management of the shunt. We have been unsuccessful in all three instances, and an experimental trial using a univentricular animal model has been initiated.

C. Surgical Technique

A midline sternotomy was used in all our patients. For left ventricular support, the outflow cannula is sewn to the aorta and exteriorized through a stab incision in the left epigastrium. Then the inflow cannula is placed through the right superior pulmonary vein, secured with two pursestring sutures, and exteriorized through the right epigastrium. Right ventricular support is established by sewing an arterial cannula to the pulmonary artery and cannulation of the right atrial appendage. With the patient in deep Trendelenburg's position, the cannulas are thoroughly deaired. With meticulous care the ventricle is filled with Ringer's solution. This step can be easily verified because the ventricles are totally transparent. Sometimes it is advisable to let the ventricle perform some strokes immersed in a large bowl filled with Ringer's solution. The ventricle is then connected to the tubing, and several single strokes are performed slowly to control for any residual air. When implantation of the device takes place with the patient on a heart-lung machine, the surgical team should be sure that the heart is completely deaired and already filled with blood and that flow from the heart-lung machine has been decreased. After another careful check for any air in the tubing and the ventricle, pumping is initiated preferably by manual actuation of the pump. Fig. 10 shows an operative site after discontination of the heart-lung machine in a 6-month-old baby supported with LVAD as a bridge to transplant. After the heart-lung machine is discontinued, the ventricle is adjusted to the desired level of support. In postcardiotomy patients, the chest is closed only temporarily. When edema is present or cannula placement was shown to compromise the heart, a sheet of Gore-Tex Surgical Membrane (W. L. Gore and Associates, Flagstaff, AZ) was used; otherwise, the skin edges were simply approximated. In all patients being bridged to transplantation, the sternum was wired and the wound closed in layers.

D. Anticoagulation and Antibiotics

In our series only nonheparin-bonded systems were used. When the implantation is done with the patient on a heart-lung machine, heparin sodium is partially

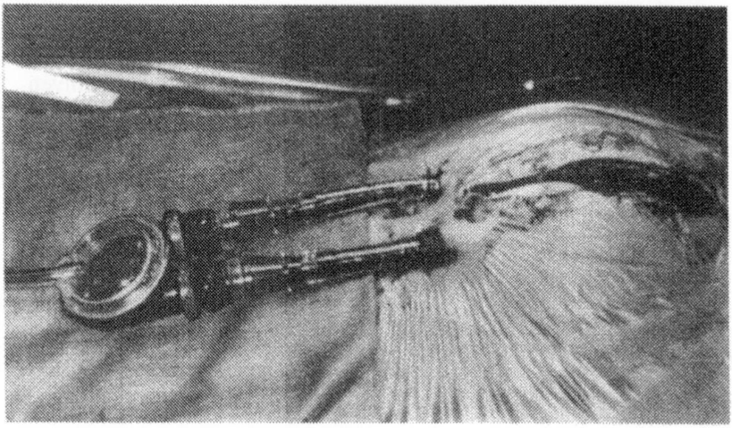

Fig. 10 Operative site after implantation of the MEDOS LVAD in a 6-month-old baby.

neutralized with protamine sulfate to an activated clotting time of 200 seconds. In the other patients, heparin is administered to achieve a comparable level of anticoagulation before placement of the outflow cannula. During the first postoperative hours, no heparin is added until chest drainage decreases; then heparin is administered to keep the activated clotting time at 180–220 seconds. In the longer runs, acetylsalicylate, 5 mg/kg/day, is added after removal of the chest tubes.

Antibiotic treatment consists initially of the routine institutional postcardiotomy treatment of children using penicillin. On the basis of blood and urine cultures and wound, tracheal, throat, or fecal swabs, the regimen should be changed later. The exit points of the VAD tubing are dressed daily under sterile conditions with povidone-iodine ointment. As soon as bleeding from chest tubes ceases and hemodynamic stability is maintained, patients are weaned from respiratory support. Patients may be safely extubated even with the wound closed temporarily. For older children, sitting in bed and walking in the room is strongly recommended. Infants are allowed to be on the parent's or nurse's arm after extubation (Fig. 11), and breast feeding is recommended, when appropriate.

E. Survival and Complications

From March 1994 to December 1998, 1000 operations for congenital heart disease were performed at the Department for Cardiovascular Surgery of the Charité University Hospital to the Humboldt University, Berlin. 48% of the patients were infants. Seventeen patients required mechanical circulatory support. In 12 the MEDOS-VAD system was used. Table 3 shows the modes in which the system was used. Four out of 5 patients in which the LVAD was used survived and were

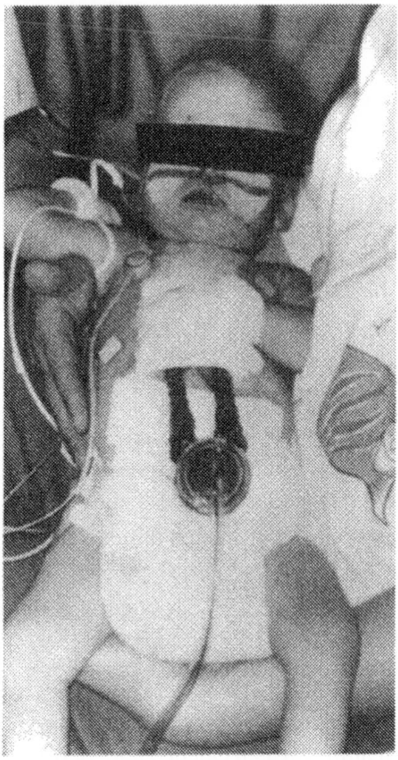

Fig. 11 Six-month-old baby at the 7th postoperative day during MEDOS LVAD support.

discharged. The shortest LVAD duration was 8 hours in a 4-month-old baby with anomalous left coronary artery arising from the pulmonary artery, and the longest run was 25 days in a 9-year-old boy in nonsurgical cardiogenic shock. This patient was weaned from the device after complete recovery of cardiac function. Intention of treatment and results are shown in Table 4. Death on the device occurred

Table 3 Results of Pediatric VAD Use at the Charité According to Mode of Support

	Total	Weaned/tx	Discharged	Survival
LVAD	5	4	4	4/5
RVAD	3	2	1	1/3
BVAD	1	0	0	0/1

Table 4 Results of Pediatric VAD Use at the Charité According to Intention of Treatment

	PCF	Bridge	Shock
No. implanted	5	3	1
No. weaned/transplanted	3	2	1
No. discharged home	2	2	1

due to multiorgan failure in two patients and retrosternal bleeding in one. Another patient died 3 days after discontinuation of right ventricular support from intractable arrhythmia.

Nonfatal complications were bleeding from the operative site requiring reexploration in four children and thrombotic formation in the sinus portion of a ventricle in one. This ventricle could be changed without difficulty in the ICU.

V. DISCUSSION

The recently available MEDOS VAD permits support of small babies as well as of adults by offering a variety of ventricular sizes that can be matched to the needs of the patient. The system has some unique features, which can be addressed best by:

Trileaflet polyurethane valves
Total transparency
Extreme powerful, reliable, quiet, and user-friendly drive unit

In small patients requiring small VAD ventricles and high pump rates, mechanical valves may be undesirable because of their closing and opening properties. These drawbacks are avoided by the design of the polyurethane valves, which are seamlessly incorporated into the VAD. The special design of the sinus portion of valves results in optimal opening and closing characteristics as well as providing "washing flow" which has been documented in extensive studies by Reul and colleagues (5). They were also able to show low gradients and negligible energy loss across the valves.

A valuable feature of the VAD is its total transparency. This allows visual control of filling and emptying and of thrombus generation on the inner surface of the device. In our series, thrombus generation at the outflow valve prompted the change of a ventricle in one patient, which could be easily managed in the intensive care unit. The special features of the drive unit were discussed in Sec.

I. The interactive touch screen monitor permits easy control of the whole system, the compressors demonstrate high performance over a large scale of heart rates up to 180/min, and during an experience of 70 pump runs in children (duration up to 97 days) no technical system failures occurred.

Successful pediatric circulatory support has been reported to be performed with ECMO or centrifugal pumps (19). Overall survival with circulatory support by means of a centrifugal pump has been reported as 50%. This rate is comparable to the experience with ECMO for cardiac support reported by the ELSO registry (20,21).

In infants and children, ECMO has been shown to be more successful than in adults (21). However, ECMO requires a complex set-up, a variety of monitoring lines, and most often endotracheal intubation, and it allows no ambulation or other physical activity. Continuous surveillance by trained personnel is mandatory. These limitations seem undesirable, especially in infants who are bridged to transplantation. Other systems that have been used in infants and children include centrifugal pumps for univentricular and biventricular support (22). However, with full unloading of the heart, they do not permit pulsatile flow. Loss of pulsatility has been blamed for capillary leakage during prolonged pump runs (23), and recovery of the heart may be improved by electrocardiogram-triggered counterpulsation of the device (24,25). Additionally, patients on centrifugal pumps are confined to bed. It would be difficult to mobilize and transport babies and small infants while they require a centrifugal pump. This can be accomplished much more easily when the pump is close to the body and wearable, as with pneumatically driven paracorporeal assist devices. Such devices are in clinical use with the Thoratec® and the Abiomed® systems, but they are currently available only for adults. The use of adult or intermediate-size pneumatic ventricles in infants and children is associated with low pump rates and large stroke volumes. Slow operation of the pump, however, increases the thromboembolic risk.

The pediatric MEDOS VAD described herein is a commercially available, CE-marked system applicable to infants and allows matching the VAD size to the patient's need.

Based on our clinical experience, we believe that pediatric LVAD and RVAD support for postcardiotomy failure, as well as for bridge to transplantation, can be performed in infants and children with a reasonable salvage rate. The system has some unique features, including VAD sizes that can accommodate small babies as well as adults. Indications for VAD are evolving in the pediatric age group. The ideal candidate for ventricular support has isolated life-threatening heart failure or dysfunction and should not have multiorgan failure or bleeding. Further experimental and clinical research addressing application of the system for pediatric biventricular support and for support of univentricular hearts is in progress.

REFERENCES

1. Reul H. The MEDOS/HIA system: development, results, perspectives. Thorac Cardiovasc Surg 1999; 47(suppl.):311–315.
2. Knierbein B, Rosarius N, Unger A, Reul H, Rau G. CAD-design, stress analysis and in vitro evaluation of three leaflet blood-pump valves. J Biomed Eng 1992; 14(7):275–286.
3. Knierbein B, Rosarius N, Reul H, Rau G. New methods for the development of pneumatic displacement pumps for cardiac assist. Int J Artif Organs 1990; 13:751–759.
4. Knierbein B, Reul H, Rau C. Entwicklung und Herstellung von Blutpumpen unter kunststofftechnischen Aspekten. Kunststoffe 1990; 80:1385–1391.
5. Reul H, Taguchi K, Herolf M, Lo HB, Reck B, Mückter H, Messmer BJ, Rau G. Comparative evaluation of disk- and trileaflet valves in leftventricular assist devices (LVAD). Int Artif Organs 1988; 2:127–130.
6. Eilers R, Harbott P, Reul H, Rakhorst G, Rau G. Design improvements of the HIA-VAD based on animal experiments. Artif Organs 1994; 18(7):473–478.
7. Rakhorst G, Hensens AG, Verkerke GJ, Blanksma PK, Bom VJJ, Elstrodt J, Magielse CPE, van der Meer J, Eilers R, Reul H. In vivo evaluation of the "HIA-VAD": a new German ventricular assist device. Thorac Cardiovasc Surg 1994; 42: 136–140.
8. Rakhorst G, Hensens AG, Blanksma PK, Bom VJJ, Elstrodt J, van der Meer J, Schakenraad JM, Verkerke GJ, Reul H. Evaluation of aprotocol for animal experiments with Helmholtz left ventricular assist devices. Cor Eur 1992; 4:155–159.
9. Waldenberger FR, Pongo E, Meyns B, Flameng W. Left-ventricular unloading with a new pulsatile assist device: the HIA-VAD system and its influence on myocardial stunning. Thorac Cardiovasc Surg 1995; 43:313–319.
10. Waldenberger FR. Novel Cardiac Assist Devices with Different Unloading Capacities. Leuven: Leuven University Press. Acta Biomedics Lovaniensia, 1995.
11. Guldner NW, Siemens HJ, Schramm U, Kraatz E, Thuaudet S, Kuppe H, Sievers HH. First clinical application of the MEDOS-HIA ventricular support system: monitoring of the thrombotic risk by means of the biomerker prothrombin fragment F + 2 and scanning electron microscopy evaluation. Heart Lung Transplant 1996; 3:291–296.
12. Konertz W, Hotz H, Schneider M, Redlin M, Reul H. Clinical experience with the MEDOS-VAD system in infants and children: a preliminary report. Ann Thorac Surg 1997; 63:1184–1244.
13. Waldenberger FR, Laube HR, Konertz W. Akute und chronische mechanische Kreislaufassistenz. Z Kardiol 1996; 85(suppl 4):61–68.
14. Kessler M, Sidiropoulos A, Halle J, Thölke R, Krause M, Konertz W. Kardiale Unterstützung im Neugeborenen- und Kindesalter. Kardiotechnik 1997; 3:64–67.
15. Busch U, Waldenberger FR, Redlin M, Hausdorf G, Konertz W. Successful treatment of postoperative right ventricular heart failure with the HIA-Medos-Assist system in a 2-year-old girl. Pediatr Cardiol 1999; 20:161–163.
16. Pennington DG, Swartz MT. Circulatory support in infants and children. Ann Thorac Surg 1993; 55:233–237.

17. Karl TR. Extracorporeal circulatory support in infants and children. Semin Thorac Cardiovasc Surg 1994; 6:154–160.
18. Weyand M, Kececioglu D, Schmid C, Kehl HG, Tandler R, Loick HM, Scheld HH. Successful briding to cardiac transplantation in a dystrophic infant with the use of a new paracorporeal pneumatic pump. J Thorac Cardiovasc Surg 1997; 114:3:505–507.
19. Sidiropoulos A, Hotz H, Konertz W. Pediatric circulatory support. J Heart Lung Transplant 1998; 17:1172–1176.
20. Delius RE, Zwischenberger JB, Cilley R, Behrend DM, Beve EL, Deeb M, Crowley D, Heidelberger KP, Bartlett RH. Prolonged extracorpored life support of pediatric and adoslescent cardiac transplant patients. Ann Thorac Surg 1990; 50:791–795.
21. Meliones IN, Custer JR, Snedecor S, Moler FW, O'Rourke PP, Delius RE. Extracorporeal life support for cardiac assist in pediatric patients. Circulation 1991; 84(suppl III):168–172.
22. Del Nido PJ. Extracorporeal membrane oxygenation for cardiac support in children. Ann Thorac Surg 1996; 61:336–339.
23. Karl TR, Sano S, Horton S, Mee RB. Centrifugal pump left heart assist in pediatric cardiac operations: indication, technique and results. J Thorac Cardiovasc Surg 1991; 102:624–630.
24. Taylor KM. Pulsatile and non-pulsatile perfusion. In: Minami K, Körfer R, Wada J, eds. Cardiac Thorac Surg, Amsterdam: Elsevier, 1992:57–65.
25. Bellotto F, Johnson RG, Watanabe J, et al. Mechanical assistance of the left ventricle. Acute effect on cardiac performance and coronary flow of different perfusion patterns. J Thorac Cardiovasc Surg 1992; 104:561–568.

17
The Use of the Berlin Heart in Children

Vladimir Alexi-Meskishvili, Roland Hetzer, Yuguo Weng, Brigitte Stiller, Matthias Loebe, and Evgenij Potapov
German Heart Institute, Berlin, Germany

I. INTRODUCTION

Ventricular assist devices (VADs) of various design and function principles have been in use over the last three decades for temporary support of the failing heart. Their aim is either for recovery of the heart postcardiotomy or postinfarct, or, more successfully, for keeping the patient alive until later transplantation, in the so-called "bridge-to-transplant" concept. Through the latter concept, which has gained wide application, assist devices have considerably evolved and have been used for periods of 2 years or more (1).

Most companies that produce such assist devices have not recommended their use in children below adult body size, and no pediatric-sized pumps were produced until 1992, when the "Berlin Heart" offered the first worldwide commercially available system with miniaturized paracorporeal pumps and cannulae. This development followed our need for a spectrum of pumps for every body size and age after our initial experience with schoolchildren, in whom we used adult-sized 'Berlin Heart' pumps, which had become available in 1988 (2).

The first reported case of an 8-year-old child supported for 8 days in intractable circulatory failure was followed by a successful transplant and an uneventful postoperative course at our institution (3). However, this was accomplished with an adult-sized 50 mL Berlin Heart left ventricular assist device (LVAD).

Most pediatric cardiac surgery departments have continued to use centrifugal pumps or extracorporeal membrane oxygenation (ECMO) as a support system for days and sometimes weeks (4). Over recent years we have preferred to use

ECMO for patients with intracardiac shunts, for very small infants, and postcardiotomy. Considering the shortage of pediatric donor hearts (5) and the tendency of increased mortality during the waiting period (6,7), VAD is preferable to ECMO for long-term circulatory support. In this group of patients we use the paracorporeal pneumatically driven, pulsatile Berlin Heart system, predominantly in a biventricular support configuration.

This report is based on experience gained with this system in 34 children under the age of 16 years between 1990 and December 1998.

II. PATIENTS AND METHODS

The Berlin Heart assist device was used in 34 children—18 boys and 16 girls—between 6 days and 16 years of age (mean 11.9 y) between 1990 and December 1998. All were in profound heart failure, and 29 had been on the respirator for more than 24 hours. All of these patients exhibited signs of acute renal failure in the form of oliguria-anuria, and 15 had elevated creatinine and serum urea levels. Twenty-six showed laboratory evidence of hepatic failure. There were three main groups of patients according to the underlying disease and the anticipated treatment concepts (see Tables 1 and 2).

A. Group I (Bridge-to-Transplant)

Group I included 22 patients with advanced chronic myocardial diseases or end stages of congenital heart disease. They were all considered for heart transplantation, but intractable life-threatening heart failure occurred before transplantation became feasible. In this group, assist pumps were implanted with the goal of achieving organ recovery until later transplantation.

Fifteen children suffered from cardiomyopathy of various origins (e.g., idiopathic, toxic, endocardial fibrosis, chronic recurrent myocarditis). One child with severe chronic left heart failure had aortic stenosis that was untreatable by conventional surgery; one child with myocardial infarction suffered from pulmonary atresia, intact ventricular septum, and coronary sinusoids; two children had transposition of the great arteries at long term after atrial corrective surgery (one Mustard, one Senning) and severe systemic ventricle failure; one suffered myocardial failure and recurrent ventricular fibrillation late after a Fontan operation; one had chronic failure of the systemic ventricle after aortic valve replacement; and one had chronic biventricular failure late after correction for tetralogy of Fallot.

B. Group II (Rescue)

This group included six children in whom heart failure occurred soon after corrective surgery for congenital heart defects. The implantation of the assist system was performed either immediately (No. 11 and 33) or between one and 8 days after the initial open heart procedure, invariably after at least one episode of cardiopulmonary resuscitation (CPR). The use of VAD support was aimed at providing support for the diseased heart in order to keep the patient alive, pending the eventual clinical course, i.e., either recovery and weaning or transplantation. The underlying defects and the operations were one Fontan operation for univentricular heart, one closure of ventricular septal defect (VSD), one Norwood operation for hypoplastic left heart syndrome, and one systemic-to-pulmonary shunt for pulmonary atresia, intact septum, and sinusoids. One child had early graft failure after heart transplantation, and one immediately after aortic valve replacement and acute endocarditis. The ages of these children ranged from 2 weeks to 12 years.

C. Group III (Acute Myocarditis)

In this group six patients were listed who presented with acute, mostly viral myocarditis. They could not be maintained by conservative means, and as an alternative either recovery or transplantation was anticipated. Four children had CPR before assist implantation and were brought to the operating room under continuous chest massage until extracorporeal circulation (ECC) was established. The duration of mechanical circulatory support in these children had been between 2 and 22 days.

D. The Assist Device

The Berlin Heart VAD system produced by Mediport Kardiotechnik, Berlin, Germany, consists of a paracorporeal air-driven blood pump, cannulae for connection of the pumps to the heart chambers and the great vessels, and electro-pneumatic driving systems (Figs. 1, 2, and 3; Table 3).

The blood pumps are now available in sizes 12, 15, 25, 30, 50, 60, and 80 mL according to their maximum blood chamber volume. The semirigid polyurethane housing the blood chamber and the air chamber are separated by a multilayer flexible polyurethane membrane. The blood-contacting membrane is seamlessly integrated within the housing. In the 50, 60, and 80 mL pumps mechanical mono-disc valves (Sorin Biomedica, Saluggia, Italy) are mounted within titanium connectors. Alternatively, these pumps are now available with polyurethane trileaflet valves (Fig. 1). Both the blood chambers and the polyurethane

Table 1 Three Groups of Patients According to Underlying Disease and Anticipated Treatment Concepts

No.	Age	Weight (kg)	Diagnosis	CPR	Type of support stroke volume (ml)	Duration of support (days)	Complications on support	Extub. during support	Support outcome	Outcome	Comments	Follow-up and late events
Bridging-To-Transplantation Group												
1	12 y	52	Idiopathic CMP	–	BVAD 50/60	6	2 × Re-thoracotomy	+	HTx	Died	Graft failure because PHT	
2	8 y	27	LV failure in AS + CoA	–	LVAD 50	8	None	+	HTx	Discharged	CoA patch plastic 18 months later	Without complications (7.5 y)
3	13 y	51	RV failure late after Mustard Op	+	LVAD 60	6	Hemothorax RV perforation	–	Died		Bleeding	
4	15 y	28.8	CMP	–	BVAD 50/60	71	Right pump exchange for thrombosis	+	Died		Intracerebral bleeding	
5	9 y	35	LV failure after AVR in endocarditis	–	BVAD 50/60	2	Re-thoracotomy	–	Died		Circulatory failure	
8	15 y	43	Toxic CMP	–	LVAD 60	34	2 × Pump exchange for thrombosis re-thoracotomy a. cer. media infarction	+	HTx	Discharged		Mild cerebral residuals (6 y)
10	15 y	45	Idiopathic CMP	–	BVAD 50/60	98	7 × Pump exchange for thrombosis	+	HTx	Discharged		Without complications (4.5 y)
12	6 d	4	Myocardial infarction in PA-atresia and coronary sinusoids	–	LVAD 12	3	None	–	Died		Circulatory failure	
14	3 y	14	Chronic recurrent myocarditis	+	BVAD 50/50	11	4 × Pump exchange for thrombosis. Brain infarction	+	HTx	Discharged		Without complications (4.5 y)
15	12 y	36	CMP in myopathy (mitochondropathy)	–	BVAD 60/60	20	Right pump exchange for thrombosis	+	HTx	Died	ECMO after HTx	
16	10 y	35	Hereditary HOCM	–	BVAD 50/60	6	Re-thoacotomy	+	HTx	Discharged		Without complications (4.5 y)
17	14 y	64	CMP	–	BVAD 60/80	72	Rethoracotomy	+	HTx	Died	Graft failure	
23	6 y	20	Chronic recurrent myocarditis	+	BVAD 25/30	21	Rethoracotomy; peritoneal bleeding	+	HTx	Discharged		Without complications (1.7 y)
24	5 y	18	Late myocardial failure after Senning Op. s/p LVOT resection: late VT/cardiac arrest	+	BVAD 30/25	13	None	+	Died		Bleeding	
25	2 y	10	CMP in endocardial fibrosis	–	BVAD 25/30	6	None	+	HTx	Discharged		Without complications (10 months)
26	15 y	43	CMP after viral myocarditis	–	LVAD 60	3	None	–	HTx	Died 3 months later	Sepsis	
27	14 y	23	CMP after viral myocarditis	–	BVAD 80/60	6	None	–	HTx	Died	Graft failure in PHT	
28	12 y	23	CMP	–	BVAD 23/30	4	None	–	Died		Circulatory failure	

29	14 y	22.5	Late myocardial failure after Fontan procedure	–	LVAD 50	0.4	None	–	Died		Circulatory failure; pulmonary edema	
30	5.5 months	6.6	CMP	–	BVAD 25/30	4	None	–	Died		Pulmonary edema	
31	11.5 y	26.6	CMP	–	BVAD 30/30	5	None	+	HTx	Discharged	Operated on in Oxford, England	Without complication (10 months)
32	13.1 y	26.7	Late myocardial failure after correction of Fallot's tetralogy	–	BVAD 25/30	111	None	+	HTx	Discharged		Without complications (10 months)
Rescue Group												
6	2 weeks	3.7	PA, IVS, coronary sinusoids, B-T shunt, LV failure after myocardial infarct	+	LVAD 12	1	None	–	Died		Circulatory failure	
7	4 y	15.7	DIRV, I-TGA, PS, Fontan Op	+	LVAD 50	0.5	Rethoracotomy	–	Died		Circulatory failure	
9	6 months	7	Myocardial failure after VSD closure	+	BVAD 12/12	1.5	Rethoracotomy	–	Died		Brain death	
11	2 weeks	3.2	HLHS, Norwood Op	+	BVAD 15	0.5	None	–	Died		Intracranial bleeding	
13	10 months	7.8	LCA ostium atresia; myocardial infarct, LIMA to LAD bypass; HTx, early graft failure	–	BVAD 12/12	8	Rethoracotomy	–	Weaned	Died	Recurrent graft failure in PHT	
33	12 y	38	AVR by endocarditis and aorto-pulmonary fistula	+	BVAD 50/50	2	Aortic cannula dislocation (2 times)	–	Died		Bleeding after aortic cannula dislocation	
Acute Myocarditis Group												
18	4 y	16.6	Acute myocarditis	+	BVAD 23/30	22	3 × Rethoracotomy, encephalopathy syndrome, pancreatitis	–	Weaned	Discharged	Weaning with ECMO	Prolonged neurological recovery, now without cerebral residuals (3.4 y)
19	3 d	2.2	Acute myocarditis	+	BVAD 12/12	2	None	–	Died		Circulatory failure	
20	8 months	7	Acute myocarditis	+	BVAD 25/30	16	2 × Rethoracotomy	–	Died		Circulatory failure	
21	5 y	23	Acute myocarditis	+	BVAD 25/30	11	Rethoracotomy	–	Weaned	Discharged	Weaning with ECMO	Without complications (2 y)
22	14 y	81	Acute myocarditis	–	LVAD 80	21	None	+	HTx	Discharged		Good cardiac function, weight loss, psychosocial problems (1.5 y)
34	13 months	10	Acute myocarditis	–	BVAD 25/30	11	None	–	Weaned	Discharged		Without complications (10 months)

AS = Aortic stenosis; AVR = aortic valve replacement; BVAD = biventricular assist device; Coa = coarctation of the aorta; CPR = cardio-pulmonary resuscitation; CMP = cardiomyopathy; DIRV = double inlet right ventricle; DORV = double outlet right ventricle; HLHS = hypoplastic left heart syndrome; HOCM = hypertrophic obstructive cardiomyopathy; HTx = heart transplantation; IVS = intact ventricular septum; LAD = left anterior descending coronary artery; LCA = left main coronary artery; LIMA = left internal mammary artery; LV = left ventricle; LVAD = left ventricular assist device; LVOT = left ventricular outflow tract; PA = pulmonary atresia; PHT = pulmonary hypertension; PS = pulmonary artery stenosis; RV = right ventricle; TGA = transposition of the great arteries; VSD = ventricular septal defect; VT = ventricular tachycardia.
Patient numbers are presented in chronological order.

Table 2 Patient Data

Group	No. of patients	Age (y)	CPR	On respirator >24 h	LVAD/ BVAD	Duration of support (d)
I	22	10 ± 5	5	17	6/16	23.2 ± 33* (0.4–98)
II	6	2.7 ± 4.3	5	6	3/3	2.3 ± 2.9* (0.5–8)
III	6	4.1 ± 5.2	4	6	1/5	14.0 ± 7.4* (2–22)
All	34	7.7 ± 5.8	14	29	10/24	17.9 ± 27.8

BVAD = Biventricular assist device; CPR = cardiopulmonary resuscitation; LVAD = left ventricular assist device. *
$p < 0.05$.

ports are transparent, which allows for transillumination detection of thrombotic deposits and for the control of chamber filling and emptying.

For the small blood pumps (12 and 15 mL) an optional modification was introduced by interposition of an elastic polyurethane reservoir between the atrial cannula and the inflow chamber port, which thus remarkably improves the cham-

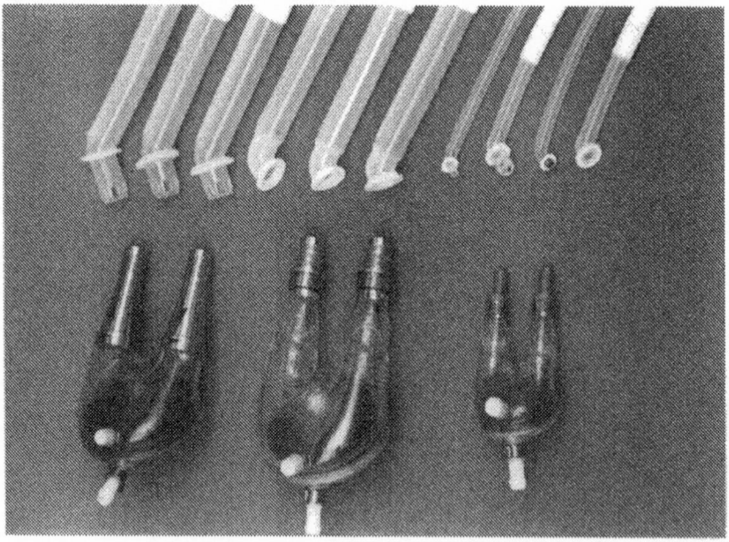

Fig. 1 Adult-size (80 mL) pump with titanium connectors (left), polyurethane ports including polyurethane trileaflet valves (center), and 12 mL pump with polyurethane ports and valves (right; bottom), spectrum of available arterial cannulae (left), arterial cannula (center) with different angles and pediatric cannulae (right; top). (From Ref. 33.)

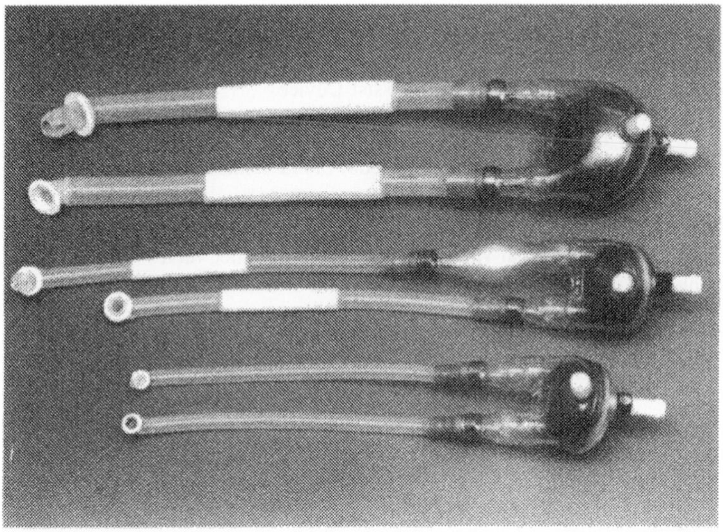

Fig. 2 Pediatric pumps and cannulae: 30 mL pump (top) with cannula showing Dacron-velour surface around central portion of skin tunnel. Miniaturized (12 mL) system with inlet port reservoir (center). Same system with reservoir equipped with smallest, infant-type cannulae (no Dacron-velour). (From Ref. 33.)

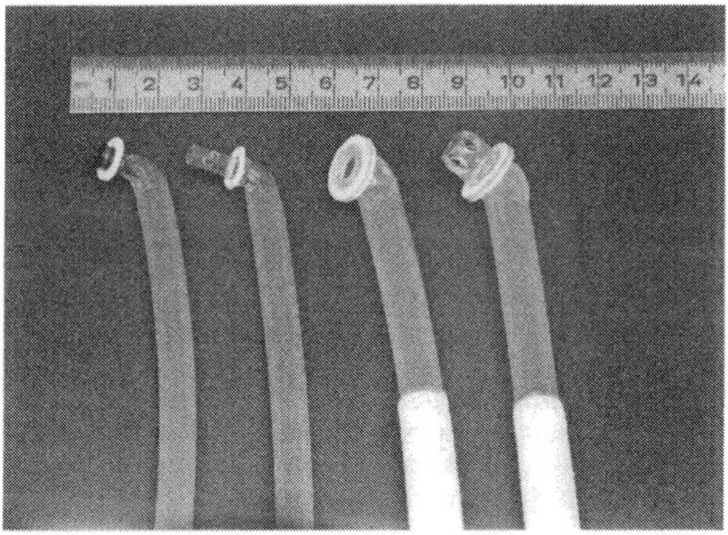

Fig. 3 Pediatric cannulae close-up: flat metal tip pushbutton-type arterial cannula with sewing ring (far left), small infant-type arterial cannula (center left), pair of cannulae tips for small children (right). (From Ref. 33.)

Table 3 Technical Data of the Berlin Heart Assist Device

Berlin Heart	Paracorporeal, pneumatically driven pump with polyurethane heparin-coated (Carmeda) blood-contacting surface (since 1994)
Pumps available	12, 15, 25, 30, 50, 60, 80 mL
	Mechanical valves, polyurethane trileaflet valves
Cannulae available	Silicone cannulae for atrial and arterial connections
	Adult, pediatric, and infant sizes
Drive units	IKUS 2000
	Heimes HD7
	Both with complete back-up

ber filling (Fig. 2). A set of atrial and arterial silicone cannulae, with inner diameters of 12.7, 9.5, 6.4, and 3.2 mm, is available that allows for individual system assembly in accordance with the individual patient's anatomy (Fig. 3).

The atrial cannulae are supplied with a basket tip at three different angles (45°, 60°, and 85°) and a sewing ring (Fig. 1). The arterial return cannulae have a Dacron-velour–covered sewing rim at their end, which allows for end-to-side anastomosis to either the aorta or the pulmonary artery. The middle portion of these cannulae is surrounded by a Dacron-velour surface, which promotes tissue in-growth, and thus provides a shield against infection migration along the skin tunnel.

In the few cases of left ventricular drainage either of the following may apply: a right-angled cannula with side holes near the tip can be inserted via the left upper pulmonary vein, the left atrium and across the mitral valve; or direct left ventricular apical drainage with a basket-tipped straight venous ECC cannula can be provided.

A variety of cannulae for infants and small children have been tried. Whereas the atrial drainage cannulae of miniaturize size have proven satisfactory, the arterial return cannulae have not done so. This is why, in most cases, indwelling regular ECC arterial return cannulae were used. However, this posed a significant resistance to the heart chambers when weaning from the pump was attempted. Only recently has a small arterial return cannula been developed that has a flat metal tip and a sewing ring at its 85° end, which resembles a push button (Fig. 3). The metal tip is inserted into the arterial lumen and allows secure fixation at the arterial wall by means of the sewing ring. This configuration ensures that there will not be any undue resistance to the natural heart output. Since 1994, all blood-contacting polyurethane surfaces have been heparin coated (Carmeda, Stockholm, Sweden), which have been used in the children Nos. 18–34.

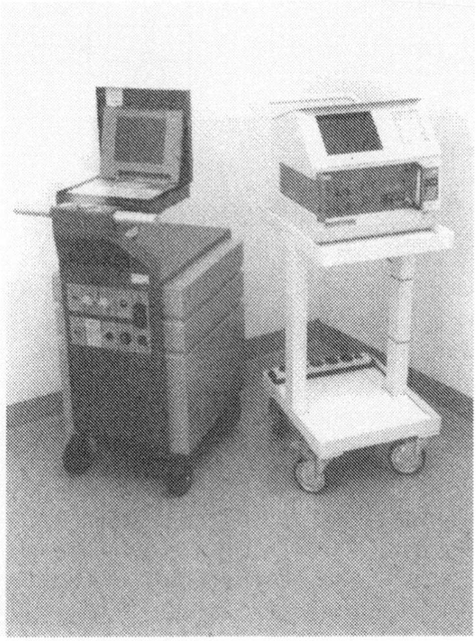

Fig. 4 Drive systems available for Berlin Heart assist device. The IKUS 2000 driver (left) is preferred in small children since it can generate high positive and negative pressures and a variety of driving modes. The lighter Heimes HD-7 driver (right) allows for a somewhat greater mobility. (From Ref. 33.)

Two different driving systems have been in use in pediatric patients (Fig. 4). Since the resistance of the small-bore cannulae is high during pump operation, positive systolic pressures of up to 350 mmHg and negative diastolic suction pressures of 100 mmHg at pumping rates of up to 140 beats/min are reached. Therefore, the power requirements are considerably higher than in the operation of the adult pump.

A drive unit that fulfills these extraordinary specifications was developed by the Institute for Artificial Hearts and Sensor Technology and produced by Mediport Kardiotechnik (Berlin, Germany)—the so-called IKUS-2000-Driver. It was specifically made for use with extracorporeal blood pumps. It was designed exclusively for operation with the Berlin Heart blood pumps sized 12, 15, 25, 30, 50, 60, and 80 mL. Characteristic of its operation are its capacity, its ease of use, as well as its technical reliability, which when combined offer the user maximum dependability.

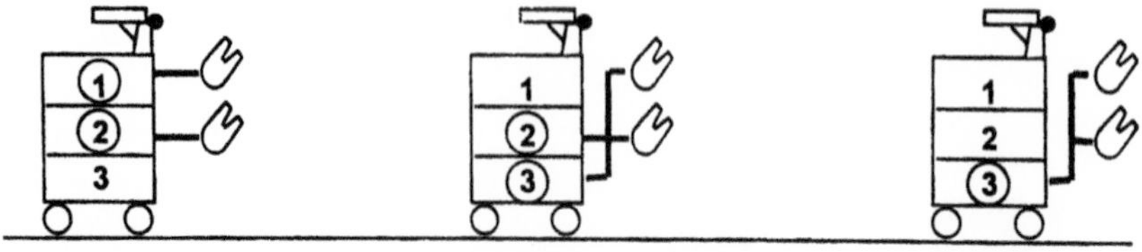

Fig. 5 Safety control of drive unit of the Berlin Heart assist device (see text).

The entire drive system essentially consists of three individual independently operating drive units. The system's safety concept is based upon this redundancy (Fig. 5). Each of these drive units consists in turn of a compressor, pressure and vacuum regulators, pressure and vacuum containers, as well as electronic controls and vents. The compressors, in conjunction with the pressure and vacuum regulators, assure constant pressure conditions in the respective containers. Control vents at the outlet of each container ensure the adjustability of the pressure and vacuum values for optimal operation of the pumps. The user controls the entire system through a laptop computer. The computers responsible for controlling the system are installed in the interior of the device's housing for security reasons and work independently of the laptop computer. As with pressure and vacuum production, the computer components were also designed to provide the required redundancy.

During operation each drive unit powers a blood pump. Accordingly, during normal biventricular operation two drive units are active while the third unit stands ready as a reserve system (Fig. 5, Case A).

If a malfunction occurs that affects operation, e.g., a drive unit ceases functioning, the inactive third unit is automatically switched on. The system's operation thus continues without interruption (Fig. 5, Case B). Even if another drive unit should cease to function, then the remaining drive unit is capable of maintaining the operation of both pumps (Fig. 5, Case C). All the necessary operating parameters for such an eventuality have been preprogrammed.

This driver can be operated by external electrical power as well as by internal batteries. The latter last for up to 2 hours and is the preferred system during the first period of assisted circulation because of the wide variety of driving modes possible.

The driving unit that has been alternatively used in our assist practice, the Heimes HD-7, weighs less and provides somewhat greater mobility. It is, however, limited by a smaller driving power. The Heimes HD-7 has an internal energy source that enables independent operation for more than 3 hours. Both drive units have completely redundant back-up systems. The semi-portable drive unit weighs less than 10 kg.

E. Implantation and Management of the Assist Devices and Treatment of Patients

The problem of limited pericardial space in infants and small children and the technical difficulties of VAD implantation after complex, reconstructive operation, especially in cases that require BVAD, which needs four cannulae, are the major surgical concerns for BVAD implantation in such patients (8). However, older children, who are awaiting a heart transplantation, often suffer chronic heart failure with resultant dilatation of the cardiac chambers, and in this group of patients implantation of VAD, even adult sized and in the biventricular configuration, is applicable.

In most cases, except for three with LVAD only, the patients were placed on conventional ECC, which greatly facilitated the assist implantation. The cannulae were secured by either pledgetted mattress sutures or, in the smaller children, by pursestring sutures and tourniquets. When the cannulae had been brought across the skin, via tight-fitting skin incisions, the pumps were connected and deaired, and assist circulation was begun and ECC stopped (Fig. 6).

Particular attention was paid to ensuring that there was a sufficient supply

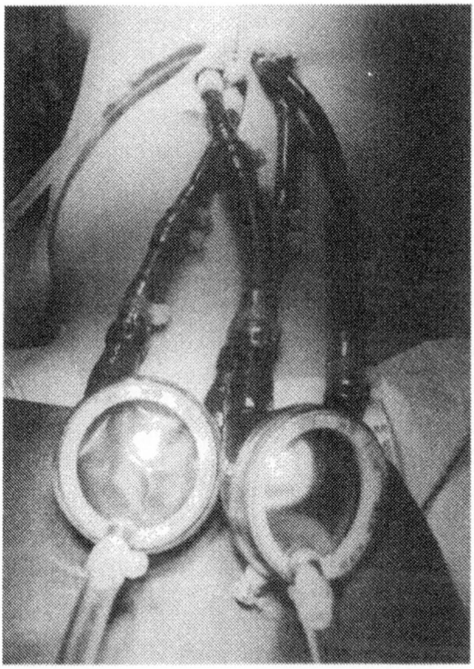

Fig. 6 External view of biventricular Berlin Heart assist device after implantation in systolic phase (patient No. 34; see Table 1).

of volume. This is important, especially during the early postoperative phase, because complete filling of the pumps is not possible because of the patient's hypovolemia. In this case an increase of the diastolic pressure will not lead to sufficient pump filling.

For sufficient filling of the circulation, venous flow to both pumps must be completely unimpeded and inlet obstruction should not occur. Nevertheless, should this occur, the only solution is an early revision of the implantation with a modification of the cannula position, since circulation assistance with venous inlet obstruction is pointless.

III. POSTIMPLANTATION CARE

Anticoagulation was maintained with continuous heparin infusion to keep an activated clotting time of 160–180 seconds. The anticoagulation regimen remained unchanged when the heparin-coated VAD was used. Pump operation was monitored daily and, if necessary, readjusted to achieve full diaphragm movement. Transillumination of the pump chambers was performed daily to detect small thrombi. In the presence of thrombi the pump was changed under sterile conditions in the operating theater. Patients who could be extubated were transferred to an intermediate ward to promote rehabilitation. Transthoracic echocardiography was performed daily to control cardiac function, especially during weaning from assist circulation. Transesophageal echocardiography is usually avoided because of the possibility of bleeding from the esophagus. Coumadin and antiplatelet agents were not used.

Antibiotic and good antistaphylococcal coverage (generally second-generation cephalosporines) was prophylactically administered in the preoperative, intraoperative, and postoperative phases. Attentive and careful searches for possible infections at the entry portals (transcutaneous lines of the blood cannulae, thorax drains, venous and arterial catheters, bladder catheter, dry smears) was absolutely essential. Blood cultures were taken daily from the venous blood and were followed by aggressive antibacterial therapy if an infection was established. Dressings were changed daily around the transcutaneous lines and were accompanied by spraying with disinfectant.

The careful removal of old blood from around the transcutaneous lines, as well as encrustations that result from wound secretions, particularly on the Dacron fabric of the blood cannulae, is strongly recommended. It is important to avoid necrosis around and particularly between the transcutaneous lines.

IV. MOBILIZATION

Older children were mobilized as soon as progress allowed, and intensive physical therapy was absolutely necessary. Even if patients are still dependent on a

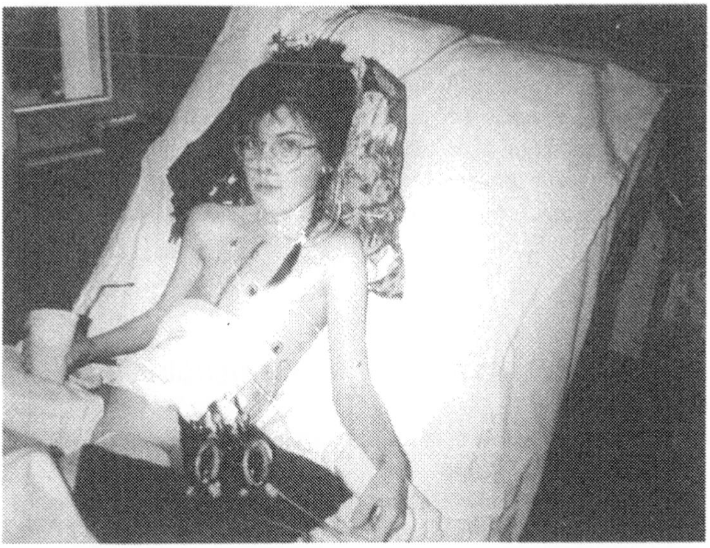

Fig. 7 Patient No. 32 (see Table 1) extubated on the biventricular system.

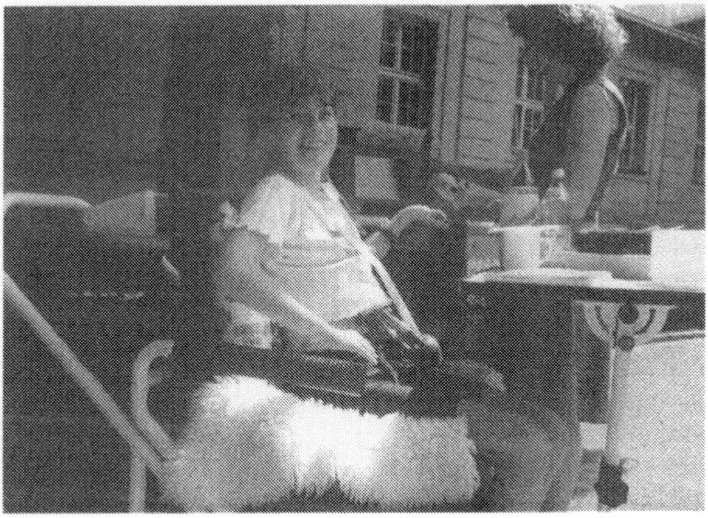

Fig. 8 Same patient as in Fig. 7 80 days after implantation of biventricular system.

respirator, they must be mobilized to the point where they are able to leave the bed. As soon as patients are weaned and extubated from the respirator, they should take shorts walks around the intensive care station and strive to improve their physical condition as much as possible for the next, and under certain circumstances, quickly approaching heart transplantation (Fig. 7 and 8).

All other children were intubated and artificially ventilated before heart transplantation was performed or the VAD was explanted (Group III, patients 18, 21, and 34).

V. TRANSPLANTATION AFTER MECHANICAL BRIDGING

Patients awaiting a heart transplant whose inotropic condition continued to deteriorate despite maximum medical therapy (catecholamine plus phosphodiesterase inhibitor = enoximon) were candidates for BVAD bridging. At the time of BVAD implantation, the patients were ordinarily in a critical circulatory condition and almost always exhibited functional limitations in one or more organs. These organ dysfunctions led to intra-, early, and late postoperative problems in the intensive care station.

All bridging patients must be cared for as if they were heart transplant patients. Particular attention must be paid to adequate peripheral resistance. As a rule, this can be achieved with low and medium doses of noradrenalin. In addition, dopamine was also given as a "renal dose" in order to improve perfusion in the splanchnic circulation. Usually additional catecholamine was not necessary.

In case of severe renal dysfunction, hemofiltration or dialysis was performed, which was dependent on the renal retention values. Respirator therapy was continued until clinical, radiological, blood gas, and breathing parameters had normalized. For most patients, our experience has shown that restoration of sufficient circulation by the assist system also leads to recovery of previously dysfunctional organs (8).

In children in whom a transplant was planned, a state called "transplantability" was defined when organ recovery was complete, the patient was without severe index, measured by thermodilution, was between 2.7 and 3.4 $L \cdot min^{-1} \cdot m^{-2}$ over the following 3 days.

In the case of patient No. 34, after an improvement of myocardial function, the BVAD was explanted on the 11th postoperative day during a short period (36 min) of normothermic cardiopulmonary bypass. Patient No. 22 was transplanted: there was a recovery of all of his organs except the heart (Table 4). On BVAD generalized edema was soon eliminated; he was extubated 2 days after implantation, regained full consciousness, and was mobilized—eating and drinking by himself and playing with his parents. When no myocardial recovery was detected by echocardiography over a period of 20 days on the BVAD, he underwent orthotopic heart transplantation with an uneventful postoperative course.

Categorical variables were evaluated using chi-squared analysis, with $p < 0.05$ considered as statistically significant. Nonparametric ordinal variables were evaluated using the Mann-Whitney U test. All statistical analyses were performed using SPSS for Windows, Release 6.0 (SPSS, Inc., 1989–1993).

VI. RESULTS

The shortest support time was 9 hours (No. 7) and the longest was 111 days (No. 32). On average the children were supported for 17.9 days (±27.8; Table 2). Nineteen were taken off the assist system, either after complete cardiac recovery or at the time of transplantation (Table 4). Fifteen patients died from either loss of peripheral circulatory resistance, which was unresponsive to α-receptor neurological deficits, was preferably awake and extubated, and was without infection. The patient was then listed as transplantable on the Eurotransplant Foundation waiting list.

Orthotopic heart transplantation was performed according to the method of Shumway-Cooley (9). Extracorporeal circulation was initiated from 30 to 45 minutes before the organ arrived in the operating room. After shutting down the assist device, the time was used to remove the cannulae and to oversew the insertion point on the left atrium. The procuring surgeon must ensure that a sufficiently long section of pulmonary artery is available (i.e., the section of the pulmonary artery used for the cannula anastomosis that can be dispensed with). The same considerations apply to the aorta. Otherwise, the transplantation was no different from primary orthotopic transplantation. Treatment after transplantation followed our usual regimen, as in other transplanted patients, except for a delay in the implantation of the intramyocardial electrogram (IMEG) rejection-monitoring system following healing of all skin incisions (10–12).

VII. THE EXPLANTATION PROCEDURE IN PATIENTS WITH ACUTE MYOCARDITIS

Continuous improvement of systolic myocardial function in three patients began after 5–14 days on the BVAD (Table 4). The BVAD was changed to ECMO for easier gradual weaning on day 21 (patient No. 18) and day 11 (patient No. 21), respectively. Over 5–6 days on ECMO the flow rate was reduced continuously. During weaning, the ventricular function was measured daily by transesophageal echocardiography, which showed continuous improvement of myocardial contractility. The pump flow was decreased in relation to systolic blood pressure

Table 4 Transplantation and Weaning After Circulatory Support with Berlin Heart Assist Device

	No.	Time of support (d)	Survivors	Late deaths
Transplanted from system				
· CMP	12	3–98	9	1
CHD	2	8 and 111	2	None
Myocarditis	1	21	1	None
Weaned from system				
After HTx	1	8	None	
Myocarditis	3	11, 12, and 22	3	None

CMP = Cardiomyopathy; CHD = congenital heart disease; HTx = heart transplantation.

and filling volumes and pressures. After successful decannulation, the cardiac stimulants due either to multiorgan damage or to sepsis, or from hemorrhagic complications while on the assist system. In these patients the decision to terminate the mechanical support was made when it became apparent that organ recovery could not be attained.

In Group I, 14 patients out of 22 reached the goal of recovery from shock sequelae and were judged "transplantable" (Table 5). Two patients died after transplantation from right heart failure due to high pulmonary vascular resistance, and two more patients died from graft failure. One of the latter was placed on ECMO and succumbed to circulatory failure with sepsis, and the other acquired a fungal disease and died from sepsis 3 months posttransplant. Causes of death for all patients are listed in Table 6. Nine patients were discharged from hospital after HTx, and one subsequently had an operation for coarctation 18 months after the transplant. The transplanted patients were treated with our triple immunosuppressive regimen (5), and rejection was monitored with the IMEG system devel-

Table 5 Results of Circulatory Support with Berlin Heart Assist Device

Group	No.	Died on system	Extubated on system	HTx/weaned	Survived	Late death
I	22	8	14	14	10	1
II	6	5	0	1	0	0
III	6	2	1	4	4	0
All	34	15	15	19	14	1

HTx = Heart transplantation.

Table 6 Causes of Death in Pediatric Patients Supported with Berlin Heart Assist Device

Peripheral circulatory failure unresponsive to α-stimulants in MOF and/or sepsis	9
Pulmonary edema	1
Hemorrhagic complications	5
Intracerebral bleeding	2
External bleeding	3

MOF = Multiorgan failure.

oped in our department (6,7). Presently all nine long-term survivors are alive, between 10 months and 8 years after transplantation, with good graft function and uneventful further developments.

All six patients in Group II died after 9 hours to 8 days of mechanical support (Table 5). In each instance this was caused by the profoundness of the preceding circulatory failure, i.e., multiorgan failure with loss of circulatory resistance, brain death, pulmonary failure, and diffuse hemorrhage. The patient with early graft failure after transplantation (No. 13) was weaned from the VAD but suffered from the rapid reoccurrence of graft failure through elevated pulmonary vascular resistance.

In Group III, two of the four patients who were brought to the operating room under continuous chest massage died after 2 and 16 days from peripheral circulatory failure. One patient was transplanted after 21 days of support; he is well and alive 1½ years after the procedure. However, he displays signs of significant psychosomatic disturbances. Two children (patients Nos. 18 and 21), who were also brought to the operation room under CPR and placed on ECC under cardiac massage, were supplied with a biventricular system with left ventricular drainage, one with a transmitral tipped cannula and another with an apical cannula. Both these children recovered and displayed a rapid restoration of their cardiac function. When the recovery from myocarditis was found to be satisfactory, after 11 and 21 days, the system was exchanged for ECMO support for 5 and 6 days, respectively, for easier stepwise weaning, after which the patients were taken off any support. Both children have since made an excellent recovery, are fully active, and have an entirely normal heart function after 2 and 3 postoperative years.

One 13-month-old child recovered 11 days after implantation of the BVAD and has normal cardiac function 10 months after the BVAD explantation (Table 5). This case illustrates the effectiveness of the BVAD in an infant with acute myocarditis.

A 13-month-old 10-kg boy 2 days after vaccination developed a respiratory infection followed by global myocardial failure and cardiogenic shock. He was admitted to another hospital where he was intubated and artificially ventilated. Due to the lack of success with conservative treatment, he was transferred to our center for further diagnostics with the suggestion that he might be a candidate for emergency mechanical circulatory support or cardiac transplantation.

The child presented with generalized edema and tachycardia (170/min). His circulation was supported by high doses of epinephrine, dobutamine, and enoximon. Echocardiography revealed the absence of cardiac defects, mitral incompetence of second degree, trivial tricuspid and pulmonary valve incompetence, poor contractility of both ventricles with a left ventricular ejection fraction (LVEF) of less than 20% and a shortening fraction (FS) of 10%.

Cardiac catheterization revealed a cardiac index of 1.9 $L \cdot min^{-1} \cdot m^{-2}$, elevated left ventricular end-diastolic pressure (LVEDP) (30 mmHg) and right ventricular diastolic pressure (18 mmHg), a pulmonary capillary wedge pressure of 30 mmHg with dilation of both ventricles and very poor contractility (LVEF of less than 10%). Myocardial biopsy, performed during cardiac catheterization, revealed extensive myocyte lysis, inflammation, and necrosis of more than 50% of the myocytes, interstitial edema with eosinophils, and a distinct vasculitis (Fig. 9).

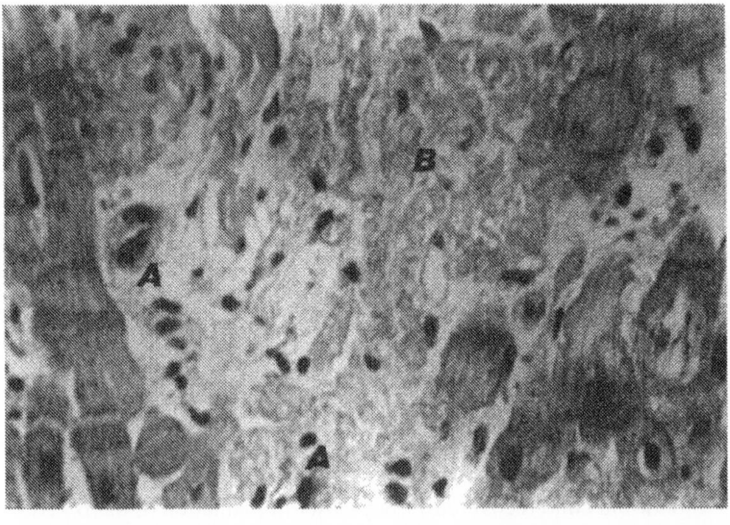

Fig. 9 Patient No. 34, biopsy of right ventricle (hematoxylin and eosin, original magnification ×400). Inflammatory process, myocardium infiltrated by lymphoid cells (A) and extensive myocytolysis necrosis (B) of more than 50% of the myocytes present.

Because of profound circulatory instability, a Berlin Heart Biventricular Assist Device was implanted via sternotomy on the same day. The cardiopulmonary bypass time was 95 minutes, and the aortic cross-clamp time was 16 minutes (Fig. 10). During support the activated clotting time was kept at 160–180 seconds and the artificial ventricle rate of 60/min.

One week after the BVAD implantation, a decrease of LVED size from 4 to 3 cm was noted together with a significant improvement of the ejection fraction to 40% and the shortening fraction to 20%, while the pump frequencies were maximally decreased. During and after implantation of the Berlin Heart Assist Device, normal flow in the arteria cerebri media was observed (Fig. 11).

Eleven days after the BVAD implantation, during a short period of total normothermic cardiopulmonary bypass (36 min), the BVAD was explanted and the sternum was primarily closed (Fig. 12). Seventeen days after the BVAD explantation the child was transferred to the referral hospital in a stable condition with no signs of infection or cardiac decompensation (Fig. 13). Before discharge echocardiography revealed significant improvement of his cardiac function: LVEF 48%, shortening fraction 28%, LVED size 2.8 cm, and no valve incompetence. Twelve months after explantation the child remains asymptomatic without any signs of myocardial damage.

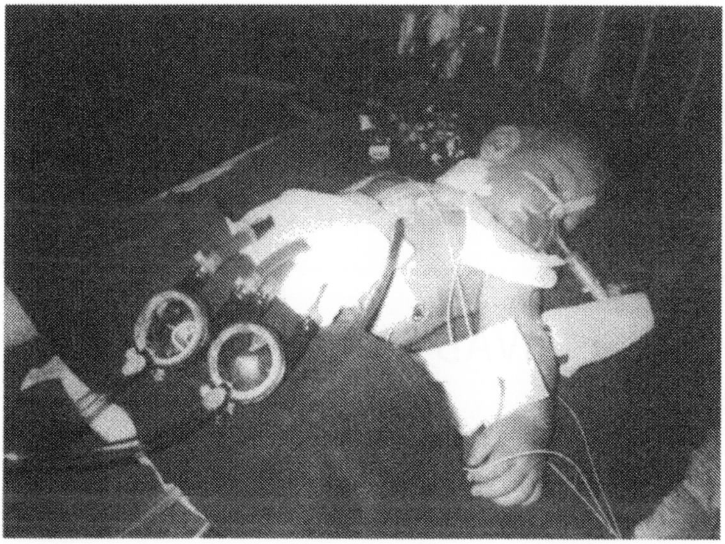

Fig. 10 Patient No. 34 with cardiomyopathy on a biventricular system with a 25 mL pump (right) and a 30 mL pump (left) early after implantation.

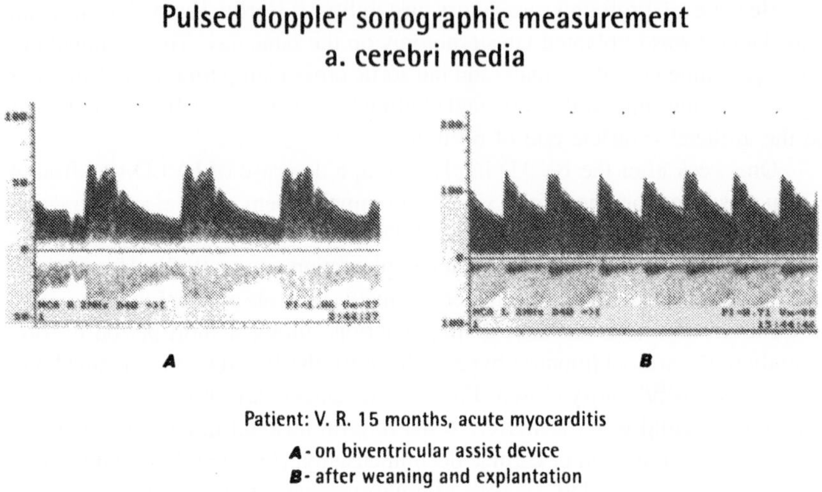

Pulsed doppler sonographic measurement
a. cerebri media
A
B
Patient: V. R. 15 months, acute myocarditis
A - on biventricular assist device
B - after weaning and explantation

Fig. 11 Pulsed Doppler sonograph measurement of flow in the arteria cerebri media during and after circulatory assist with the Berlin Heart in patient No. 34. Note the normal flow patterns during ventricular assist.

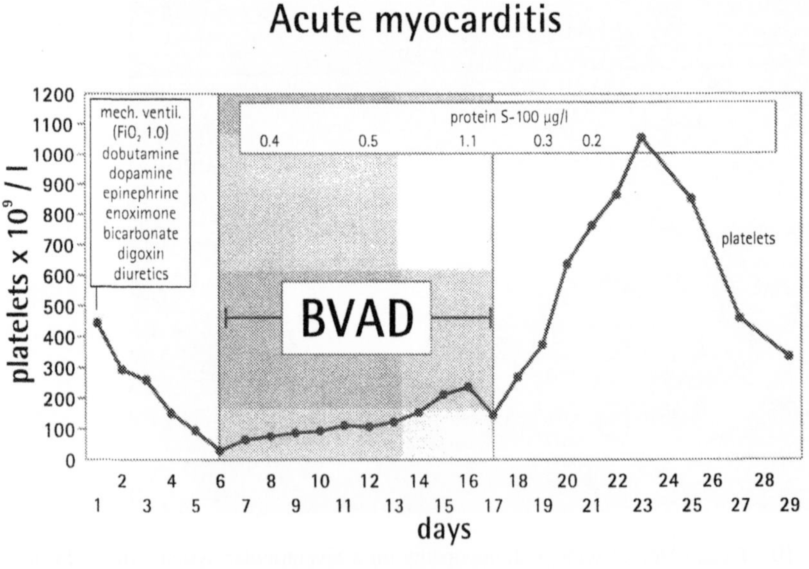

Fig. 12 Clinical course of patient No. 34 with acute myocarditis. No platelet transfusion was performed before, during, or after circulatory assist with the Berlin Heart assist device.

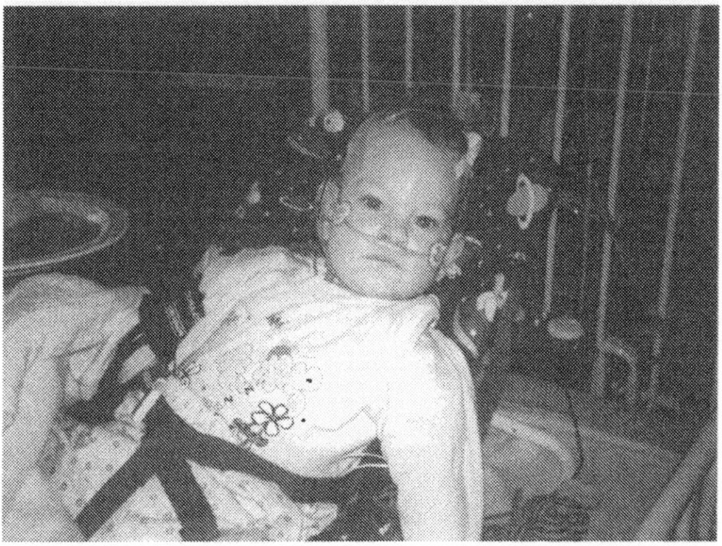

Fig. 13 The same patient as in Fig. 10 after explantation of the Berlin Heart assist device shortly before discharge.

VIII. COMPLICATIONS DURING SUPPORT

During the support period a number of aspects deserve more detailed description. There was no significant hemolysis detectable during the support period. Two patients suffered cerebral thromboembolism on the device. One (No. 8) had a significant arteria cerebri media infarction that 5½ years after transplantation still showed some minor compensated residuals. This patient had a history of previous cerebrovascular accidents, probably due to thrombus formation in the dilated heart. In another patient (No. 14) signs of less severe cerebral embolism totally disappeared after 6 weeks (Table 7).

In five children, invariably supported by the nonheparinized pumps during our earlier experience, thrombi were detected in the blood pumps which necessitated repeated pump exchanges (Table 7). Since heparin-coated pumps became available, no such instances have occurred and there have been no instances of thromboembolic organ damage.

Bleeding after assist implantation has been the most frequent complication that required surgical reexploration in 11 patients. Arterial cannula dislocation and leaking, which caused terminal bleeding, was observed in one child (No. 33).

Except for those patients who died very early from circulatory failure, none

Table 7 Complications During Circulatory Support with a Berlin Heart Assist Device in Children

Complication	No. of patients
Thrombi in pump chambers[a]	5
Pump exchange[a]	15 instances
Thromboembolism (cerebral)[a]	2
Hemorrhage req. reexploration	11
Arterial cannula dislocation	1
Mediastinitis	0
Technical failure	0

[a] No thrombotic complications since heparin-coating (1994).

of the children suffered de novo infection, and, most importantly, no instance of mediastinitis was observed, even in the patients after reexplorations (Table 7). There was no instance of technical failure, neither of the blood pump components, nor of the drive system. The recovery of organ function from shock sequelae was quite variable. In particular, no significant differentiation could be made according to laboratory data prior to assist implantation as to the potential of later recovery (8).

Fifteen of the patients on the assist system in Group I and Group II were taken off the respirator and were mobilized. Out of this group 13 were transplanted. Three patients in Group III were successfully weaned and later extubated.

IX. COMMENTS

The experiences presented in this report indicate that children with advanced heart failure or even in profound cardiogenic shock, who would otherwise immediately die, may be kept alive and either completely recover or qualify for successful heart transplantation with the aid of a pediatric version of the ventricular assist device.

While the first such applications in children were made at our institution with adult-sized devices as early as 1990 with long-term survival, after subsequent heart transplantation of 7½ years (3), 34 children were supported predominantly with the smallest adult pump (50 mL) or with miniaturized pediatric pump systems for up to 111 days. Meanwhile, other pediatric-type pneumatic systems, which closely resemble our Berlin Heart model, have been introduced into clinical practice with some instances of short-term use (13,14).

The 'Berlin Heart' system may completely substitute cardiac-output in a mono-ventricular or, more frequently, in a biventricular configuration (2). Widely used alternatives are either centrifugal pumps or even ECMO, which may sustain the circulation for several days or sometimes for a few weeks (4,14–18). These systems, and particularly ECMO, apart from greater damage to the blood components and the profound disarray of the coagulation system, require continuous intensive care with only a theoretical chance of extubation and mobilization of the patient. However, ECMO seems invaluable when intracardiac shunts persist or when profound respiratory insufficiency accompanies heart failure. ECMO, in our hands, or left ventricular support with a centrifugal pump are the methods of choice for these conditions and for prolonged support for some days after open heart surgery when immediate weaning from the extracorporeal circulation cannot be accomplished and when myocardial recovery can be expected (19).

This mode of treatment has proved to be successful at our institution, in particular in infants with myocardial impairment such as in Bland-White-Garland's syndrome, after arterial switch operation and total anomalous venous drainage correction (20,21). Even heart transplantation from ECMO has been successful in complex cardiac defects with a shunt after as long as 17 days of support in individual cases (19).

Whereas the extracardiac pneumatic blood pump chambers in their miniaturized form, in particular with the inner surfaces now heparin coated, pose little or no technical problems and complications, the cannulae for small children and infants have undergone several modifications. Today a configuration of the cannulae has been reached which seems to be satisfactory and does not necessarily hinder blood flow within the native great vessels of the patient.

Cerebral infarction related to thrombus formation in the VAD was observed in two patients. This can be avoided by the use of the appropriate-sized pump, which provides a good washout of the blood-contacting inner surface of the pump and thus prevents thrombus formation. The beneficial effect of the heparin-coating system was demonstrated in patient No. 32, in whom no thrombus formation in the system was noted over the 111 days of assist with the BVAD, which was followed by successful heart transplantation.

The high rate of hemorrhagic complications in the assist patients is a major problem and is related to systemic anticoagulation, impaired coagulation in shock, and to the fact that the intrathoracic assist cannulae prevent surface contact of the heart and the intrathoracic structures, a factor that is most important in patients who have undergone previous cardiac surgery.

The interposition of a flexible polyurethane reservoir into the inflow limb of the small 12-mL pumps has helped with the adequate filling of the pump chamber, which may otherwise be impaired in the light of high suction pressures. The drive system has not created any technical problems, and it has been in routine use in several hundred adult cases for periods of up to 1½ years in some patients (22).

The overall survival rate in our 34 pediatric patients has been 41.2%. This result in patients with very advanced disease can certainly be improved upon in the future and must be seen in the light of technical developments, growing experience in the treatment of the patients on the device, and, most importantly, with respect to adequate patient selection. Meanwhile, the accumulated amount of knowledge is well documented by the fact that of the 14 patients supported since 1996, 10 patients (71.4%) have successfully reached transplantation or weaning.

Recovery from profound heart failure and even cardiac arrest has been somewhat better in the children when compared with adults. This is underlined by the surprisingly complete recovery of some patients who were brought to the operating room under chest massage and in cardiac arrest.

Our experience shows that even when major organ dysfunctions (hepatic and renal) occur before VAD implantation, patients can still undergo successful heart transplantation after recovering hepatic and renal function (8). Recently it was shown that the recovery of liver function is the most predictive factor of adult patient survival in bridging to transplantation (23). Severe respiratory failure, which requires mechanical ventilation, seems to have a negative impact on the outcome of pediatric heart transplantation after VAD support (8).

On the other hand, some conditions must be considered as unsuitable for implantation of an assist device. All patients in Group II, where the VAD was implanted in the postoperative period some time after open-heart corrective operations and after the application of high-dose catecholamines, eventually succumbed to multiorgan failure or intracerebral hemorrhage. This small patient group was treated during 1992 and one in 1998 (No. 33). At our institution, their condition has since been considered to be an indication, if at all, for the use of centrifugal pump support or ECMO.

Termination of mechanical support in the face of progressive multiorgan failure and sepsis has opened up a new and ethically difficult problem (24), since the mechanical system can supply a patient with a full cardiac output even when the patient is in a state of extensive tissue damage, which would otherwise have caused intractable heart failure. While weaning, heart transplantation and brain death are clear indications for the termination of mechanical support, but this decision is not otherwise as easily made. The final observation was invariably that of a profound loss of peripheral resistance that was unresponsive to any medication, i.e., α-receptor stimulants.

Initially, heart transplantation was considered early after mechanical support was started. Also, as derived from our adult experience with bridge-to-transplant in up to 108 patients, we would now wait long enough to give the patient the chance for full recovery of all the organs (2,25,26) and the immune system (27) on the mechanical support device prior to a state of "transplantability" being declared and the patient then being listed for organ relocation.

A very exciting experience, which opens up an entirely new treatment concept, has been made with acute myocarditis and intractable heart failure. World experience with VAD or ECMO in patients with acute myocarditis is very limited (28,29). The ECMO Registry reported in 1998 50 patients with acute myocarditis supported by ECMO with a 54% survival rate (30). Whereas in the past children with this condition have been regarded as bridge-to-transplant candidates, three children demonstrated complete and lasting recovery of the heart function after 11 and 22 days of VAD support, which was then terminated in two patients via ECMO, gradual weaning, and the final taking-off of any mechanical system after a few more days.

It was suggested that "mechanical circulatory assist in severe acute myocarditis can allow the metabolic energy of the heart to be used for repair, rather than work" (29). A similar mechanism of myocardial recovery is also reported by our group in patients after reimplantation of anomalous left coronary artery during mechanical circulatory support (21,31).

In two children with acute myocarditis in Group III, left ventricular drainage and unloading had been carried out through the right upper pulmonary vein and in one child through direct left ventricular apical cannulation, which appears to be mandatory in order to provide a state of complete "rest" to allow myocardial resting and recovery (32). In none of the cases with the atrial drainage configuration was such an impressive recovery observed. This is in agreement with our experience in adults with chronic dilated cardiomyopathy, where we have now explanted LVAD pumps between 2 months and 26 months after support with apical left ventricular drainage and where 13 patients out of 19 have undergone complete cardiac function restoration for up to almost 4 years (24,25). Acute myocarditis, even moreso than cardiomyopathy, obviously has, at least in a substantial proportion of the cases, an excellent predisposition to aim for such a recovery.

X. CONCLUSION

It now seems well established that the beneficial effects of VAD treatment, as demonstrated in the adult patient group, may well be transposed to children of any age where longer support periods are anticipated. Earlier implantation in the course of progressive heart failure now appears to be justified since the systems, such as the Berlin Heart, have undergone the necessary modifications and since the accumulation of clinical knowledge that makes the use of this system highly reliable and safe.

REFERENCES

1. Hetzer R, Hennig E, Loebe M. Mechanical Circulatory Support. Darmstadt: Steinkopf-Verlag, 1997.
2. Hetzer R, Hennig E, Schiessler A, Friedel N, Warnecke H, Adt M. Mechanical circulatory support and heart transplantation. J Heart Lung Transplant 1992; 11: 175–181.
3. Warnecke H, Berdijis F, Hennig E, Lange P, Schmitt D, Hummel M, Hetzer R. Mechanical left ventricular support as bridge to cardiac transplantation in childhood. Eur J Cardiothorac Surg 1991, 5:330–333.
4. Bartlett RH. Extracorporeal membrane oxygenation for cardiac support in children. Semin Thorac Cardiovasc Surg 1994, 6:154–160.
5. Kelly D. Pediatric transplantation comes of age. Br Med J 1998, 317:897.
6. Sable CA, Shaddy RE, Suddaby EC, Hawkins JA, Sell JE, Martin GR. Impact of prolonged waiting time of neonates awaiting heart transplantation. J Perinatol 1997, 17:481–488.
7. Boucek MM, Novick RJ, Bennet LE, Fiol B, Keck BM, Hosenpud JD. The Registry of the International Society of Heart and Lung Transplantation: second official pediatric report—1998. J Heart Lung Transplant 1998; 17:1141–1160.
8. Ishino K, Loebe M, Uhlemann F, Weng Y, Hennig E, Hetzer R. Circulatory support with paracorporeal pneumatic ventricular assist device (VAD) in infants and children. Eur J Card-Thorac Surg 1997; 11:965–972.
9. Shumway NE, Lower RR, Stofer RC. Transplantation of the heart. Adv Surg 1996; 2:265–284.
10. Hetzer R, Potapov E, Müller J, Hummel M, Wenig Y, Stiller B, Loebe M, Warnecke H, Lange PE. Daily non-invasive rejection monitoring improves long-term survival in pediatric heart transplantation. Ann Thorac Surg 1998; 66:1343–1349.
11. Müller J, Warnecke H, Spiegelsberger S, Hummel M, Cohnert T, Hetzer R. Reliable noninvasive rejection diagnosis after heart transplantation in childhood. J Heart Lung Transplant 1993; 12:189–198.
12. Warnecke H, Müller J, Cohnert T, Hummel M, Spiegelsberger S, Sinawski H, Lieback E, Hetzer R. Clinical heart transplantation without routine endomyocardial biopsy. J Heart Lung Transplant 1992; 11:1093–1102.
13. Konertz W, Hotz H, Schneider M, Redlin M. Reul H. Clinical experience with the MEDOS HIA-VAD System in infants and children: preliminary report. Ann Thorac Surg 1997; 63:1138–1144.
14. Weyand M, Kececioglu D, Schmid C, Kehl H, Tandler R, Loick H, Scheld H. Successful bridging to cardiac transplantation in dystrophic infant with the use of a new paracorporeal pump. J Thorac Cardiovasc Surg 1997; 114:505–507.
15. Del Nido P. Extracorporeal membrane oxygenation for cardiac support in children. Ann Thorac Surg 1996; 61:336–339.
16. Karl T. Extracorporeal circulatory support in infants and children. Semin Thorac Cardiovasc Surg 1994; 6:154–160.
17. Pennington D, McBride L, Miller L, Swartz M. Eleven years' experience with the

Pierce-Donachy ventricular assist device. J Heart Lung Transplant 1994; 13:803–810.
18. Klein M, Withlesey G. Extracorporeal membrane oxygenation. Pediatr Clin North Am 1994; 41:365–384.
19. Alexi-Meskishvili V, Hetzer R, Weng Y, Ishino K, Potapov E, Loebe M, Hennig E, Uhlemann F, Lange PE. Extracorporeal circulatory support in pediatric patients—the Berlin experience. In Hetzer R, Hennig E, Loebe M, eds. Mechanical Circulatory Support. Darmstadt: Steinkopf-Verlag, 1997:33–52.
20. Alexi-Meskishvili V, Nurnberg JH, Werner H, Lange PE, Hetzer R. Long-term extracorporeal membrane oxygenation in a newborn child after arterial switch operation. Cardiovasc Surg 1996; 4(2):258–260.
21. Alexi-Meskishvili V, Hetzer R, Weng Y, Loebe M, Lange PE, Ishino K. Successful extracorporeal circulatory support after aortic reimplantation of anomalous left coronary artery. Eur Cardio-Thorac Surg 1994; 8:533–536.
22. Loebe M, Hennig E, Müller J, Spiegelsberger S, Weng Y, Hetzer R. Long-term mechanical circulatory support as a bridge to transplantation, for recovery from cardiomyopathy and for permanent replacement. J Heart Lung Transplant 1997; 16: 1176–1179.
23. Renhartz O, Farar DJ, Hershon JH, Avery GJ, Haeusslein A, Hill JD. Importance of preoperative liver function as a predictor of survival in patients supported with THORATEC ventricular assist devices as a bridge to transplantation. J Thorac Cardiovasc Surg 1998; 116:633–640.
24. Powell TP, Oz MC. Discontinuing the LVAD: ethical considerations. Ann Thorac Surg 1997; 63:1223–1224.
25. Müller J, Wallukat G, Weng Y, Dandel M, Spiegelsberger S, Semrou S, et al. Weaning from mechanical cardiac support in patients with dilated cardiomyopathy. Circulation 1997; 96:542–549.
26. Hetzer R, Müller J, Weng Y, Wallakat G, Spiegelsberger S, Loebe M. Cardiac recovery in dilated cardiomyopathy by unloading with a left ventricular assist device. Ann Thorac Surg 1999; 68:742–749.
27. Hummel M, Czerlinski S, Friedel N, Liebenthal C, Hasper D, von Baer R, Hetzer R, Volk HD. Interleukin-6 and interleukin-8 concentrations as predictors of outcome in ventricular assist device patients before heart transplantation. Crit Care Med 1994; 22(3):448–454.
28. Khan A, Gazzaniga AB. Mechanical circulatory assistance in pediatric patients with cardiac failure. Card Surg 1995; 4:43–49.
29. Marelli D, Laks H, Amsel B, Kimble Jett G, Couper G, Ardehali A, Galindo A, Drinkwater DC. Temporary mechanical support with BVS 5000 Assist Device during treatment of acute myocarditis. J Card Surg 1997; 12:55–59.
30. Conrad SA, Rycus PT. Extracorporeal life support 1977. ASAIO J 1988; 44:848–852.
31. Jin Z, Bergen F, Uhlmann F, Schröder C, Hetzer R, Alexi-Meskishvili V, Weng Y, Lange PE. Improvement in the left ventricular dysfunction after aortic reimplantation in 11 consecutive pediatric patients with anomalous origin of the left coronary artery from the pulmonary artery. Eur Heart J 1994; 15:1044–1049.

32. Moreno-Cabral CE, Moreno-Cabral RS, McNamara JJ, Dembitsky RM, Adamson RM. Prolonged extracorporeal circulation for acute myocarditis. Int J Artific Org 1992; 15:475–480.
33. Hetzer R, Loebe M, Potapov EV, Weng Y, Stiller B, Hennig E, Alexi-Meskishvili V, Lange PE. Circulatory support with pneumatic paracorporeal ventricular assist device in infants and children. Ann Thorac Surg 1998; 66:1498–1506.

18
Experimental Development of the Medos-HIA Ventricular Assist Device in Children

Dominique Shum-Tim
Montreal Children's Hospital and McGill University, Montreal, Quebec, Canada

I. INTRODUCTION

Mechanical circulatory support using ventricular assist devices (VADs) has been shown to benefit many patients in whom the pumping function of the heart is inadequate. Mechanical VADs restore tissue perfusion by supporting the circulation and allow the failing myocardium to rest by decreasing preload and thereby reducing end-diastolic and end-systolic ventricular size. It has become a standard option of circulatory support in adult patients with cardiac failure refractory to pharmacological therapy. A variety of devices have been successfully used clinically as a bridge to recovery of ventricular function or cardiac transplantation with acceptable morbidity and mortality (1–5). Aggressive extracorporeal circulatory support has been increasingly applied in infants with severe cardiopulmonary dysfunction in the hope that survival can be improved even in pediatric patients with complex congenital cardiac anomalies undergoing extensive surgical repair. While the indications and outcome of pediatric patients requiring circulatory support are preliminary and still evolving, the clinical experience at the Children's Hospital in Boston is encouraging and favorable (6). However, fewer treatment options for mechanical circulatory support are available for infants and small children who experience profound ventricular dysfunction. At the present time, extracorporeal membrane oxygenation (ECMO) is the support method of choice in the pediatric cardiac patients if there is severe pulmonary dysfunction either preoperatively or postoperatively. In small neonates (<5 kg) with isolated biventricular failure, ECMO also facilitates cannulation. On the other hand, regardless of patient size, when single-ventricle dysfunction is present or isolated biventricular failure without pulmonary dysfunction in larger-size infants exists, VAD is preferable. The isolated VAD simplifies the ECMO circuit and offers an advantage in that it reduces blood cell trauma, hemorrhagic complications, and capillary leak that attend total cardiopulmonary bypass (CPB) and ECMO. The development of a pulsatile VAD for children, however, has been limited by size constraints and the requirement of multiple pumps with different volumes to accommodate a wide range of pediatric sizes. At present, there is no pulsatile VAD available in United States for pediatric patients.

II. PULSATILE VERSUS NONPULSATILE PERFUSION

The benefits of pulsatile circulatory support have not been unequivocally demonstrated. In addition, good clinical outcome has been reported using nonpulsatile VADs in short-term circulatory support (7,8). Yet subtle physiological benefits have been overwhelmingly documented by many studies leading to the exclusive use of pulsatile devices in long-term mechanical circulatory support. Theories for improved physiological parameters during pulsatile arterial flow focus on the effect of pulsation on microcirculatory patency (9,10). Capillary perfusion is facilitated by the increased energy contained in the pulsatile flow pattern, which is translated to a longer period of microcirculatory patency during peak systolic pressure (9,10). Nonpulsatile perfusion, on the other hand, resulted in increased systemic vascular resistance (SVR) when compared with pulsatile perfusion (11,12). This is, in part, attributed to the renin-angiotensin system (13). Specific angiotensin II inhibitors have been shown to reduce SVR during nonpulsatile blood flow (14). Therefore, increased SVR associated with nonpulsatile flow produced an increase in ventricular afterload, thereby increasing left ventricular work and impairing cardiac performance. While maintaining similar total arterial blood flow and mean arterial pressure, the presence of pulsatility reduced tissue oxygen consumption, metabolic acidosis, and lactate accumulation (15,16).

Organ structure and function studies further substantiate the metabolic benefits of pulsatile flow. In a clinical study evaluating the cerebral effect of pulsatile and nonpulsatile circulation, Murkin and Farrar demonstrated that the cerebral blood flow (CBF) is augmented with pulsatile perfusion (17). The observed reduction in CBF associated with the lack of pulsatility is consistent with the hypothesis of functional capillary closure during nonpulsatile perfusion. Cerebral cellular integrity reflected by creatine kinase isoenzymes in cerebrospinal fluid is also better preserved with pulsatile perfusion than nonpulsatile flow (18). Yet, the difference in patient outcome in the setting of short-term circulatory support is difficult to conclude because the neurological and neuropsychological outcomes after hypothermic CPB were similar in a cohort of patients managed with pulsatile and nonpulsatile blood flow (19).

On the other hand, renal excretory function is disturbed during nonpulsatile perfusion (20). Optimal intrarenal blood flow distribution associated with preserved outer cortical flow and renal function as well as reduced renin release was observed with pulsatile perfusion (20,21). Hepatic arterial flow and oxygen consumption are decreased by 50% during nonpulsatile but are well maintained with pulsatile circulatory support (22). Superior increases in aortic pressure, cardiac output, and myocardial perfusion were also observed with pulsatile left ventricular assist device (LVAD) flow in an acute ischemic canine model (23). Other studies suggested that pulsatile, compared to nonpulsatile, blood flow during cardiac surgery and CPB improved hemodynamic parameters with associated reduced inotropic requirement and intra-aortic balloon pump (IABP) support (24–26). In the pulmonary circulation, elevated pulmonary vascular resistance and increased lung water content have been experimentally shown during nonpulsatile circulatory support (27–29).

III. THE MEDOS-HIA VENTRICULAR ASSIST DEVICE

The Medos®-HIA VAD (Medos-Helmholtz Institute, Aachen, Germany) is a pneumatically driven pulsatile blood pump (Fig. 1). The disposable blood pump incorporates a multilayered diaphragm, which separates the blood flow chamber from the pneumatic drive chamber of the device. There are two integral trileaflet, polyurethane valves at the inflow and outflow connectors (30). The pumps, when used as LVAD, are available in a number of sizes with stroke volumes of 10, 25, 60, and 80 mL. For RVAD, there is 10% reduction in stroke volume for each pump size (9, 22.5, 54, and 72 mL, respectively), which was found to be optimal in a right-left ventricular output balance. The polyurethane pumps are pneumatically activated by an integrated driving system, which consists of a solid-state electronic control console with digital readout. The control console allows adjustment of pulse rate, drive pressure, and percentage systole to optimize hemodynamics. The system can be triggered by the electrocardiogram for operation in a synchronous mode to provide counterpulsation. The second component of the Medos drive system is an electrically powered internal pneumatic compressor and vacuum. An internal back-up battery facilitates transportation, and, in case of power failure, a manually operated pneumatic pump is available.

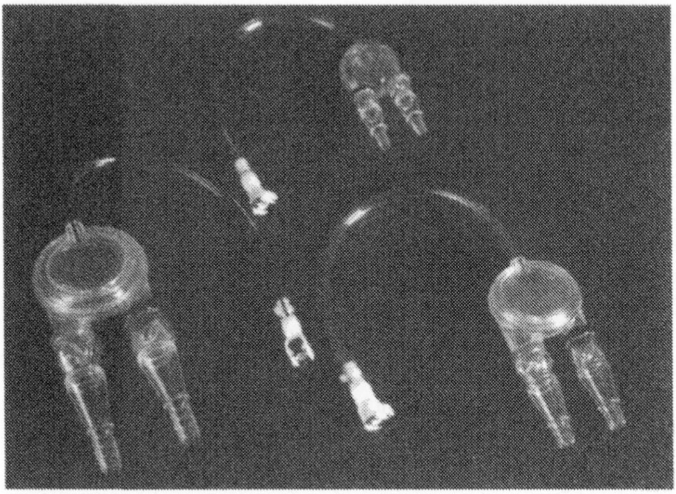

(a)

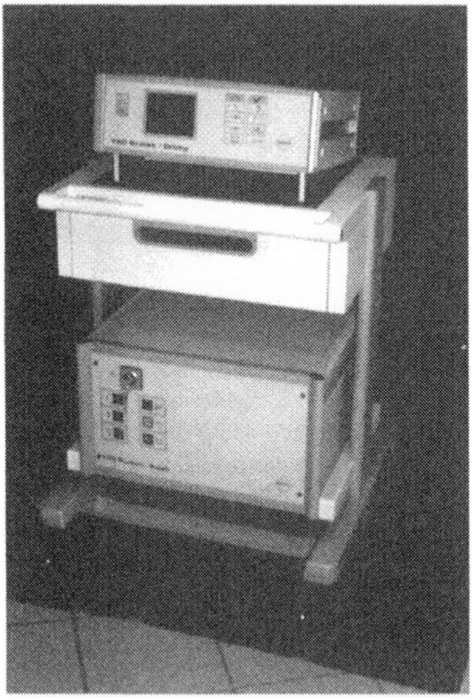

(b)

Fig. 1 (a) The Medos®-HIA VAD system consists of pneumatically driven polyurethane blood pumps. Pumps with stroke volumes of 10, 25, and 60 mL are shown. (b) Top: Integrated control unit with touch screen monitor for the Medos®-HIA VAD. Bottom: Internal power supply unit and pneumatic compressor and vacuum. (From Ref. 31.)

IV. EXPERIMENTAL DESIGN

In order to evaluate the Medos®-HIA pulsatile VAD, a lamb model of acute right ventricular (RV) failure was created and supported with a 9 mL right ventricular assist device (RVAD) (31). The hemodynamic effects of this new pulsatile pediatric VAD were evaluated with the device on and off over a 6-hour period until the experiment was electively terminated.

A. Anesthesia and Instrumentation

Three-week-old lambs (average weight 8.6 ± 0.9 kg) were used for the following studies. All animals were sedated with intramuscular Ketamine hydrochloride (50 mg/kg), then intubated and mechanically ventilated. Anesthesia was maintained with intravenous Fentanyl (30 μg/kg/h), and Midazolam (0.3 μg/kg/h). Body temperature was maintained between 37.5 and 38.0°C using a warming blanket and heat lamp. Catheters were inserted into the femoral artery and vein for blood sampling, fluid infusion, and monitoring of systemic arterial pressure. The femoral venous line was advanced into the right atrium (RA) for pressure monitoring. A median sternotomy was then performed and the main pulmonary artery (PA) and left atrial (LA) appendage were catheterized for pressure monitoring. An electromagnetic flow probe (MFV-3200, Nihon Kohden Corporation, Tokyo, Japan) was placed around the distal main PA to record the cardiac output at baseline and 10-minute timepoints after the induction of RV failure in all animals. The flow probe was removed from the PA and placed in-line with the outflow cannula for animals supported by RVAD (see below).

B. Right Ventricular Injury and Hemodynamic Measurements

Acute RV failure was surgically induced in Group I animals ($n = 5$) without subsequent mechanical circulatory assistance. In Group II ($n = 5$) animals, RV support using the Medos®-HIA VAD was instituted after the completion of RV injury. The RVAD was maintained in asynchronous mode for 6 hours postinjury until the experiment was electively terminated.

After placement of monitoring lines and recording of baseline parameters, all animals were fully heparinized (300 units/kg). A 14 French arterial cannula (DLP, Inc., Grand Rapids, MI) was inserted into the main PA and secured with pursestring sutures. This PA cannula allowed blood transfusion in all animals and provided outflow cannulation for RVAD-supported Group II animals. A patent foramen ovale (PFO), which was invariably present in lambs at this age, was closed primarily with inflow occlusion. A ventriculotomy was

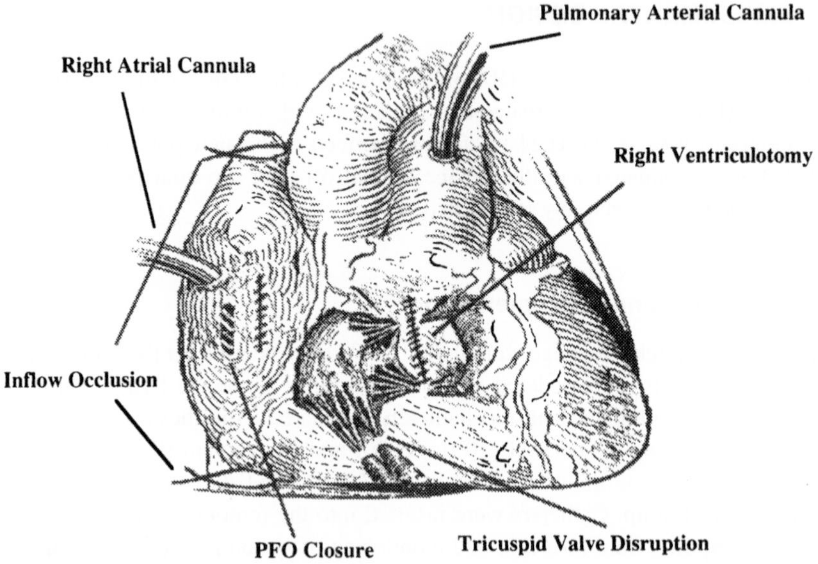

Fig. 2 The operative procedures to create acute right ventricular failure and cannulation sites for RVAD are shown. After inflow occlusion of both vena cava, the patent foramen ovale is primarily closed through an atriotomy. A ventriculotomy is performed in the RV outflow tract. Through this ventriculotomy, complete disruption of the tricuspid valve chordal attachments is performed.

then performed along the RV outflow tract. Through this incision, the tricuspid valve was disrupted by division of all chordal attachments (Fig. 2). Lethal RV injury was reliably produced by right ventriculotomy and tricuspid regurgitation.

Following the induction of RV failure, the absence of shunting at the atrial level was confirmed by measurement of RA and LA blood gases. For animals supported by RVAD, a 24 French right-angled cannula (Polystan, Varlose, Denmark) was inserted through the RA appendage. The RVAD settings were adjusted to reestablish baseline cardiac output and systemic pressure. Hemodynamic parameters were recorded after 10 minutes of stabilization postinjury in all animals. Hemodynamic measurements were repeated every 2 hours for 6 hours in Group II animals with RVAD support. During the measurement period, the RVAD was turned off for 5 minutes. In this way, each animal served as its own control for hemodynamic measurements on and off RVAD. Pulmonary vascular resistance (PVR in mmHg·min/L) was calculated as follows: (Mean PA pressure − Mean LA pressure)/Cardiac output.

V. STATISTICAL ANALYSIS

All values are expressed as the mean ± standard deviation. The baseline and postinjury values were compared within and between groups by the paired and unpaired Student's *t*-tests, respectively. Subsequent serial measurements of all parameters between assisted and nonassisted modes of the same animals were compared by paired *t*-test. Differences were considered statistically significant when the *p*-value was less than 0.05.

VI. RESULTS

A. Baseline Hemodynamics

The following baseline hemodynamic parameters were recorded in Groups I and II prior to RV injury: mean systemic arterial pressure (SAP), heart rate (HR), right atrial pressure (RAP), mean pulmonary arterial pressure (PAP), left atrial pressure (LAP), and mean pulmonary arterial cardiac output (CO). The pulmonary vascular resistance (PVR) was calculated for each animal. Baseline measurements are summarized in Table 1.

B. Effect of Right Ventricular Injury

Right ventriculotomy and surgically induced tricuspid regurgitation resulted in lethal acute RV failure. Severe RV dysfunction developed in both groups, characterized by systemic hypotension, increased RA pressure, decreased LA pressure, and decreased CO (Table 1 and Fig. 3). All the animals in control Group I died at a mean period of 71.4 ± 9.4 minutes after surgery. The RVAD-supported Group II hemodynamics were not significantly different from control Group I after RV injury. All Group II animals survived the 6 hours of planned RVAD support.

C. Effect of Right Ventricular Assist Device on Right Ventricular Failure

Institution of RVAD resulted in significant improvements in all hemodynamic parameters. The hemodynamic effects of RVAD support for Group II animals are summarized in Table 1 and illustrated in Fig. 4–10. Hemodynamic values shown reflect the mean values for all Group II animals on full RVAD support compared with the mean values obtained from the same animals with the device off for 5 minutes at 2 hours, 4 hours, and 6 hours after RV injury.

Table 1 Hemodynamic Parameters in Groups I and II at Baseline, Post–Right Ventricular Injury, and the Effects of RVAD

	Mean SAP (mmHg)	Mean RAP (mmHg)	Mean PAP (mmHg)	Mean LAP (mmHg)	CO (L/min)	PVR (mmHg · min/L)	HR (beat/min)
Group I Baseline	88.4 ± 9.2	4.5 ± 1.6	17.0 ± 2.9	4.9 ± 1.4	1.4 ± 0.2	8.8 ± 2.5	120.6 ± 21.6
10 min Postinjury	34.8 ± 5.9*	17.8 ± 9.7*	23.4 ± 3.6*	1.7 ± 0.6*	0.5 ± 0.2*	43.8 ± 13.4*	134.0 ± 31.2*
Group II Baseline	80.6 ± 12.7	4.6 ± 2.1	15.6 ± 4.2	4.8 ± 0.8	1.4 ± 0.2	7.6 ± 3.0	127.2 ± 18.8
10 min Postinjury	38.8 ± 10.4*	16.8 ± 2.3*	23.2 ± 3.8*	1.4 ± 0.5*	0.6 ± 0.1*	40.8 ± 10.9*	147.0 ± 14.6*
10 min RVAD on	75.0 ± 13.7**	6.0 ± 3.0**	20.6 ± 2.3	5.0 ± 1.6**	1.0 ± 0.3**	16.5 ± 2.9**	168.4 ± 32.2
2 h RVAD on	75.2 ± 12.5	5.6 ± 2.3	25.8 ± 5.6	5.6 ± 2.1	0.9 ± 0.1	22.8 ± 6.9	171.2 ± 25.2
2 h RVAD off	34.6 ± 9.6**	12.6 ± 0.5**	15.2 ± 2.2**	2.4 ± 1.5**	—	—	177.2 ± 31.6
4 h RVAD on	73.2 ± 11.6	6.6 ± 2.6	25.4 ± 4.3	4.6 ± 2.1	1.0 ± 0.2	22.0 ± 8.5	183.0 ± 31.2
4 h RVAD off	32.8 ± 4.9**	14.0 ± 1.0**	13.8 ± 2.8**	2.2 ± 1.3**	—	—	175.2 ± 31.7
6 h RVAD on	68.0 ± 13.0	8.2 ± 2.3	24.8 ± 6.5	6.4 ± 2.1	1.0 ± 0.2	18.6 ± 8.2	190.4 ± 7.0
6 h RVAD off	33.4 ± 6.7**	15.0 ± 2.3**	15.6 ± 3.1**	2.6 ± 0.9**	—	—	166.2 ± 50.9

* $p < 0.05$ versus baseline; ** $p < 0.05$ RVAD on versus off.

CO = Cardiac output; HR = heart rate; LAP = left atrial pressure; PAP = pulmonary arterial pressure; PVR = pulmonary vascular resistance; RAP = right atrial pressure; RVAD = right ventricular assist device; SAP = systemic arterial pressure.

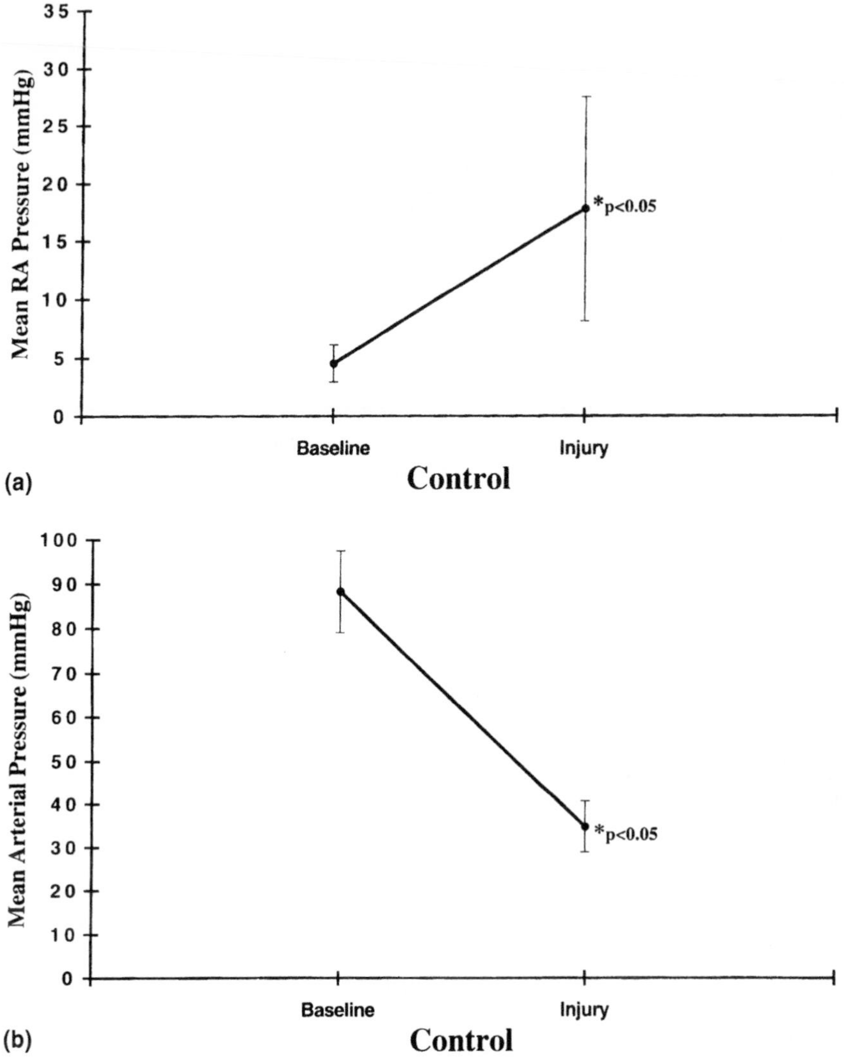

Fig. 3 Hemodynamic measurements after acute right ventricular failure were characterized by significantly elevated right atrial pressure (a), as well as significant decreases in systemic pressure (b), left atrial pressure (c), and cardiac output (d). (From Ref. 31.)

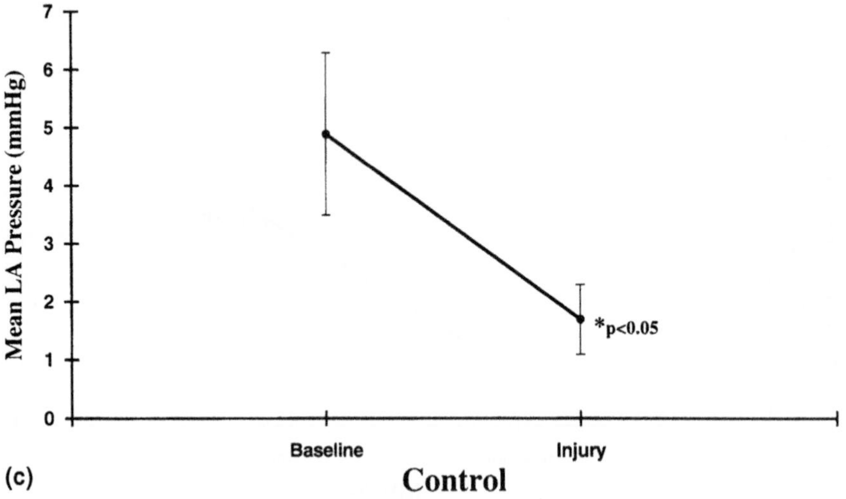

(c)

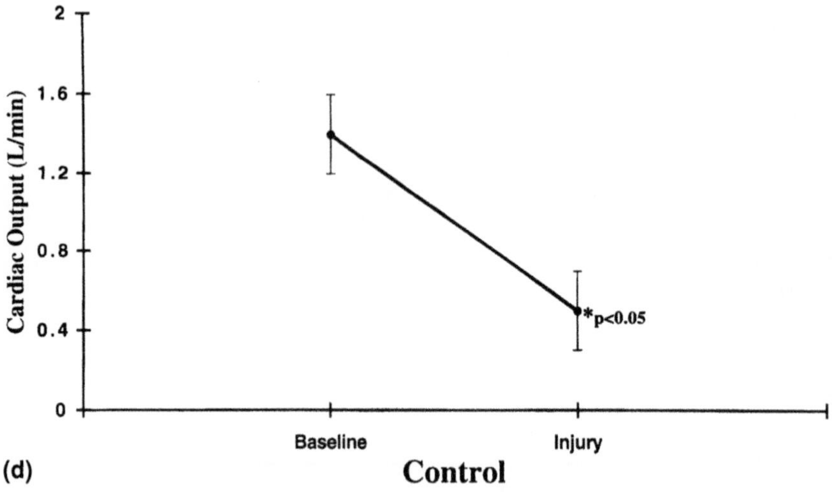

(d)

Fig. 3 Continued

With the initial RV injury, expected decreases were observed in mean SAP (Fig. 4), LAP (Fig. 5), and CO (Fig. 6). Right atrial pressure increased significantly (Fig. 7). All hemodynamic parameters were subsequently normalized by RVAD support as demonstrated. Values for CO off RVAD are demonstrated only at 10 minutes. As described above, in Group II animals the CO flow probe was removed from the PA and placed in-line with the outflow cannula after measuring baseline hemodynamics due to size constraints.

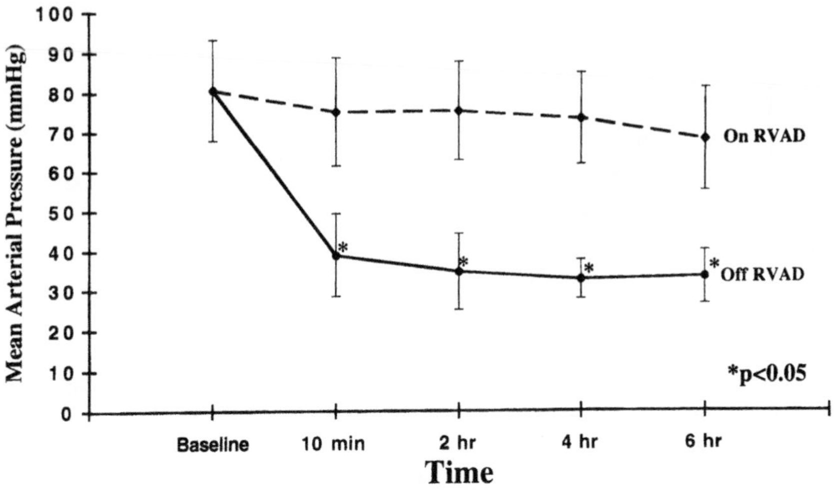

Fig. 4 Normalization of systemic mean arterial pressure in Group II was maintained over 6 hours by the Medos®-HIA RVAD. (From Ref. 31.)

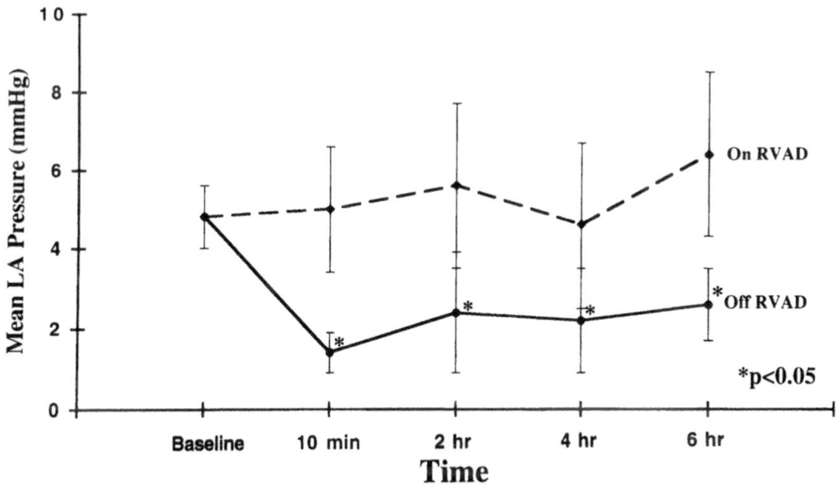

Fig. 5 Left atrial filling pressure was significantly reduced by RV failure and effectively normalized by the institution of RVAD support. (From Ref. 31.)

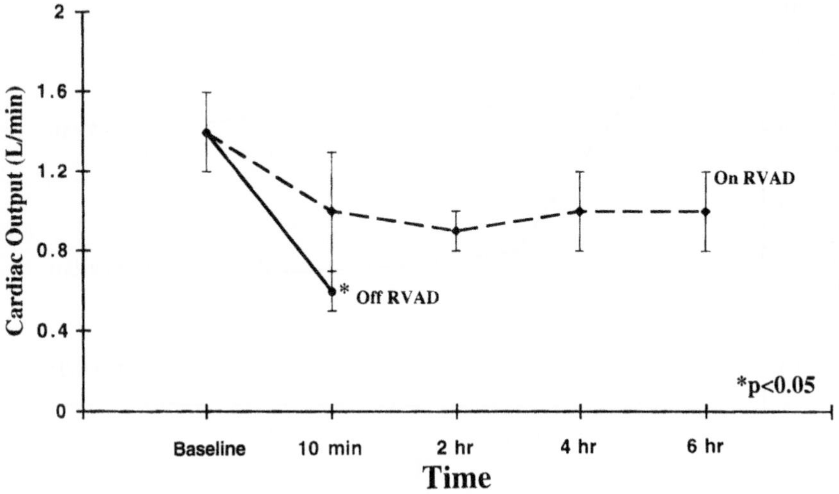

Fig. 6 Low cardiac output induced by acute right ventricular failure was reversed by the pulsatile Medos®-HIA RVAD system. (From Ref. 31.)

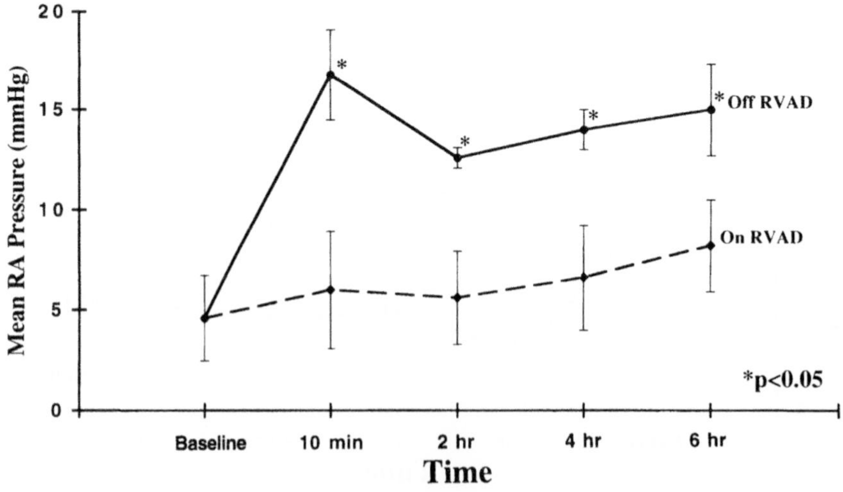

Fig. 7 Significant reduction of the elevated mean right atrial pressure following RV injury in Group II was observed after the onset of RVAD. (From Ref. 31.)

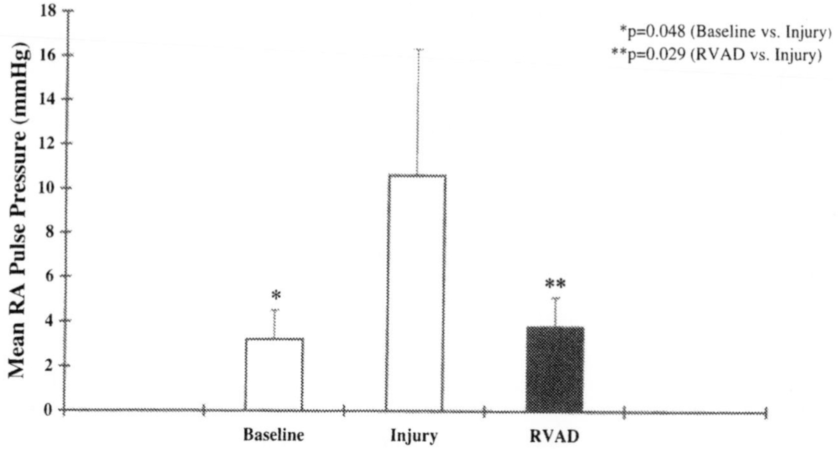

Fig. 8 Evidence of severe tricuspid regurgitation after surgical induction of RV failure was shown by significantly elevated right atrial pulse pressure compared with baseline value. Note the effect of RVAD in ameliorating the hemodynamic characteristics of severe tricuspid regurgitation. (From Ref. 31.)

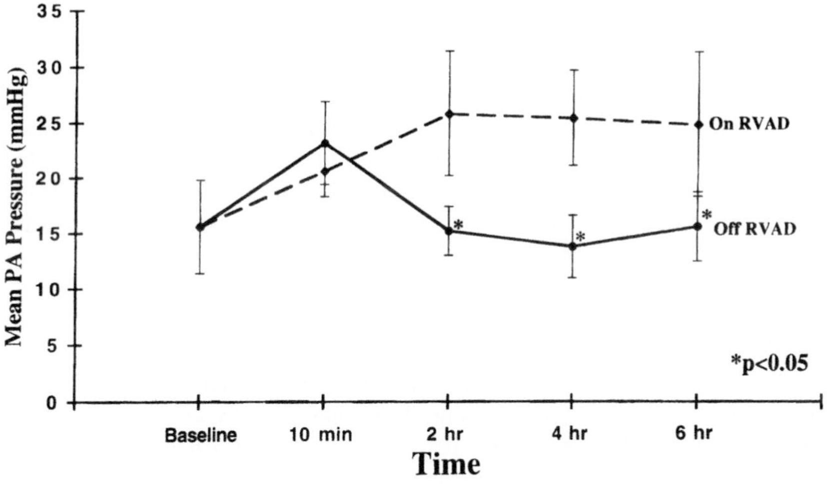

Fig. 9 Following the RV injury, there was a transient elevation of mean pulmonary pressure possibly secondary to reactive pulmonary vasoconstriction after surgical injury. Significant reduction of pulmonary blood flow characterized by reduction of mean pulmonary pressure was observed after 2 hours when RVAD was turned off and the onset of RVAD preserved pulmonary arterial pressure. (From Ref. 31.)

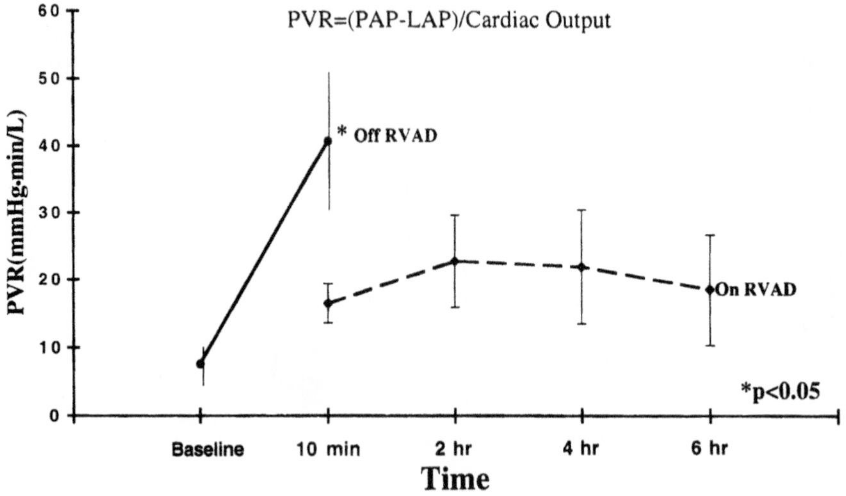

Fig. 10 Pulmonary vascular resistance was acutely elevated by the surgical procedure of inflow occlusion, blood transfusion, and reduced left-sided pressure. The RVAD partially offset this elevated pulmonary vascular resistance and maintained the same level throughout the 6-hour period of experiment. (From Ref. 31.)

Severe tricuspid insufficiency was demonstrated by a dramatic increase in mean RA pressure with a pulsatile waveform in all animals. The mean pulse pressure of the RA increased from a baseline of 3.2 ± 1.3 to 10.6 ± 5.7 mmHg (p = 0.048) immediately after the induction of RV injury (Fig. 8). The mean RA pressure was rapidly reduced, and the pulsatility of the waveform was obliterated by the onset of RVAD. These hemodynamic characteristics were maintained throughout the duration of study. Upon termination of mechanical support, the animals in Group II survived for 58.2 ± 28.2 minutes (p = NS vs. Group I).

The pulmonary artery pressure was observed to increase immediately after the surgical insult to the RV (Fig. 9) accompanied by an increase in the calculated PVR in all animals (Fig. 10). These changes in PAP and PVR normalized after 2 hours of circulatory support. Initial increases in PAP probably represent the animals' response to rapid transfusion, inflow occlusion, and catecholamine surge associated with the surgical procedure. Elevations in the calculated PVR were magnified by accompanying decreases in LA pressure and cardiac output.

VII. COMMENTS

A variety of mechanical circulatory assist devices have been successfully employed for adults with severe ventricular dysfunction (1–5). Intra-aortic balloon counterpulsation as well as VADs from several different manufacturers are currently available. The effectiveness of IABP is limited in pediatric patients due to their increased aortic elasticity, rapid heart rates with small stroke volumes, and technical difficulties related to insertion in small femoral vessels (32). The development of VAD for pediatric patients has been limited by size constraints and differences in the pathophysiology of cardiac failure in children. A pulsatile pediatric VAD requires multiple pump sizes to provide stroke volumes in the range of patients from newborns to young adults. In contrast to predominant left ventricular failure secondary to coronary artery disease in adults, children are more likely to demonstrate right ventricular, biventricular, and pulmonary failure. These factors, in addition to the favorable experience in treating life-threatening pulmonary conditions in children, have led to the widespread use of ECMO for cardiac support in many pediatric centers (7,8).

However, there are several potential advantages that a pulsatile VAD designed specifically for children would provide. This device would ideally provide pulsatile flow with a range of pump volumes capable of supporting small neonates through adolescents. The complexity of the ECMO circuitry with the presence of an oxygenator requires increased anticoagulation and larger priming volume and produces more blood cell trauma. For these reasons, ECMO may not always be the optimal methodology for prolonged circulatory support in pediatric patients. The potential disadvantages of hemorrhagic complication and capillary leak, may limit its application to early postoperative periods. In addition, pulsatile flow might confer advantages for end-organ preservation during long-term support.

The Medos®-HIA VAD system provides pulsatile circulatory support with pumps available in a variety of stroke volumes to accommodate newborn to adult patients. The circuit is simple, with the disposable blood pump connected directly to the inflow and outflow cannulas. This minimizes the surface area of blood contact and reduces priming volumes. The priming volume for the circuit in this study, utilizing the 9 mL blood pump, was less than 20 mL. Deairing the device is facilitated by its transparent design. Two trileaflet polyurethane valves integrated into the device have been shown to result in excellent hemodynamic properties and minimal hemolysis with low thrombogenicity (33–35). Due to the simplicity of the circuit, set-up can be performed within minutes in an emergency situation. Furthermore, the simple circuit with its self-contained power console minimizes intensive personnel surveillance and facilitates transportation of patients during support.

In this study, we created an acute pediatric model (<10 kg) of RV failure. The surgical technique was a combination of those reported in larger animals (36–38). This model created RV dysfunction by making a right ventriculotomy and disrupting the tricuspid valve. The RV failure produced was progressive and rapidly fatal without mechanical assistance. The Medos®-HIA VAD system employed as an RVAD was able to normalize systemic arterial pressure and cardiac output while reducing the dramatically elevated right atrial filling pressure seen in this model. In contrast to previous studies employing right ventricular apical cannulation, the insertion of RVAD itself did not accelerate RV dysfunction (37). All the experimental animals in Group II survived for a mean of 58.2 ± 28.2 minutes after the discontinuation of RVAD support, which was not significantly different from that of the control Group I. The absence of deterioration of RV function in this report may reflect RA cannulation rather than RV apical cannulation in previous studies.

The benefits of pulsatile circulatory support have not been demonstrated in short-term application, and good clinical outcome has been reported using nonpulsatile VADs (39–42). Yet substantial physiological differences have been suggested by many studies (17,18,20–29). The difference in patient outcome between pulsatile and nonpulsatile flow in the setting of long-term circulatory support is probably significant but remains unproved clinically. Although conclusive data are not available, most agree that pulsatile circulation is necessary for long-term assistance and most devices in use for long-term support employ pumps that provide pulsatile flow. It is likely that the physiological benefits of pulsatility accrue over time, and its significance is proportional to the duration of assistance. The present study did not aim to address the potential benefits conferred by pulsatile circulatory assistance because of the acute nature of the experimental design.

There are several limitations that merit further discussion. First of all, this study represents an acute model to assess the feasibility and reliability of the pulsatile pediatric RVAD. The long-term effects of this device remain to be evaluated. Second, the current protocol utilized full anticoagulation simulating the clinical situation of RVAD support following cardiopulmonary bypass. In addition, we used heparinized fresh blood transfusion obtained from another donor lamb for the creation of RV injury. Therefore, the anticoagulation regimen and hematological effects of this device could not be evaluated by this particular study.

In conclusion, there is currently no pulsatile VAD available in the United States for pediatric patients, although this device has been used successfully in children in Europe (43). The ability to supply pulsatile circulatory assistance for a range of patient sizes from small newborns to young adults makes this a potentially valuable system. This initial in vivo study demonstrates the ability of the pulsatile Medos®-HIA VAD to maintain satisfactory hemodynamics in a pediatric lamb model of acute RV failure. Further studies will be required to evaluate its longer-term hemodynamic and metabolic effects. Implantation in the systemic circulation will further challenge the reliability of this promising pediatric VAD prior to clinical application.

REFERENCES

1. Pae WE, Miller CA, Matthews Y, Pierce WS. Ventricular assist devices for postcardiotomy cardiogenic shock. J Thorac Cardiovasc Surg 1992; 104:541–553.
2. Chen JM, Levin HR, Rose EA, et al. Experience with right ventricular assist devices for perioperative right-sided circulatory failure. Ann Thorac Surg 1996; 61:305–310.
3. Champsaur G, Ninet J, Vigneron M, Cochet P, Neidecker J, Boissonnat P. Use of the Abiomed BVS system 5000 as a bridge to cardiac transplantation. J Thorac Cardiovasc Surg 1990; 100:122–128.
4. Pennington DG, Samuels LD, Williams G, et al. Experience with the Pierce-Donachy ventricular assist device in postcardiotomy patients with cardiogenic shock. World J Surg 1985; 9:37–46.
5. Buckley MJ, Craver JM, Gold HK, Mundth ED, Daggett WM, Austen WG. Intraaortic balloon pump assist for cardiogenic shock after cardiopulmonary bypass. Circulation 1973; 47,48(Pt 2); III90–94.
6. Duncan BW, Ibrahim AE, Hraska V, et al. Use of rapid-deployment extracorporeal membrane oxygenation for the resuscitation of pediatric patients with heart disease after cardiac arrest. J Thorac Cardiovasc Surg 1998; 116(2):305–311.
7. Del Nido PJ. Extracorporeal membrane oxygenation for cardiac support in children. Ann Thorac Surg 1996; 61:336–339.
8. Klein MD, Shaheen KW, Whittlesey GC, et al. Extracorporeal membrane oxygenation for the circulatory support of children after repair of congenital heart disease. J Thorac Cardiovasc Surg 1990; 100:498–505.
9. Takeda J. Experimental study of peripheral circulation during extracorporeal circulation with a special reference to a comparison of pulsatile flow with nonpulsatile flow. Arch Jpn Chir 1960; 29:1407–1412.
10. Shepard RB, Simpson DC, Sharp JF. Energy equivalent pressure. Arch Surg 1996; 93:730–740.
11. Taylor KM. Vasopressor release and multiple organ failure in cardiac surgery. Perfusion 1988; 3:1–16.
12. Minami K, Körner MM, Vyska K, et al. Effects of pulsatile perfusion on plasma catecholamine levels and hemodynamics during and after cardiac operation with cardiopulmonary bypass. J Thorac Cardiovasc Surg 1990; 99:82–91.
13. Taylor KM, Bain WH, Morton JJ. The role of angiotensin II in the development of peripheral vasoconstriction during open-heart surgery. Am Heart J 1980; 100:935–937.
14. Taylor KM, Casals J, Morton JJ, et al. The haemodynamic effects of angiotensin-converting enzyme inhibition after cardiopulmonary bypass in dogs. Cardiovasc Res 1980; 14:199–205.

15. Shepard RB, Kirklin JW. Relation of pulsatile flow to oxygen consumption and other variables during cardiopulmonary bypass. J Thorac Cardiovasc Surg 1969; 58:694–702.
16. Jacobs LA, Klopp EH, Seamore W, et al. Improved organ function during cardiac bypass with a roller-pump modified to deliver pulsatile flow. J Thorac Cardiovasc Surg 1969; 58:703–712.
17. Murkin JM, Farrar K. The influence of pulsatile vs nonpulsatile cardiopulmonary bypass on cerebral blood flow and cerebral metabolism. Anesthesiology 1989; 71: A41.
18. Taylor KM, Devlin BJ, Mittra SM et al. Assessment of cerebral damage during open-heart surgery. A new experimental model. Scand J Thorac Cardiovasc Surg 1980; 14:197–203.
19. Murkin JM, Martzke JS, Buchan AM, Bentley C, Wong CJ. A randomized study of the influence of perfusion technique and PH management strategy in 316 patients undergoing coronary artery bypass surgery. II. Neurologic and cognitive outcomes. J Thorac Cardiovasc Surg 1995; 110(2):349–362.
20. Many M, Soroff HS, Birtwell WC, et al. The physiologic role of pulsatile and non-pulsatile blood flow: II. Effects on renal function. Arch Surg 1967; 95:762–766.
21. Many M, Soroff HS, Birtwell WC, et al. The physiologic role of pulsatile and non-pulsatile blood flow: III. Effects of unilateral renal artery depulsation. Arch Surg 1968; 97:197–223.
22. Mathie R, Desai J, Taylor KM. Hepatic blood flow and metabolism during pulsatile and non-pulsatile cardiopulmonary bypass. Life Support Syst 1984; 2:303–305.
23. Hirofumi I, Yamaguchi A, Takashi I, et al. Evaluation of the pulsatility of a new pulsatile left ventricular assist device—the integrated cardioassist catheter—in dogs. J Thorac Cardiovasc Surg 1994; 107:569–575.
24. Bregman D, Bowman FO, Parodi EN, et al. An improved method of myocardial protection with pulsation during cardiopulmonary bypass. Circulation 1977; 56(suppl II):157–161.
25. Maddoux G, Pappas G, Jenkins M, et al. Effect of pulsatile and non-pulsatile flow during cardiopulmonary bypass on left ventricular ejection fraction early after aorto-coronary bypass surgery. Am J Cardiol 1976; 37:1000–1006.
26. Taylor KM, Bain WH, Davidson KG, et al. A comparative study of pulsatile and non-pulsatile cardiopulmonary bypass in 325 patients. Proc Eur Soc Artif Org 1979; 6:238–242.
27. Raj JU, Kaapa P, Anderson J. Effect of pulsatile flow on microvascular resistance in adult rabbit lungs. J Appl Physiol 1992; 72:73–81.
28. Clarke PC, Kahn DR, Dufek JH, Sloan H. The effects of nonpulsatile blood flow on canine lungs. Ann Thorac Surg 1968; 6:450–457.
29. Richenbacher WE, Pierce WS, Jurmann M, et al. Pulmonary vascular effects of pulsatile and nonpulsatile mechanical right ventricular assistance. Surg Forum 1989; 40:254–255.
30. Knierbein B, Rosarius N, Reul H, Rau G. New methods for the development of pneumatic displacement pumps for cardiac assist. Int J Artif Organs 1990; 13:751–759.
31. Shum-Tim D, Duncan BW, Hraska V, Friehs I, Shin'oka T, Jonas RA. Evaluation

of a pulsatile pediatric ventricular assist device in an acute right heart failure model. Ann Thorac Surg 1997; 64:1374–1380.
32. Del Nido PJ, Swan PR, Benson LN, et al. Successful use of intra-aortic balloon pumping in a 2-kilogram infant. Ann Thorac Surg 1988; 46:574–576.
33. Eilers R, Harbott P, Reul H, Rakhorst G, Rau G. Design improvements of the HIA-VAD based on animal experiments. Artif Organs 1994; 18:473–478.
34. Rakhorst G, Hensens AG, Verkerke GJ, et al. In-vivo evaluation of the ''HIA-VAD'': a new German ventricular assist device. Thorac Cardiovasc Surg 1994; 42: 136–140.
35. Reul H, Taguchi K, Herold M, et al. Comparative evaluation of disk and trileaflet valves in left ventricular assist devices. Int J Artif Organs 1988; 11:127–130.
36. Jett KG, Applebaum RE, Clark RE. Right ventricular assistance for experimental right ventricular dysfunction. J Thorac Cardiovasc Surg 1986; 92:272–278.
37. Jett KG, Picone AL, Clark RE. Circulatory support for right ventricular dysfunction. J Thorac Cardiovasc Surg 1987; 94:95–103.
38. Fischer SIC, Willshaw P, Armentano RL, Delbo MIB, Pichel RH, Favaloro RG. Experimental acute right ventricular failure and right ventricular assist in the dog. J Thorac Cardiovasc Surg 1985; 90:580–585.
39. Sakaki M, Teanaka Y, Tatsumi E, Nakatani T, Takano H. Influences of nonpulsatile pulmonary flow on pulmonary function: evaluation in a chronic animal model. J Thorac Cardiovasc Surg 1994; 108:495–502.
40. Reddy RC, Goldstein AH, Pacella JJ, Cattivera GR, Clark RE, Magovern Sr. GJ. End organ function with prolonged nonpulsatile circulatory support. ASAIO J 1995; 41:M547–M551.
41. Karl TR, Sano S, Horton S, Mee RBB. Centrifugal pump left heart assist in pediatric cardiac operations: indications, technique, and results. J Thorac Cardiovasc Surg 1991; 102:624–630.
42. Louis PT, Bricker JT, Frazier OH, et al. Nonpulsatile total left ventricular support in pediatric patients. Crit Care Med 1992; 20:704–707.
43. Konertz W, Hotz H, Schneider M, Redlin M, Reul H. Clinical experience with the HIA-Medos VAD system in infants and children: a preliminary report. Ann Thorac Surg 1997; 63:1138–1144.

19

Development of the Nimbus/ University of Pittsburgh Pediatric Rotary Blood Pump

Harvey S. Borovetz, Mahendar Macha, Marina V. Kameneva, Bartley P. Griffith, and Philip Litwak
McGowan Center for Artificial Organ Development, University of Pittsburgh, Pittsburgh, Pennsylvania

Kenneth C. Butler, Timothy R. Maher, Lynn P. Taylor, and Douglas C. Thomas
Nimbus Inc., Rancho Cordova, California

I. INTRODUCTION

The subject of this chapter involves the development of a mechanical circulatory support system (MCSS) intended specifically for use in pediatric care, covering the needs of patients ranging from neonates to small children. A common opinion regarding devices currently approved for this class of patients is that they are disproportionately large and, in general, lack technical innovation associated with MCSSs used in adult care. The work described herein represents a long-term effort conducted jointly by Nimbus Inc. (Rancho Cordova, CA) and its development partner the University of Pittsburgh (UOP) McGowan Center for Artificial Organ Development.

The long-term objective of this collaborative effort was to complete the development of an extracorporeal rotary blood pump capable of providing either steady or pulsatile flow to neonatal and pediatric (N/P) patient populations. The device is a miniature centrifugal pump capable of uninterrupted operation for approximately 7 days and likely beyond. A console controller generates either steady or pulsatile flow, the latter via programmed oscillation of the motor current. The benefits of such a product for circulatory support include physiologically similar flow, a very low priming volume, and device operating parameters appropriate for N/P rather than adult patients. Other competitive advantages that this product offers include the absence of one-way flow-directing valves, no polyurethane pumping bladders or use of other raw materials whose continued supply is in question, and control of pump operation and generation of pulsatile flow via a console that incorporates important safety features for this patient group.

II. PRODUCT DESCRIPTION

A. Overview

The basis for this new technology is Nimbus's experience with miniature centrifugal blood pumps and breakthroughs the company has made over the years in applying these to create a safe, effective, and low-cost clinical product for adult cardiopulmonary bypass. The pediatric pump concept is adapted from the adult design and uses a disposable, miniature extracorporeal blood pump connected into the circulation via inflow and outflow cannulae. This pump mates to a relatively small power module placed in close proximity to the patient. A remote console powers and controls the blood pump.

B. Centrifugal Blood Pump

The N/P blood pump (Fig. 1) is a one-time-use item, which mates to a small power module as shown in Fig. 2. With the pump placed in the module as shown,

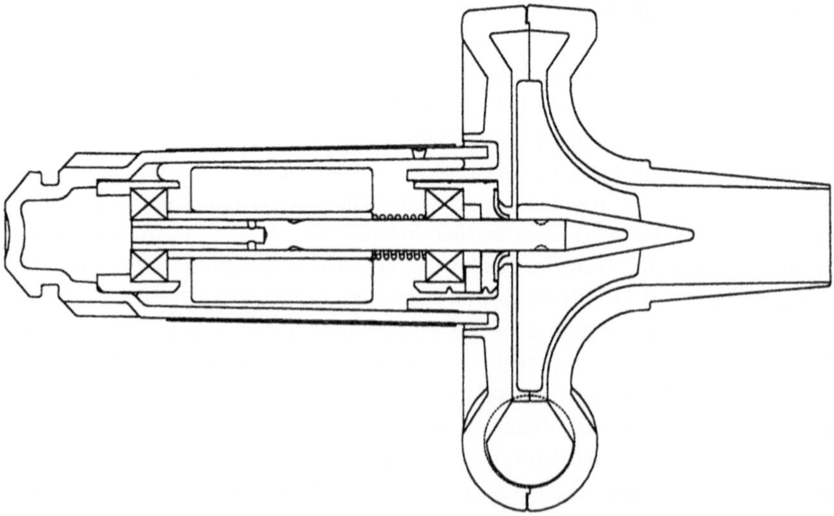

Fig. 1 N/P centrifugal blood pump.

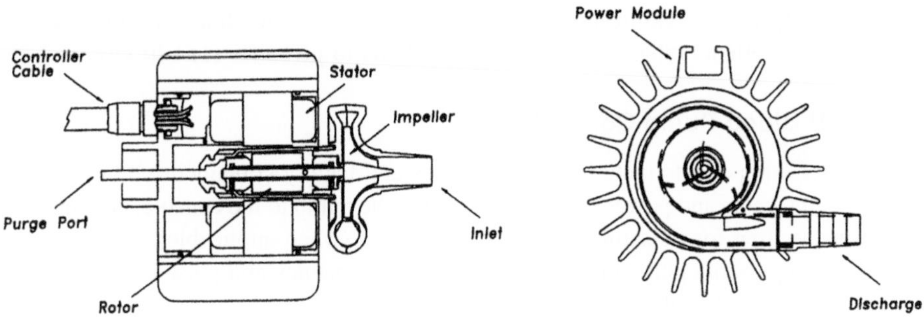

Fig. 2 N/P centrifugal blood pump installed in power module.

the motor's rotor, which is incorporated into the pump bearing housing, is centered within the bore of the motor coil set. Torque to drive the pump is developed by three-phase electrical current in the coils imparting electromagnetic forces to the motor rotor. This rotor, a two-pole permanent magnet, is fixed to the pump drive shaft, which in turn is mounted to an impeller comprised of three open, backward-curved blades. Two bearing assemblies support the drive shaft loads radially and axially. A lip-type seal prevents blood products from entering the bearing housing. To extend the potential use life of the N/P centrifugal pump, versions of the pump were designed that incorporate a purge fluid assembly to continuously wash the impeller seal.

The key design specifications associated with the N/P centrifugal blood pump are:

Flow range	0.3–3.0 L/min
Differential pressure range	60–400 mmHg
Speed range	3000–6500 rpm
I/O Port size	0.25 inch diameter
Impeller	1.25 inch diameter, 3 blades
Volute diameter	2.0 inch
Priming volume	13 cc
Housing material	Polycarbonate
Impeller material	Polycarbonate
Seal type, material	Lip seal, polyurethane
Shaft material	304 Stainless steel
Magnet material	Neodymium iron boron
Sterilization	EtO or radiation
Purge fluid (when applicable)	Physiological solution

The hemodynamic pressure-flow range cited above indicates that this product can support patients ranging from newborn infants to juveniles (15–20 kg).

C. N/P Blood Pump Controller

Controller components include the electronics and battery contained within the console, the cable and power module that couple the pump to the console, and the software written for pulsatile waveform generation (when applicable). Features essential to pulsatile pump operation such as beat frequency and pulse amplitude were incorporated in the basic console design.

The N/P console delivers three-phase excitation current to the pump motor via the power module. The power module consists of a motor stator bonded to a finned cooling chamber. The motor rotor is fixed directly to the impeller shaft, thus pump rotation is induced once the pump assembly is installed into the power module and the drive signal applied. Constant motor speed is adjusted manually at the front panel, and pulsatile flow is achieved by selecting a pulse frequency and amplitude. Available pulse rates are 30, 60, and 90 beats per minute. Pulse amplitude settings are 25%, 50%, 75%, and 100% of the constant motor speed, which represent the magnitude of the motor speed variation above and below the average speed during one beat cycle.

Figure 3 shows examples of pulsatile flow generation possible with the N/P centrifugal pump. It is possible to change the character of the wave pulse (e.g.,

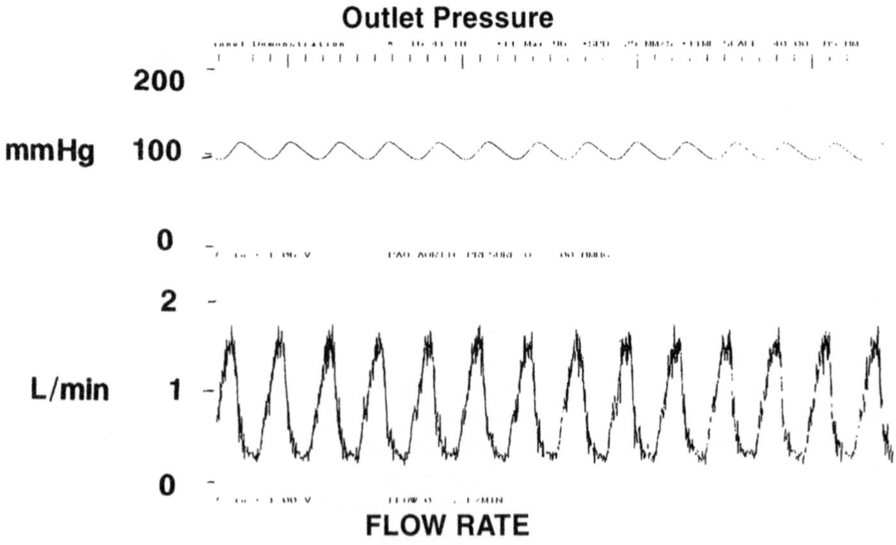

Fig. 3 Typical pulsatile output resulting from sine wave input signal.

from sine wave to square wave) by manipulation of the aforementioned parameters and application of Fourier signal analysis.

III. IN VITRO TESTING

Tests were conducted to quantify the performance of the N/P centrifugal pump as regards hydraulic output and the propensity to liberate hemoglobin from red blood cells (hemolysis). These tests were carried out in a recirculating flow loop using fresh bovine blood as the working fluid. The N/P centrifugal pump was installed directly upstream of a metal-tipped cannula, which was sized to match the cannula used for the in vivo tests. The loop was instrumented for pump inlet and outlet pressures, cannula outlet pressure (equivalent to arterial pressure), and volumetric flow rate. Prior to use, the blood was filtered, adjusted for percentage hematocrit with normal saline, and anticoagulated with heparin. The volume of the test circuit is 1 L.

A. Hydraulic Performance

Flow characteristics were mapped as follows. For specified pump beat per minute (bpm) and flow pulse amplitude (when applicable), loop flow resistance was set with a clamp, and delivered pump flow and corresponding pressure differential were measured for various clamp settings, up to full shut-off. This process was repeated over a range of bpm and flow pulse magnitudes (from zero or steady flow up to 100% of the constant motor speed).

The resultant hydraulic characteristics are recorded in Fig. 4. These curves depict the differential pressure versus flow rate characteristics covering a speed range between 2500 and 6000 rpm. From the span of flow rates included in this data—0.3–3.0 L/min—it is clear that the pump adequately achieves the hemodynamic requirements for the intended patient population.

B. Hemolysis

Hemolysis testing involved operating the N/P pump at a specified flow rate and afterload in the mock circulatory loop. Further, the effect of pulsatile flow on hemolysis was determined by comparing data collected during pulsatile testing with data from a continuous (steady) flow test. Physiological aortic pressure was maintained at 100 mmHg for all tests, with a corresponding simulated pulse rate of approximately 100 bpm. Blood samples were drawn every 15 minutes for analysis; results are shown in Table 1 as average values (in several different units) over a 1-hour experiment. In the case of a 1 L/min mean flow rate, the

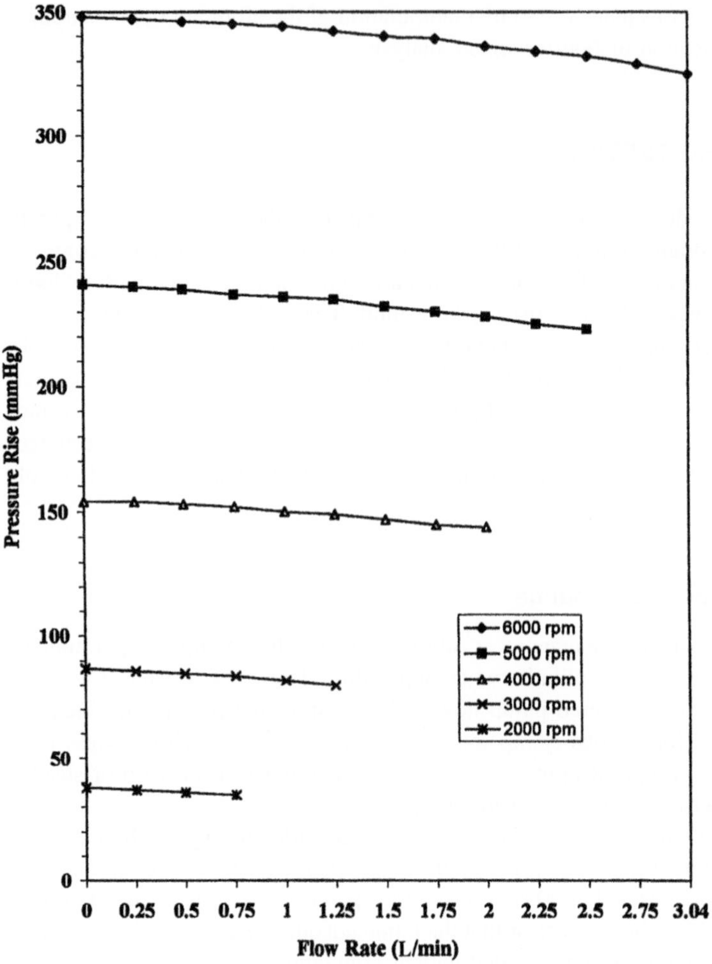

Fig. 4 In vitro hydraulic characteristics—pump pressure differential versus volumetric flow rate.

amplitude of the flow pulse spanned 1.2 L/min. For 0.3 and 1.5 L/min, the individual flow rate oscillations were 0.6 and 2.2 L/min.

All of these values represent very low levels of hemolysis and indicate that the N/P centrifugal flow blood pump is atraumatic to red blood cells over the range of hemodynamics anticipated for this patient population, whether delivering steady or pulsatile flow.

Table 1 In Vitro Hemolysis

	Average flow rate (L/min)	Aortic pressure (mmHg)	Hemolysis (g/d)	Hemolysis (mg/dL)	Hemolysis index (mg%/h)
Continuous, pre-test					
	1.0	100	0.73	4.2	0.051
Pulsatile					
	0.3	100	0.6	3.4	0.138
	1.0	100	0.78	4.4	0.054
	1.5	100	1.51	8.6	0.070
Continuous, post-test					
	1.0	100	0.87	5.0	0.060

IV. IN VIVO TESTING

A. Animal Model/Surgical Procedure

We chose to use sheep (juvenile lambs) as the species in which to test the prototype N/P extracorporeal blood pumps.

Surgical implantation of the flow cannulae in the lamb involves performing a thoracotomy and establishing pump inflow via cannulation of the left atrium or left ventricle; pump outflow (arterial return) is via a cannula placed in the descending thoracic aorta. For the aortic cannula we adapted an 18 Fr. DLP, Inc. (Grand Rapids, MI) curved metal-tipped cannula, in which we drill an additional hole to allow more flow into the distal aorta. The pump is positioned very close to the animal in order to minimize priming and overall circulatory volume. Figure 5 illustrates the extracorporeal pump placement in a typical 10 kg lamb. We were able to devise a sling method of restraint in order to avoid having to keep the lambs anesthetized and ventilated during the observation period.

In all juvenile lamb experiments, anticoagulation was accomplished using heparin, which is started before the cannulae are implanted. After a loading dose of 3.0 mg/kg, activated clotting times (ACT) were monitored every 2 hours for the first 48 hours. Additional heparin was administered to keep the ACT at 1.5–1.75 times the pre-heparin control value (mean of 162 s). This required about 1200 IU/h.

B. Results—Hemodynamics

Table 2 summarizes the results of the N/P centrifugal pump animal trials using lambs. The first five experiments evaluated the suitability of the N/P centrifugal pump to deliver steady flow in the lamb model. Perfusion times ranged between

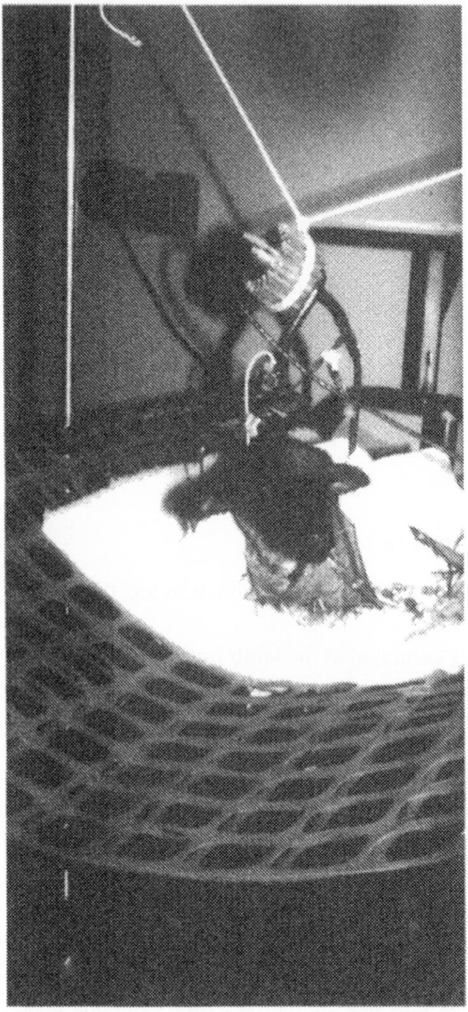

Fig. 5 Placement of pump and power module relative to typical 10 kg lamb. (From Ref. 5.)

8 and 148 hours. The longest experiment continued for 6 days. Two of these cases were electively terminated after 8 and 76 hours. Three lambs died due to respiratory failure, the cause of which was considered to be ventilator-induced barotrauma in two lambs and acute pneumonia in the other.

The remaining four experiments verified the capability of the pump to deliver pulsatile flow. The second animal had to be terminated at 24 hours due to

Table 2 Summary of N/P Centrifugal Pump Lamb Trials

Weight (kg)	Duration (h)	Pulsatile flow	Flow rate (L/min)	Results
21	8	No	0.5–0.8	Acute experiment, elective sacrifice
5.5	33	No	0.4–0.6	Experiment stopped due to respiratory failure
8.8	76	No	0.8–1.3	Elective sacrifice
6.3	44	No	0.3–0.6	Animal death due to respiratory failure
18.4	148	No	0.7–2.0	Pump functioned flawlessly for 140 hours; death due to acute pneumonia
10.3	8	Yes	1.3	Acute experiment, elective sacrifice
9.3	24	Yes	1.0–1.2	Pump adhesive failure
7.5	96	Yes	0.8–1.5	Elective sacrifice
10	72	Yes	1.2–1.5	Elective sacrifice

a blood leak around the adhesive seal joining the two polycarbonate molded pump components. Nimbus subsequently modified its pump assembly and inspection procedures, which eliminated this problem in all subsequent in vivo trials. The third and fourth animals achieved their perfusion goals, at which time the experiments were electively terminated.

Overall, pump function has been remarkably good and, from a hemodynamic viewpoint, the pumps have functioned as designed. Figure 6 presents typical hemodynamic data from the 96 hour juvenile lamb pulsatile flow experiment (Table 2). As pump flow was increased from near 0 to a mean flow rate of approximately 1.3–1.5 L/min, one notes concomitant rises in the pump outlet pressure and the animal's arterial pressure. The pulsatile nature of the pump outlet pressure and flow waveforms is apparent. The mean left ventricular pressure in this animal during the 3-second period of this example approached 20 mm Hg, which suggests that the N/P pump was supplying essentially all of the animal's systemic flow during this brief observation period.

C. Results—Physiology

In both the steady and pulsatile flow experiments, the animals tolerated the N/P centrifugal pump well. Table 3 summarizes the laboratory values that were monitored at least daily for the five steady flow experiments. Plasma free hemoglobin remained below 20 mg/dL following the perioperative period, a finding also documented in the two lamb pulsatile flow experiments that continued for 72 and 96 hours. For both the pulsatile and steady-flow trials there were transient increases in white cell counts, which were believed to be associated with the

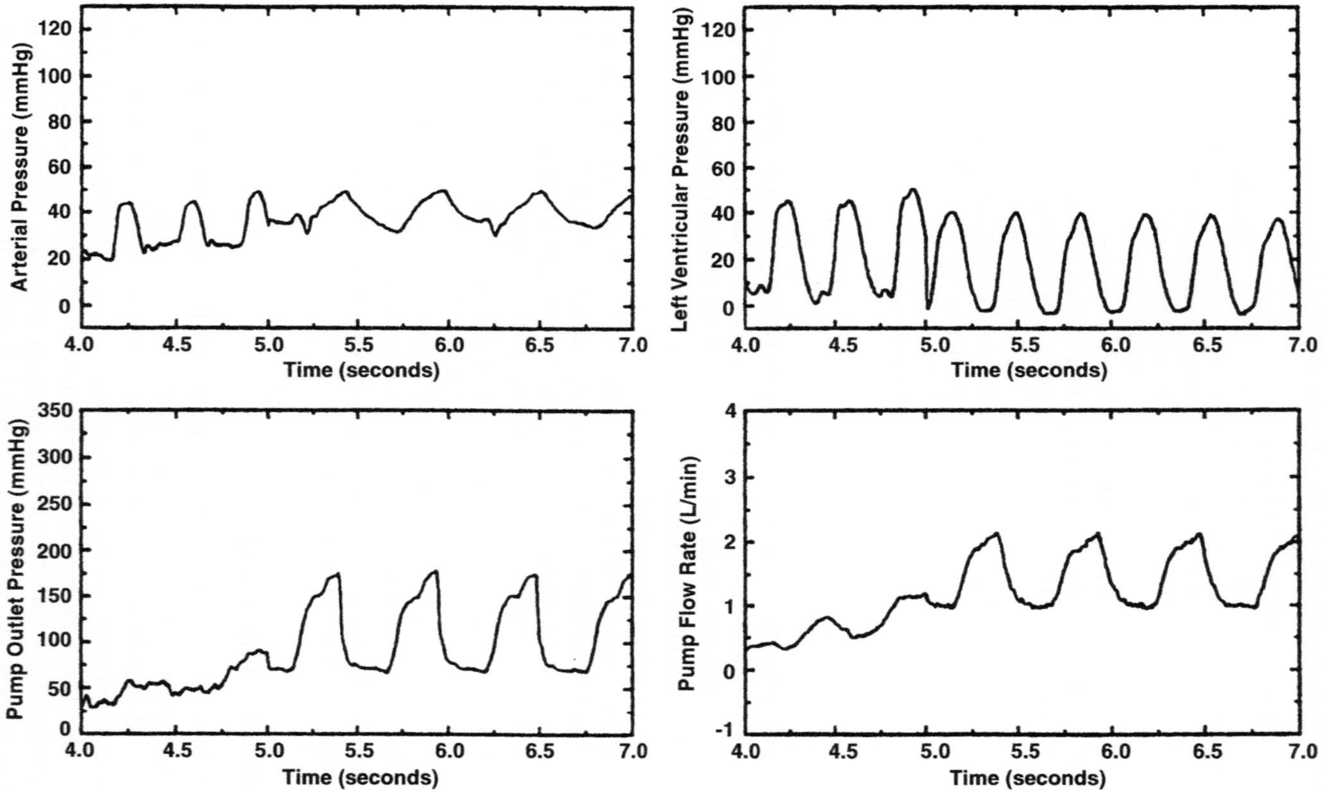

Fig. 6 Hemodynamic tracing taken from 96-hour pulsatile flow lamb experiment.

Table 3 Mean ± SEM Laboratory Values for Five Steady-Flow Lamb Experiments

	ACT (s)	HCT (%)	PfHb (mg/dL)	WBC ($\times 10^3$/mm^3)	PLT ($\times 10^5$/mm^3)	Creatinine (mg/dL)	BUN (mg/dL)
Mean	250 ± 30	26 ± 1	13 ± 3	11 ± 1	6 ± 1	0.7 ± 0.02	16 ± 3
Range	134–1000	17–31	3–46	5–15	3–10	0.6–0.7	11–32
Baseline	120 ± 9	34 ± 2	6 ± 1	7 ± 2	6 ± 1	[a]	18 ± 2

[a] Incomplete data.
ACT = Activated clotting time; HCT = hematocrit; PfHb = plasma free hemoglobin; WBC = white blood cell count; PLT = platelet count.
Source: Ref. 5.

surgical procedure. Platelet counts were in the normal physiological range in all animals (steady and pulsatile flow models). Likewise, after the expected postoperative decline due to hemodilution, hematocrit and hemoglobin remained stable thereafter.

Finally, there were only minor transient alterations in kidney and liver function. The lambs awoke, ate, and drank (nursed) as would nonoperated similarly aged animals.

D. Results—Necropsy

Among the steady and pulsatile flow lamb models, none had thrombus within the pump itself. Two animals (8.8 and 18.4 kg lambs) had bilateral renal cortical infarcts, which were associated with small amounts of thrombus in the pump inflow and/or outflow cannulae. Among the four pulsatile flow experiments, one lamb had single infarcts in both kidneys, but there was no evidence of more widespread thromboembolic complications to the liver, spleen, gastrointestinal tract, or brain. The three lambs that succumbed to respiratory failure had evidence of pulmonary edema and areas of consolidation, but no evidence of infection. Several of the pulsatile flow lamb models also had small patches of atelectasis and pneumonia. As noted above, respiratory complications are believed to be associated with ventilator-associated barotrauma occurring intraoperatively.

E. Results—Pump Seal Integrity

In the five steady-flow experiments pump seal integrity was noted to be intact. In the longest experiment (148 h) there was some evidence of moisture accumulation within the rotor housing, but the pump continued to function well. In the several pulsatile flow experiments, pump versions were used that incorporate a purge fluid assembly to continuously wash the impeller seal. In these experiments, blood was not observed within the motor rotor cavity.

V. DISCUSSION

This project was originally motivated by the perceived lack of mechanical circulatory support systems intended specifically for use in pediatric care, covering the needs of patients ranging from neonates to small children. As noted in the various chapters of this text, mechanical circulatory support occupies an increasingly important role in the treatment of neonates and pediatric patients requiring cardiac support. Clearly, the need for innovative products to treat these special patients remains a considerable challenge to physicians and engineers alike in this area.

A review of the literature indicates that for N/P cardiac support, most groups have investigated pneumatic devices in which one-way valves direct flow into and out of a flexible blood sac. One example is the device developed at Washington University, which is a scaled-down version of the Pierce-Donachy ventricular assist device (VAD) with specially designed ball valves. In vivo testing with this unit revealed flow-related thrombosis on the blood sac surface with peripheral microembolization. The cause of these events was postulated to be hemodynamically inferior valves that produced fluid dynamics in the device conducive to thrombus formation (1).

Another interesting pediatric N/P concept along these lines is the tubular VAD of Kung et al. (2). This concept features an integrally formed inflow valve, pump chamber, and outflow valve. The inflow and outflow valves and the pump chamber are all actuated pneumatically. Acute in vivo studies were conducted in newborn lambs and focused on the hemolysis characteristics of the VAD. The authors believe that these first in vitro and in vivo studies demonstrate the feasibility of the tubular VAD for N/P support.

Two chapters in this book describe the Medos®-HIA VAD, and hence this product will not be discussed in detail here. This device is also actuated pneumatically and is available in sizes as low as 25 and 10 mL maximum stroke volume, suitable for N/P cardiac support. Polyurethane tri-leaflet valves direct flow into and out of the blood sac (3).

The Nimbus-UOP device differs from these other concepts and features a miniature centrifugal pump of very low priming volume, which is also easy to manufacture. A console controller generates either steady or pulsatile flow, the latter via programmed oscillation of the motor current. From the data presented above, the clinical use life of this product is approximately 7 days and likely longer for pump versions that incorporate a purge fluid assembly to continuously wash the impeller seal and thereby prevent blood products from entering the motor rotor cavity.

The results presented herein (see also Refs. 4 and 5) indicate the strong potential of this pump for N/P cardiac support. From a hemodynamic viewpoint, pump performance spanned the range of flow rates required for such a device. Even more importantly, the N/P pump was well tolerated physiologically. Consistent with in vitro measurements, hemolysis was also acceptably low in the aforementioned lamb trials. There were no pump-related infections or thromboembolic organ failure. While several animals demonstrated renal infarcts at autopsy, these did not appear to affect renal function during pump operation as evidenced by serum creatinine and BUN levels. Further, there was no evidence of more widespread thromboembolic complications to the liver, spleen, gastrointestinal tract, or brain.

These encouraging results have convinced the present authors that this product is worthy of continued development and qualification, leading to clinical trials. Current efforts are focused on identifying a corporate partner to spearhead this development effort.

ACKNOWLEDGMENT

This work was supported in part by NIH Small Business Innovative Research (SBIR) grants HL51667 and HL53131.

REFERENCES

1. Pettitt TW, Lourenco LM, Daily BB. High resolution quantitative flow maps of a pediatric VAD. Ann Biomed Eng 1994; 22(suppl 1):22.
2. Kung RTV, Champsaur GL. A tubular ventricular assist device—design considerations and system characteristics. ASAIO J 1996; 42:255–262.
3. Konertz W, Hotz H, Schneider M, Redlin M, Reul H. Clinical experience with the MEDOS HIA-VAD system in infants and children: a preliminary report. Ann Thorac Surg 1997; 63:1138–1144.
4. Litwak P, Butler KC, Thomas DC, Taylor LP, Macha M, Yamazaki K, Konishi H, Kormos RL, Griffith BP, Borovetz HS. Development and initial testing of a pediatric centrifugal blood pump. Ann Thorac Surg 1996; 61:448–451.
5. Macha M, Litwak P, Yamazaki K, Kameneva M, Butler KC, Thomas DC, Taylor LP, Griffith BP, Borovetz HS. In vivo evaluation of an extracorporeal pediatric centrifugal blood pump. ASAIO J 1997; 43:284–288.

20

Myocardial Remodeling and Thyroid Regulation in the Developing Heart During Mechanical Circulatory Support

Michael A. Portman
Children's Hospital and Regional Medical Center and University of Washington School of Medicine, Seattle, Washington

The preceding chapters reveal the many technical innovations in mechanical circulatory support that have been developed over the past several years. Emerging technologies offer several new therapies for patients in this area. However, the rapid technical advances have not been accompanied by comparable research into many basic mechanisms, which may be altered by these therapies. Indeed, review of the medical and scientific literature reveals a paucity of research regarding ventricular remodeling and/or disruption of hormonal and metabolic homeostasis during prolonged support through extracorporeal membrane oxygenation (ECMO) or left ventricular assist devices (LVADs) in the pediatric population. In this chapter, we will review findings related to myocardial remodeling during mechanical circulatory support in adult patients. These findings and specific theories related to them will be considered with respect to their possible relevance in the pediatric patient.

LVADs reduce both preload and afterload, evidenced by closure of the aortic valve throughout the cardiac cycle during the device functioning (1). This unloading of the heart through mechanical circulatory support appears to reverse pathological ventricular remodeling, which occurs in dilated cardiomyopathies (1–4). This alteration provides restructuring of cellular and fibrous architecture, which improves the functional capacity of the failing heart (2,3,5). However, remodeling and its signals may vary according to the antecedent cardiac morphology, the presence or absence of ventricular hypertrophy or dilation, the etiology of myocardial damage, and the degree of unloading.

I. LEFT VENTRICULAR GEOMETRY AND HISTOLOGY

Changes in left ventricular geometry have been described in adult patients during LVAD. Near immediate and progressive reductions in left ventricular volume decrease wall stress during the support period and may contribute to arrest of progressive cell damage and loss in ischemic cardiomyopathy (5). Prolonged left ventricular assist produces a reduction in left ventricular mass and a leftward shift in the end-diastolic pressure volume relation in isolated explanted hearts after LVAD (1). These findings imply that LVAD produces elevations in diastolic compliance as well as improvement in systolic function.

Morphometric studies have revealed that LVAD reduces myocardial injury. Geometric changes are caused in part by reductions in myocardial injury and fibrosis. Florid changes of acute myocardial necrosis including prevalent wavy fibers and contraction band necrosis, present in both dilated and ischemic cardiomyopathy, substantially decrease during chronic ventricular support (5).

II. MYOCYTE GEOMETRY AND FUNCTION

Geometric reductions in left ventricular mass and volume during LVAD are accompanied by alterations in myocyte size and shape (3,5,6). In particular, Zafeiridis et al. (6) demonstrated that the marked increases in myocyte width, length, and volume in ischemic and nonischemic cardiomyopathic hearts are abrogated in cardiomyopathic hearts supported by prolonged LVAD. Although a reduction in fibrosis might explain elevations in diastolic compliance, myocytes from LVAD-supported hearts also demonstrate enhanced diastolic as well as systolic function compared to cells from untreated cardiomyopathic hearts. Dipla and colleagues isolated cardiomyocytes from ventricular myocardium at the time of orthotopic cardiac transplantation (2). Myocytes from hearts supported by prolonged LVAD demonstrated superior performance by several systolic and diastolic contractile indices, including elevated percent shortening, reduced time to peak contraction, and reduced time to 50% relaxation.

III. MITOCHONDRIAL FUNCTION

Deficits in myocardial bioenergetics and mitochondrial function have been linked to heart failure in several animal models. Zhang et al. showed in a porcine model of postinfarction left ventricular remodeling that the severity of bioenergetic abnormality in the form of decreased phosphocreatine/ATP ratio in situ is directly related to the severity of left ventricular dysfunction (7). Lee et al. measured the effect of LVAD on respiratory control indices in heart failure patients (8). Though respiratory control indices have limited applicability to the heart in situ (9,10), mitochondria from LVAD-supported hearts demonstrated significantly higher values than mitochondria isolated from nonsupported hearts. These studies imply that deficits in mitochondrial function and perhaps structure occur during left ventricular remodeling. LVAD seems to improve mitochondrial function during regression of left ventricular hypertrophy. However, investigations of mitochondrial function during prolonged mechanical circulatory support have been limited technically. Further research in this area is required to clarify the effects of mechanical circulatory support on mitochondrial function during left ventricular remodeling. In summary, mechanical circulatory support in the adult heart reverses pathological myocardial remodeling, which is a central feature in the progression of myocardial failure.

Studies investigating changes in left ventricular morphology induced by mechanical circulatory support have been restricted to adult populations. No similar study involving infants or children has been published to date. Thus, theories regarding potential for left ventricular remodeling in the pediatric population must be based on the data acquired in adults as well as limited echo data from infants during extracorporeal life support (ECLS). In general, echocardiographic studies in pediatric populations have only examined infants undergoing ECLS for noncardiac indications (11,12). Martin and Short (11) and Strieper et al. (12) performed longitudinal M-mode echocardiographic studies in relatively small populations of neonates during arteriovenous or venovenous ECMO, respectively. These studies were not directed towards evaluation of geometric changes or ventricular remodeling during ECMO. Although M-mode measured left ventricular end-diastolic volume trended upwards, no significant increase occurred in either of these small neonatal groups during 96 hours of ECMO. These findings must be considered keeping in mind that Martin's group recently reported a near 12% incidence of myocardial stunning in a retrospective review of 500 ECMO patients (13). Stunning was defined by the reversible near-total absence of ventricular shortening and aortic valve opening on two-dimensional echocardiogram and/or by clinical criteria including narrowing of pulse pressure. Left ventricular dilation also occurred in patients exhibiting this phenomenon (14). The presence of stunning adversely affected survival rate in this population. The same group reported a separate early decrease in load-dependent measures of cardiac performance including shortening fraction and cardiac output (15). Myocardial stunning was felt to be a distinct phenomenon, which the authors attributed to possible mismatch between afterload and contractility (13). However, attempts at pharmacological or mechanical reduction of afterload did not result in improved myocardial performance during ECMO (16).

Conceivably, a relationship exists between stunning and ventricular unloading with remodeling during ECMO. However, this possibility has not yet been investigated. Myocardial remodeling stimulated by partial or complete ventricular unloading in the normal heart, which may occur during ECMO, might cause myocardial atrophy and diminish contractile function. Experimental evidence supporting this suggestion is provided by Tomanek and Cooper (17), who demonstrated progressive atrophy of feline right ventricular papillary muscles mechanically unloaded through transection of the chordae tendinae. Atrophy was characterized first by disorientation and then loss of contractile filaments as well as a marked increase in connective tissue. Similarly, heterotopic cardiac isografts in rats are hemodynamically unloaded and undergo atrophy (18). Some changes associated with atrophy can occur within only 3 days of mechanical unloading but are rapidly reversible with reloading (19). These particular experimental preparations provide models of complete ventricular loading and therefore only remotely resemble the normal infant heart partially unloaded by ECMO. However, these experiments do raise specific concerns regarding ventricular atrophy induced by unloading. It is unclear whether stunning represents a maladaptive response to hemodynamic unloading or results from other factors such as coronary perfusion via the left ventricle with deoxygenated blood returning from nonaerated lungs.

The response of the developing human heart to ventricular unloading has not been closely investigated. Studies performed in infants with transposition of the great arteries do reveal the potential for rapid changes in myocardial mass in young patients. Clinical studies indicate that correction for simple transposition of the great arteries (TGA) should occur within the first 2 weeks of life (20). Beyond this period, the left ventricle presumably loses its ability to accommodate the acute increase in workload of systemic pressure (21). Rates of left ventricular mass regression or atrophy have not been reported in infants with TGA who have not undergone correction. However, the reverse—acquisition of ventricular mass—has been demonstrated in infants undergoing pulmonary artery banding as a rapid two-stage arterial switch operation (22). Accordingly, Boutin et al. (22) demonstrated that pulmonary artery banding results in a 95% increase in left ventricular mass over 7 days, with the vast majority of the hypertrophic response occurring during the first 2 days. These studies reveal the developing heart's potential for rapid increases and perhaps decreases in ventricular mass in response to changes in loading.

The mechanisms through which reversal of pathological myocardial remodeling occurs during mechanical circulatory support have not been totally defined but have been a focus of intense interest in basic science and adult cardiology literature (23). A complete review of the mechanisms for remodeling and hypertrophy is not the intention of this chapter. However, certain of these mechanisms are also developmentally regulated and should be considered with respect to the pediatric-age heart undergoing mechanical circulatory support and some degree of unloading. Results obtained from basic studies imply that alterations in mechanical stretch induce myocardial hypertrophy. Hemodynamic loading may be simulated in vitro by stretching individual cardiomyoctyes on a silastic membrane (24). Stretch in this model causes hypertrophy accompanied by an induction of early response genes (c-fos, c-jun, and c-myc) and ''fetal genes'' such as skeletal alpha-actin, atrial natriuretic factor, and beta-myosin heavy chain. Stretching myocytes inherently emulates increases in preload. Accordingly, some studies indicate that preload influences expression of these genes more than afterload (25). However, hypertrophy and changes in gene expression, which approximate those found during myocyte stretching, also occur during the pressure overload induced in rat LV myocardium by acute aortic constriction in vivo (26) Paradoxically, some of the ''early response'' and fetal genes increase expression during unloading manifested in the heterotopic transplanted heart (23). Switching of myosin heavy chain expression to the beta isoform in both hypertrophied and mechanically unloaded hearts occurs coordinately with induction of specific genes regulating myocardial energetics. In particular, reductions in transcript levels for the glucose transporter isoform 4 (GLUT4) and carnitine palmitoyl transferase I occur coordinately with the myosin heavy chain isoform switching (23). Depre et al., (23) have suggested that improvements in contractile function elicited by mechanical circulatory support relate to changes in proteins regulating energy production and/or consumption. Coordinate expression of these multiple genes is regulated in part by paracrine/autocrine peptides, such as transforming growth factor β (TGF-β). With respect to the developing heart, myocardial transcripts for TGF-β1 and its associated cell surface receptor have been shown to increase in response to aortic banding in the postnatal rat. The response of gene transcripts to mechanical unloading has not been described in the developing heart and remains an area for future research (27). Since expression of multiple genes can be modified by environmental factors, such as hormones, their importance is of clinical relevance in addition to academic interest. Thyroid hormone levels in particular respond to mechanical circulatory support and might provide a mode to alter gene responses.

IV. THYROID HORMONE

Thyroid hormones (THs) influence cardiac contractile performance through several mechanisms, which might be relevant to patients under mechanical circulatory support. This hormone can elicit rapid changes in contractile function and mediate promotion of specific proteins related to cardiac energy utilization and production. Both animal and clinical studies have documented decreases in circulating thyroid hormone levels during and after cardiopulmonary bypass (28–30). Mechanisms responsible for low levels have been suggested but are not yet substantiated. These include (a) dilution effects induced by the cardiopulmonary bypass circuit, (b) accelerated peripheral uptake and metabolism of thyroxine (T4), (c) inhibition of T4 to triiodothyronine (T3) conversion, and (d) central inhibition of thyrotropin-releasing hormone by nonpulsatile flow (30–32).

Regardless of the mechanisms involved in decreasing T3 and T4 levels, triiodothyronine supplementation provides acute increases in cardiac performance after cardiopulmonary bypass in both animal and humans (28,29). T3 produces improvements in contractile function after coronary artery bypass, which result from direct cardiac inotropic effects as well as decreases in systemic vascular resistance (28,29,33,34). However, investigators have been unable to demonstrate changes in clinical outcome parameters such as length of mechanical ventilation, postoperative intensive care unit stay, or hospital stay in patients receiving triiodothyronine after coronary artery bypass surgery (29). The relatively uncomplicated postoperative course in control patients that occurs with standard management after coronary artery bypass would make it difficult to establish a benefit using any adjunct therapy.

Conceivably deficits in circulating thyroid hormones cause postoperative dysfunction in infants and children. Circumstantial evidence relating low levels to postoperative recovery supports this hypothesis. Infants and children exhibit more persistent and severe suppression of the pituitary-thyroid axis postoperatively than their adult counterparts (31,35). Depressed T3 and T4 levels in pediatric age groups are associated with prolonged myocardial dysfunction leading to greater use of inotropic agents and to extension of the intensive care treatment period (31,35,36). Delayed rebound to normal levels coincides with contractile recovery, although direct causation is yet to be proven. Mainwaring et al. published the only study to date, which attempted to examine the effects of thyroid repletion in children after cardiopulmonary bypass (37). Thyroid hormone supplementation appeared to reduce the length of hospitalization in children who have undergone a modified Fontan operation (37). However, significant problems in design and execution, such as nonrandomization of the study population, diminish the validity of the results. Nevertheless, that study offers promising results and provides the basis for developing hypotheses related to thyroid repletion in postbypass pediatric patients.

Similarities between cardiopulmonary bypass and extracorporeal life support provide reasons for thinking that prolonged mechanical circulatory support can disrupt thyroid hormone homeostasis. Depression of thyroid levels persists in infants for several days after even a brief period of cardiopulmonary bypass.

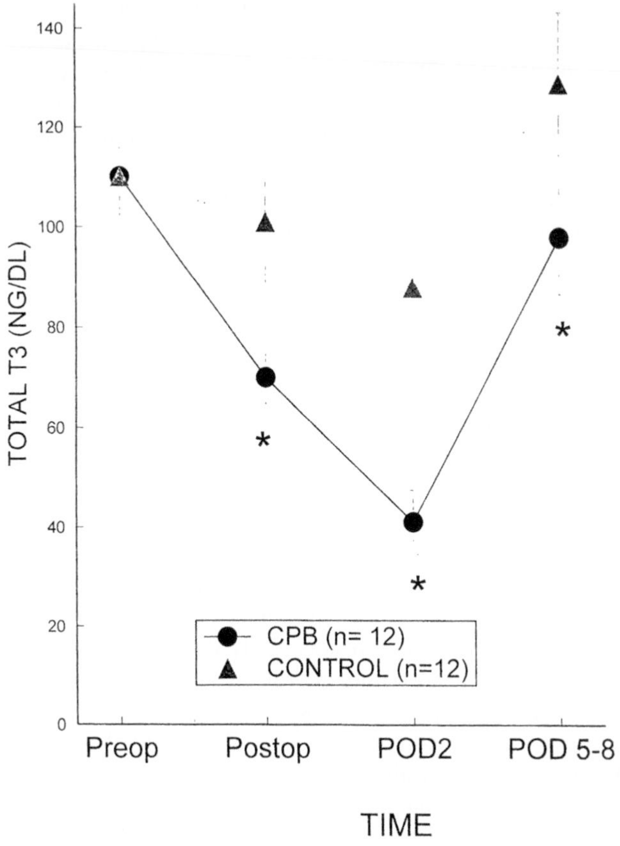

Fig. 1 Total T3 values are plotted for infants, who underwent thoracic surgery with cardiopulmonary bypass (CPB) or without (CONTROL). $*p < 0.03$ versus preoperative value. (Adapted from Ref. 36.)

Figure 1 illustrates this phenomenon with the delay in rebound of circulating total T3 levels in infants. To date, no reports of thyroid levels during prolonged mechanical circulatory support have been published in either pediatric or adult age groups. Preliminary data collected from several patients in this institution suggest that similar persistent depression of circulating T3 and T4 levels occurs throughout the duration of extracorporeal life support.

Thyroid hormones regulate protein synthesis through transcriptional and translational mechanisms. Thus, persistent disruption of thyroid hormone homeostasis might alter T3-promoted gene and protein expression during or after mechanical circulatory support. Although the acute actions of T3 supplementation during bypass have been investigated (28,29), the more persistent influences on gene and protein expression have not been studied in these clinical situations. Some of the proteins, which undergo alterations during myocardial remodeling, are also under thyroid control.

Myosin heavy chain expression has been particularly well studied with regards to thyroid regulation and myocardial remodeling. Thyroid promotes the developmental shift in myosin heavy chain isoforms from beta to alpha, which occurs in some species (38–40). Changes in relative isoform distribution can affect the myocardial contractile velocity and efficiency of ATP utilization. A reversal of this developmental shift occurs during conditions of hypertrophy or unloading, which simulate changes during mechanical circulatory support. Thyroid does not alter protein content, protein synthesis, or total myosin content in the mechanically unloaded heterotopic transplanted heart, which demonstrate this reversal (18). However, thyroxine treatment does shift myosin heavy chain isoform expression back towards the alpha subtype in that particular model.

Several studies have indicated that isoform shifts do not occur in human ventricular myocardium because the alpha subtype remained less than 5% of total myosin throughout development. These results imply that myosin isoform distribution plays no role in human heart failure and/or myocardial remodeling. However, recent studies using quantitative RT-PCR and human specific cDNA probes found that the alpha isoform comprises nearly 30% of total myosins (41,42). Furthermore, downregulation of alpha-myosin and reciprocal upregulation of the beta isoform occurs during human heart failure and hypertrophy. In a single patient with hypothyroid cardiomyopathy, Ladenson et al reported an 11-fold increase in alpha-myosin expression with thyroid replacement and a pronounced increase in left ventricular ejection fraction (43). Thus, changes in myosin isoform distribution, in part thyroid-regulated, probably contribute to contractile dysfunction noted during remodeling.

Specific studies of mechanical unloading and thyroid state have not been investigated in the developing heart. Thyroid regulation of protein synthesis is not restricted to the myosin heavy chains. Cardiac growth and maturation of contractile fibers, sarcoplasmic reticulum, and mitochondrial proteins depend on the neonatal surge of thyroid hormone (44,45). Preliminary data in our laboratory indicate that extracorporeal life support can attenuate the neonatal thyroid hormone surge normally present during the first few days of life. The importance of this disruption needs further clarification.

The clinical relevance of myocardial remodeling and disruptions in thyroid hormone homeostasis during mechanical circulatory support is not proven. Further study in these areas is warranted.

ACKNOWLEDGMENT

This work is supported in part by a National Institutes in Health Grant 1R01-HL-60666.

REFERENCES

1. Levin HR, Oz MC, Chen JM, Packer M, Rose EA, Burkhoff D. Reversal of chronic ventricular dilation in patients with end-stage cardiomyopathy by prolonged mechanical unloading. Circulation 1995; 91:2717–2720.
2. Dipla K, Mattiello JA, Jeevanandam V, Houser SR, Margulies KB. Myocyte recovery after mechanical circulatory support in humans with end-stage heart failure [see comments]. Circulation 1998; 97:2316–2322.
3. Altemose GT, Gritsus V, Jeevanandam V, Goldman B, Margulies KB. Altered myocardial phenotype after mechanical support in human beings with advanced cardiomyopathy. J Heart Lung Transplant 1997; 16:765–773.
4. McCarthy PM, Nakatani S, Vargo R, et al. Structural and left ventricular histologic changes after implantable LVAD insertion. Ann Thorac Surg 1995; 59:609–613.
5. Nakatani S, McCarthy PM, Kottke-Marchant K, et al. Left ventricular echocardiographic and histologic changes: impact of chronic unloading by an implantable ventricular assist device. JACC 1996; 27:894–901.
6. Zafeiridis A, Jeevanandam V, Houser SR, Margulies KB. Regression of cellular hypertrophy after left ventricular assist device support [see comments]. Circulation 1998; 98:656–662.
7. Zhang J, Wilke N, Wang Y, et al. Functional and bioenergetic consequences of postinfarction left ventricular remodeling in a new porcine model. MRI and 31 P-MRS study. Circulation 1996; 94:1089–1100.
8. Lee SH, Doliba N, Osbakken M, Oz M, Mancini D. Improvement of myocardial mitochondrial function after hemodynamic support with left ventricular assist devices in patients with heart failure. J Thorac Cardiovasc Surg 1998; 116:344–349.
9. Nichols D, Ferguson S. Bioenergetics 2. San Diego: Academic Press Limited, 1992.
10. Portman MA, Heineman FW, Balaban RS. Developmental changes in the relation between phosphate metabolites and oxygen consumption in the sheep heart in vivo. J Clin Invest 1989; 83:456–464.
11. Martin GR, Short BL. Doppler echocardiographic evaluation of cardiac performance in infants on prolonged extracorporeal membrane oxygenation. Am J Cardiol 1988; 62:929–934.
12. Strieper MJ, Sharma S, Dooley KJ, Cornish JD, Clark RH. Effects of venovenous extracorporeal membrane oxygenation on cardiac performance as determined by echocardiographic measurements. J Pediatr 1993; 122:950–955.
13. Becker JA, Short BL, Martin GR. Cardiovascular complications adversely affect survival during extracorporeal membrane oxygenation. Crit Care Med 1998; 26:1582–1586.

14. Martin GR, Short BL, Abbott C, O'Brien AM. Cardiac stun in infants undergoing extracorporeal membrane oxygenation. J Thorac Cardiovasc Surg 1991; 101:607–611.
15. Karr SS, Martin GR, Short BL. Cardiac performance in infants referred for extracorporeal membrane oxygenation. J Pediatr 1991; 118:437–442.
16. Martin GR, Chauvin L, Short BL. Effects of hydralazine on cardiac performance in infants receiving extracorporeal membrane oxygenation. J Pediatr 1991; 118:944–948.
17. Tomanek R, Cooper IV GC. Morphological changes in the mechanically unloded myocardial cell. Anat Rec 1981; 200:271–280.
18. Klein I, Hong C, Schreiber SS. Cardiac atrophy in the heterotopically transplanted rat heart: in vitro protein synthesis. J Mol Cell Cardiol 1990; 22:461–468.
19. Thompson EW, Marino TA, Uboh CE, Kent RL, Cooper Gt. Atrophy reversal and cardiocyte redifferentiation in reloaded cat myocardium. Circ Res 1984; 54:367–377.
20. Castaneda AR, Trusler GA, Paul MH, Blackstone EH, Kirklin JW. The early results of treatment of simple transposition in the current era. J Thorac Cardiovasc Surg 1988; 95:14–28.
21. Jonas RA, Giglia TM, Sanders SP, et al. Rapid, two-stage arterial switch for transposition of the great arteries and intact ventricular septum beyond the neonatal period. Circulation 1989; 80:I203–208.
22. Boutin C, Jonas RA, Sanders SP, Wernovsky G, Mone SM, Colan SD. Rapid two-stage arterial switch operation. Acquisition of left ventricular mass after pulmonary artery banding in infants with transposition of the great arteries [see comments]. Circulation 1994; 90:1304–1309.
23. Depre C, Shipley GL, Chen W, et al. Unloaded heart in vivo replicates fetal gene expression of cardiac hypertrophy. Nat Med 1998; 4:1269–1275.
24. Sadoshima J, Jahn L, Takahashi T, Kulik TJ, Izumo S. Molecular characterization of the stretch-induced adaptation of cultured cardiac cells. An in vitro model of load-induced cardiac hypertrophy. J Biol Chem 1992; 267:10551–10560.
25. Slinker BK, Stephens RL, Fisher SA, Yang Q. Immediate-early gene responses to different cardiac loads in the ejecting rabbit left ventricle. J Mol Cell Cardiol 1996; 28:1565–1574.
26. Izumo S, Lompre AM, Matsuoka R, et al. Myosin heavy chain messenger RNA and protein isoform transitions during cardiac hypertrophy. Interaction between hemodynamic and thyroid hormone-induced signals. J Clin Invest 1987; 79:970–977.
27. Engelmann GL, Campbell SE, Rakusan K. Immediate postnatal rat heart development modified by abdominal aortic banding: analysis of gene expression. Mol Cell Biochem 1996; 163–164:47–56.
28. Novitzky D, Human PA, Cooper DKC. Inotropic effect of triiodothyronine (T3) following myocardial ischemia and cardiopulmonary bypass: an experimental study in pigs. Ann Thorac Surg 1988; 45:50–55.
29. Klemperer JD, Klein I, Gomez M, et al. Thyroid hormone treatment after coronary-artery bypass surgery [see comments]. N Engl J Med 1995; 333:1522–1527.
30. Holland FW, Brown PS, Clark RE. Acute severe postischemic depression reversed by triiodothyronine. Ann Thorac Surg 1992; 54:301–305.

31. Mainwaring RD, Lamberti JJ, Carter TL, Jr., Nelson JC. Reduction in triiodothyronine levels following modified Fontan procedure. J Card Surg 1994; 9:322–331.
32. Robuschi G, Medici D, Fesani F. Cardiopulmonary bypass: a low T4 and T3 syndrome with blunted thyrotropin (TSH) response to thyrotropin releasing hormone (TRH). Hormone Res 1986; 23:151–158.
33. Ojamaa K, Klemperer JD, Klein I. Acute effects of thyroid hormone on vascular smooth muscle. Thyroid 1996; 6:505–512.
34. Khoury SF, Hoit BD, Dave V, et al. Effects of thyroid hormone on left ventricular performance and regulation of contractile and CA(2+)-cycling proteins in the baboon. Implications for the force-frequency and relaxation frequency relationships. Circ Res 1996; 79:727–735.
35. Bettendorf M, Schmidt KG, Tiefenbacher U, Grulich-Henn J, Heinrich UE, Schonberg DK. Transient secondary hypothyroidism in children after cardiac surgery. Ped Res 1997; 41:375–379.
36. Brogan TV, Bratton SL, Lynn AM. Thyroid function in infants following cardiac surgery: comparative effects of iodinated and noniodinated topical antiseptics. Crit Care Med 1997; 25:1583–1587.
37. Mainwaring RD, Lamberti JJ, Nelson JC, Billman GF, Carter TL, Schell KH. Effects of triiodothyronine supplementation following modified Fontan procedure. Cardiol Young 1997; 7:194–200.
38. Lompre AM, Nadal-Ginard B, Mahdavi V. Expression of the cardiac ventricular alpha- and beta-myosin heavy chain genes is developmentally and hormonally regulated. J Biol Chem 1984; 259:6437–6446.
39. Schwartz K, Lompre AM, Bouveret P, Wisnewsky C, Whalen RG. Comparisons of rat cardiac myosins at fetal stages in young animals and in hypothyroid adults. J Biol Chem 1982; 257:14412–14418.
40. Lompre AM, Mercadier JJ, Wisnewsky F, et al. Species- and age dependent changes in the relative amounts of cardiac myosin isoenzymes in mammals. Dev Biol 1981; 84:286–290.
41. Lowes BD, Minobe W, Abraham WT, et al. Changes in gene expression in the intact human heart. Downregulation of alpha-myosin heavy chain in hypertrophied, failing ventricular myocardium. J Clin Invest 1997; 100:2315–2324.
42. Nakao K, Minobe W, Roden R, Bristow MR, Leinwand LA. Myosin heavy chain gene expression in human heart failure. J Clin Invest 1997; 100:2362–2370.
43. Ladenson PW, Sherman SI, Baughman KL, Ray PE, Feldman AM. Reversible alterations in myocardial gene expression in a young man with dilated cardiomyopathy and hypothyroidism. Proc Natl Acad Sci USA 1992; 89:5251–5255.
44. Portman M, Xiao Y, Ning X-H. Thyroid regulates maturation of mitochondria and myocardial respiratory control in vivo. Pediatr Res 1998; 43:26A.
45. Boerth SR, Artman M. Thyroid hormone regulates Na+-Ca+ exchanger expression during postnatal maturation in adult rabbit ventricular myocardium. Cardiovasc Res 1996; 31:E145–152.

Index

Printed and bound by CPI Group (UK) Ltd, Croydon, CR0 4YY
23/10/2024
01778262-0002